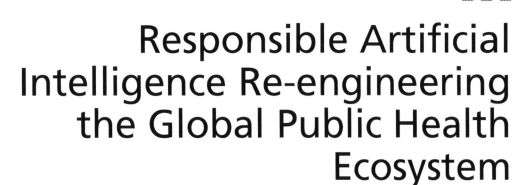

Responsible Artificial Intelligence Re-engineering the Global Public Health Ecosystem

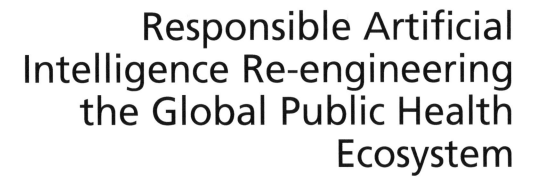

Responsible Artificial Intelligence Re-engineering the Global Public Health Ecosystem

A Humanity Worth Saving

Dominique J. Monlezun

UT MD Anderson Cancer Center, Houston, TX, United States

ELSEVIER

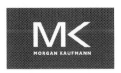

ISBN: 978-0-443-21597-1

For Information on all Morgan Kaufmann publications
visit our website at https://www.elsevier.com/books-and-journals

Publisher: Mara Conner
Acquisitions Editor: Chris Katsaropoulos
Editorial Project Manager: Himani Dwivedi
Production Project Manager: Fizza Fathima
Cover Designer: Miles Hitchen

Typeset by MPS Limited, Chennai, India

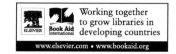

Working together
to grow libraries in
developing countries

www.elsevier.com • www.bookaid.org

Dedication

To Mary, who first started me on this journey.

To Susan, Lucy, André, and Jude, who are the whole reason for it.

To my parents, siblings, and extended family, for helping me remain on it.

To my medical and public health colleagues, for letting me serve our patients shoulder to shoulder with them through it.

To Dr. Colleen Gallagher, Dr. Cezar Iliescu, Dr. Alberto Garcia, Dr. Oleg Sinyavskiy, Dr. Lorenzo Berra, Dr. Francesco Nordio, Matthew O'Brien, Dr. Timothy Harlan, Dr. Richard Velkley, Dr. Rebecca Mark, Dr. Shane Courtland, Dr. Charles Monlezun, and Dr. B., as I hope your mentorship is faithfully honored in its pages.

Contents

About the author

Dominique J. Monlezun is a practicing physician-data scientist and ethicist. He earned his first AI-focused PhD in global health management and policy and his second PhD in bioethics (with the latter recognized by Microsoft as producing the world's top AI ethics doctoral dissertation). He serves as an academic physician for the world's top-ranked hospital, professor of cardiology for two American academic medical institutions, professor of bioethics for two United Nations–affiliated universities, and the principal investigator and senior data scientist and biostatistician for more than 50 research studies associated with Harvard University, the National Institutes of Health, and the European Union among others. He has authored more than 400 peer-reviewed manuscripts, conference abstracts, and book chapters, in addition to the first five comprehensive AI textbooks on bioethics, metaphysics, healthcare systems, public health, and quantum health. He created BAM-PS AI-statistics and Personalist Social Contract ethics after cofounding Culinary Medicine. He has provided medical care for thousands of immigrant, imprisoned, and underserved patients while teaching bioethics and health policy to graduate students in four continents.

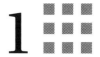

1

Power and artificial intelligence: transformation of the global public health ecosystem

1.1 Part I: History

1.1.1 Power versus justice: why artificial intelligence and global public health matter

There is no humanity without health, and no modernity without artificial intelligence (AI). In just the first two decades of the 21st century, we are increasingly witnessing how they are transforming our global civilization—and in some ways even threatening its survival. Global public health at the intersection of modern healthcare, political economics, and the global digital ecosystem is emerging as one of modernity's most transformative societal trends, while AI is driving this ecosystem as our world's most disruptive technology (Monlezun 2023). Our lives are increasingly digitalized, globalized, and interdependent at such a rapid rate and at such a scale and degree that what happens somewhere and to someone likely will inevitably ripple outward to affect us wherever we are. For me, these macrotrends were manifested in the moment that generated the idea for this book, caught in a hospital between a hurricane and a pandemic. I was grasping the hands of one of my frail patients before we had to rush dozens of other critically and acutely sick people onto helicopters and ambulances to escape an approaching hurricane in 2021, bearing down on our rural under-served hospital already overwhelmed with COVID-19 cases. Our best technology, knowledge, and teamwork versus a monster pandemic and storm amid severe staff shortages swirled into a microcosm of our larger global health challenges, which our era increasingly is realizing we must face down as they quickly approach us.

Yet amid these developments, growing empirical evidence supports how we have never been as healthy, happy, and peaceful as we are now (Veenhoven 2010). In just the first two decades since 2000, humanity witnessed its fastest surge in health, economic, and technological growth, with the global economy tripling in this timeframe alone (including especially fast growth in low-income countries [LICs]; Woetzel et al. 2021). But by 2022, we also reached the historical point in which there has never been a smaller group of individuals with more power and less accountability who can challenge the world's nations for greater dominance or with greater disruption (including those controlling the biggest economies and nuclear arsenals; Eurasia 2023; Lusigi 2022; Woetzel et al. 2021). Concurrently, we face the rising risk

Responsible Artificial Intelligence Re-engineering the Global Public Health Ecosystem. DOI: https://doi.org/10.1016/B978-0-443-21597-1.00001-9

of postpandemic global stagflation and debt crises imperiling in particular the LICs (worsened by the growing global food-, energy-, and water-shortage crises following a nuclear armed state in 2022 invading its smaller nation reportedly to erase its identity and sovereignty, ultimately erasing 5 years of progress in global human development). Further, just 5 out of nearly 200 countries internationally—the United States, China, Japan, Germany, and India—account for nearly 60% of the wealth worldwide. Finally, these trends are colliding at the same time that AI-powered technologies are increasingly becoming the "weapons of mass disruption," exerting greater autocratic societal control while further polarizing and fragmenting democracies. At this modern inflection point caught between colliding crises, the COVID-19 pandemic crystalized how AI and global public health are the technological and societal tools with unprecedented influence over our lives. Yet to bring out the best and avoid the worst in this polycrisis moment, we need a common understanding of this new reality that informs our common values and solutions. This book, therefore, is the first known comprehensive work to explain how AI is transforming the global public health ecosystem, how it is reengineering our future, and how we can make tomorrow a common home worth saving.

But before we get to know why you need this book instead of others (and what makes it unique, relevant, and actionable), let us establish why the focus of this book is critical for our era: why does AI and global public health essentially matter? Power. And making it work for our common good, the central aim of justice as the age-old counterweight to it. Power can compel us to adhere to (or avoid) a minimum set of behaviors required for a healthy, prosperous, and stable society for the good of all. Yet power unrestrained by justice can quickly become control by the powerful few for their own gain over (and at the expense of) the weak many. Societies generally have no pushback when they ban murder, sex trafficking, and theft for national security; they are generally seen as clear immediate harms committed against others, contributing to unstable internal political economics undermining national resilience to external political economic threats. Yet there is typically much greater resistance when societies try to mandate, punish, or incentivize individual health behaviors that may be less well defined or their long-term benefits demonstrated (i.e., vaccines, healthy diet, and exercise). The scale and complexity of this resistance can become exponentially greater when requirements or prohibitions are implemented across state borders, expanding public health locally to global public health internationally as a powerful few can dictate or determine the individual behaviors for the many, even outside their borders. But if the states lack either national or human security, their stability, prosperity, and equality can be undermined. Global public health, thus, is about the just use of power for the common good. Its emerging AI-empowered evolution set to increasingly dominate the future is about finding the most effective, efficient, and equitable ways of optimizing it (especially in the face of limited resources or public goods required for it). Who gets the power, how it is used, and why it is used—according to what definition of health—become fundamentally critical questions the responsible AI and governance must answer for the global public health ecosystem. So, let us briefly examine the (1) technical, (2) societal, and (3) historical dimensions of this central tension of power and justice underexplored in both AI and health and how this book can uniquely address them in actionable ways relevant to you.

1.1.2 Technical dimensions

AI is widely acknowledged already to be the defining technology of our era. It fuels the Fourth Industrial Revolution in which AI accelerates global digitalization, increasingly integrating the physical, digital, and biological dimensions into cyber-physical systems (like with individuals via smartphones linked with social media networks, healthcare systems, companies, and governments; Schwab 2016; Allison and Schmidt 2020). AI is also the primary battleground for modernity's military-business arms race, especially between the United States and China who dominate AI global investments and breakthroughs. AI has been heralded as "our final invention," given its extraordinary potential and progressive successes lowering prediction costs and thus accelerating efficient productivity through virtually every economic and societal sector (Barrat 2013; Agrawal et al. 2018). It increasingly gets us to receive better answers faster, typically by analyzing large amounts of information (or "Big Data") to better inform decisions. Any human action typically is meant to achieve a desired effect through the means we expect is the most likely to achieve that end. You may take one street rather than another, as your reasoning based on prior experience will get you to your school or business faster amid the traffic. A drug company may develop Drug A over Drug B because prior studies suggest one will deliver more effective and affordable results than the other. Thus influential proponents argue that AI may be our final creation as it progressively empowers us to develop subsequently more smarter inventions. And yet there is a dark side to that technological prediction (which some describe is hype and many nonetheless assert is dangerous enough to consider)—AI may also be our ultimate invention that ultimately ends us (Bostrom 2014; Barrat 2013). Current AI is "weak AI," mostly consisting of machine learning (ML), in which we code, program, or instruct an algorithm exactly what to do and how to "learn" to do tasks better over time. But there are rapidly expanding efforts to achieve artificial general intelligence (AGI) or "strong AI," in which an algorithm can "teach itself" any intellectual task a human can do. "Superintelligence," according to the University of Oxford philosopher, Nick Bostrom, is the final evolutionary step of strong AI in which the algorithm may continue developing to the point it exceeds human cognitive performance in practically all domains. The question then becomes, how do we control something that is smarter than use? Consider how 69% of the United Nations (UN) Digital Library focuses on nuclear war among the existential threats challenging humanity (Boyd and Wilson 2020). The Manhattan Project's Albert Einstein and the scientists of the University of Chicago who created the first atomic bomb that generated the existential threat of nuclear war went on to create the *Bulletin of the Atomic Scientists*, followed by the Doomsday Clock to highlight existential risks annually. Since 2019, its board members (including 11 Nobel laureates) have kept the clock no further than 100 seconds to the apocalyptic "midnight," the closest the clock has ever been (Mecklin 2022). The *Bulletin*'s board highlighted not just the long-running existential threat of nuclear war, but also increasingly of the new threat from AI-driven disruptive technology, especially its risk of catalyzing (even unintended) nuclear war and wider conflict. The Stanford University political scientist and Eurasia Group President, Ian Bremmer, echoes these concerns by emphasizing the trifecta of crises defining our modern era: AI-driven disruptive technologies and their interlinked "global health emergencies" and "transformative climate change," with all worsening each other and disproportionately harming the sicker and poorer communities rather than the healthier and wealthier ones (Bremmer 2022).

Now consider global health. On the one hand, coordinated health efforts at the national level as with the United States in the 20th century generated 25 out of the 30 years of improved life expectancy (nearly doubling it), particularly through improved vaccination, sanitation, noncommunicable disease prevention, workplace safety, mother and child health, and diet (Groseclose 1999). Similar efforts at the international level from the 1990s to the 2000s, especially with the Millennium Development Goals (MDGs) of the UN, saved upward of 29.7 million lives especially in sub-Saharan Africa, China, and India, while raising nearly half a billion extra people out of extreme poverty (McArthur and Rasmussen 2017). The latter finding is particularly notable, given how poverty appears to be the leading fundamental driver of death globally and how it negatively impacts education, social support, and inequality, while also worsening the burden of infectious or communicable diseases (or CDs, through decreased healthcare prevention and treatment resources) and noncommunicable diseases (NCDs) or chronic comorbidity diseases (compounded by decreased healthcare access and worse health behaviors; Galea et al. 2011; WHO 2010). The Nobel Prize—winning economist and theorist in integral human development, Angus Deaton, demonstrated how such 20th-century public health advances manifested the interdependent explosion of health and wealth in scientific-capitalist states (Deaton 2022; Bondarenko 2021). The technological innovations of these predominantly North American and European nations empowered them to get richer and healthier much faster than the rest of the world, while globalization of economic activity was followed by globalization of its societal effects for the rest of the world. Yet Deaton also stresses how this global progress may have also advanced entrenched international structures of ideological and political economic colonialism by deepening the subservience of poorer, sicker, and thus weaker countries to the wealthier, healthier, and stronger countries.

It should be also noted that despite all these advances, NCDs like cardiovascular disease and cancer remain the leading medical causes of death worldwide, accounting for nearly two-thirds of all deaths (WHO 2010). They are growing fastest in LICs while driving up significant mortality disparities, as almost 80% of NCDs occur in LICs and middle-income countries (MICs) according to the WHO, the UN's main international health agency. Yet over 80% of NCDs are caused by modifiable health behaviors according to the WHO, including unhealthy diet, insufficient physical activity, excessive alcohol consumption, and tobacco use. A *Lancet* systematic evaluation of 195 nations showed how excessive sodium and insufficient whole grains and fruit were the top modifiable risk factors for death, and that fixing them could prevent one of every five deaths annually or 11.5 million globally (GBD 2017 Diet Collaborators 2019). In the United States, which spends the most on healthcare, less than 3% of healthcare expenditures are for these public health and prevention efforts (Himmelstein and Woolhandler 2016). Social disparities accelerated, compounded, and perpetuated by poverty exacerbate these structural issues, meaning that poorer populations bear an unequal burden of bad health outcomes (OECD 2011). As a recent example of global health disparities, the cost to the global economy from COVID-19 vaccine nationalism may be upward of $9.2 trillion, as high-income countries (HICs), including North America and Europe, withheld their highly effective mRNA-based vaccines from low- and middle-income countries (LMICs) in the early pandemic period (Çakmaklı et al. 2021). Equitable health investments in low-cost behavioral and capacity changes can have outsized improvements in health, its inequities, and thus overall economic productivity, political stability, and national security. But instead, it appears that we throw 97% of our efforts to fix 20% of health outcomes, while making minimal improvements to their related inequities or rampant individual and societal costs.

1.1.3 Societal dimensions

Consider the power—justice tension from the technical dimension of AI-enabled global public health applied to the concrete case of high-profile strategic pivots. The historic successes and threats of these twin transformative tools—AI and global public health—may be illustrated with China's COVID-19 response from 2019 to 2022. At least in the two decades leading up to it, China progressively sought strategically to demonstrate its reportedly superior Marxist—Leninist communist "state capitalist" model by dethroning the United States with its liberal democratic capitalist model as the global hegemon or dominant power (Khalil 2020; Allison and Schmidt 2020). China emerged by the late 2010s as what its critics describe as the world leader in "digital authoritarianism," describing how authoritarian governments deploy digital technologies to influence and control populations through surveillance, manipulation, repression, and censorship to ultimately increase the government's power. Proponents counter that by the COVID-19 pandemic in 2020, China leveraged its digital capacities to enact what became the most successful infectious disease lockdowns (government-mandated and enforced restriction or prevention of travel to reduce infectious disease spread), receiving international initial praise from the medical, public health, and scientific communities for "its rapid containment of COVID-19" (Huang 2022, p. 26). The rest of the world, particularly the US-led democratic Global "West" (of North America, Europe, Oceania, and East Asia), conversely were criticized for their supposed initial dysfunction and division resulting in a higher early COVID impact. Yet amid that early criticism, the West developed and deployed in record time the first mRNA-based vaccines with unparalleled safety and efficacy, accelerating the West and South's opening up of their populations and economies—while China doubled down on its seeming indefinite "zero-COVID" policy for 3 years amid mounting domestic and global critique of its politicization of public health that was more about control than health (Owens and Parry 2022; Khalil 2020). Shunning the more effective Western vaccines while failing to vaccinate its elderly and most vulnerable population, China's AI-driven digital surveillance state faced a popular crisis by November 2022. International corporations had been accelerating their capital and labor flight from the country after rolling lockdowns became increasingly too costly. Meanwhile, Chinese citizens gained growing glimpses of the world's largely maskless countries crowded together celebrating soccer's World Cup, until an apartment fire finally sparked widespread outcry and protests (Wright et al. 2022). In the Chinese city of Urumqi, where the communist government has been accused of imprisoning up to 2 million ethnic and religious minorities, particularly the Muslim Uyghurs, social media reports broke through the internet censorship to share reports how an apartment fire killed at least 10 people, as their apartment building was alleged by multiple witnesses to not only be physically locked due to COVID-19 lockdowns (including by locks and doors welded shut), but also firefighters were not physically able to reach the building or its inhabitants trapped in the building blaze. After the largest national protests since the 1980s, the government suddenly reversed zero-COVID with "whipsaw speed," with the resultant surge in infections overwhelming the already strained national healthcare system; up to "half" of the healthcare workers in hard-hit areas were out sick, as the nation faced "wave after wave of shocks," leaving consumer demand, international exports, external investments, and recovery prospects blunted at best (at least as of the 2023 writing of this book; Buckley et al. 2022).

What is stopping AI from transforming and empowering not just governments and their public health, but also global public health? What happens if AI continues to increasingly enable a shrinking number of centralized government and corporate leaders to exert outsized control on the data, products, and services populations consume not just inside their borders and sectors but also worldwide? What happens if AI continues to allow such actors growing influence over the global digital ecosystem that informs, incentivizes, and restricts what we value, demand, and believe (while catalyzing the effectiveness and efficiency with which such actors coordinate efforts including under the banner of global public health to shape collective actions)? Up to 70% of AI leaders, policymakers, and researchers, according to a 2021 Pew Research study, do not believe health AI will be ethical, or able to facilitate human good or the common good (Rainie et al. 2021). Echoed by the Institute of Electrical and Electronics Engineers (IEEE), a global AI standard setter, Stanford University (Institute for Human-Centered Artificial Intelligence), and the US National Security Commission on AI, the general consensus is the world's main AI actors are focused on economic and/or political (and military) dominance, while AI's rapidly and pervasively disruptive influence globally is moving faster than societal efforts to prevent or mitigate its unethical, unfair, and damaging effects. Essentially, AI and its takeover of global public health may seem to many critics to be increasingly and simply about raw power as a unifying strategy unto itself, explaining much of how our current era's major AI and health actors understand themselves, our world, and their actions toward us in it. But to understand what is driving it—and how to orientate it to a mutually desirable future—let us consider the final historic dimension.

1.1.4 Historic dimensions

"The strong do what they can, and the weak suffer what they must," according to the ancient Greek-Athenian historian-general, Thucydides, over 24 centuries ago (Thucydides and Warner 1972).

He is credited with founding scientific history (systematic attempts at impartial evidence-based accounting and analysis) and political realism (international relations theory arguing that self-interested states ultimately seek power as the capacity for national security, required for self-preservation in an anarchic world of no global authority enforcing fair rules of state behavior). By 375 BCE, Athens as the world's first democracy executed arguably the first philosopher, Socrates, for arguing the justice is over even power itself, because it is ruled by the Good, which is what the philosopher and the just ruler ultimately seek (Plato and Jowett 1991):

Until philosophers are kings, or the kings and princes of this world have the spirit and power of philosophy...cities will never have rest from their evils—nor the human race, as I believe—and then only then will this our State have a possibility of life and behold the light of day.

The Athenian ruling elites charged rather that Socrates was "corrupting the youth" by challenging their power and authority. According to this mysterious thinker, a good tool or good ruler or good health were only such if they conformed to the type of good that the thing is meant to be in its ideal form to achieve its end or fulfillment (conforming to its excellent form or its "virtue"). A good tool like a knife achieves the end it is meant for, i.e., cutting well. A good ruler achieves their end, i.e., justice or the good ordering and governance of society. Developed further by his student, Plato, and his student, the physician philosopher, Aristotle, good health enables a person to be free from disease and disability that may hamper them reaching humanity's highest good of *eudaemonia*, the state of "good spirit," "happiness," perfection, or fulfillment (Aristotle et al. 2012). Ethics and political philosophy, therefore, respectively are the scientific studies of good human actions and societal governance. What ultimately makes anything good is what Socrates and Plato described as the highest good, goodness itself, or "the Good," which is desired for its own sake, and for its sake we desire all other intermediary goods or ends that brings us closer to it (by knowing and being united to it like knowing, loving, and being united with a spouse). In this line of argument before and ever since, there has been the historic human struggle between the strong and weak, with the only force other than power resolving the dispute between them being the appeal to this seemingly amorphous but still substantively real conception of justice (as reason restraining and dictating force as appropriate).

This brings us to the final consideration of the historic dimension of this defining struggle underlying AI and the modernization of global public health: why do we want power? (And thus, how is its pursuit determining so much of the present and future of AI-empowered global public health that is muscling itself increasingly into our daily lives?) Recent modern psychological studies challenge old assumptions about this. They show that we generally want power, not to control others but to be free of others controlling us in ways we do not want (Lammers et al. 2016). Power is not just influence (controlling others by directing them to the strong's end), but also autonomy (resilient resistance to the influence of others that enables one to pursue their own self-chosen end). We may like influence, but we need autonomy according to such empirical research. The psychological theory of "self-determination" similarly emphasizes how such autonomy complements relatedness (belonging with others) and competence (mastery of one's goals or end-directed actions) as humanity's basic psychological needs (Deci and Vansteenkiste 2004). Accordingly, attaining power as a good means or tool appears to enable us to become happy as the ultimate end by reaching our self-determined fulfillment (Kifer et al. 2013). Power may allow prestige, pleasure, and wealth, but modern science generally supports classical philosophy that what we ultimately want is the good life. Such research suggests that we seek power (as autonomy) to enable self-authenticity (being "true" to ourselves and our unique pursuits of happiness), which reaches its end or destination in self-fulfillment (in what Aristotle would describe as knowing the Good and thus living the good life, and what the modern sense would emphasize as living the good life unique to you) as the abiding state of well-being. In the classical sense developed by Socrates (and through Plato, Aristotle, and the related philosophical tradition), the Good governs justice. It does so by defining and safeguarding the individual's good life (fulfillment through the virtuous life including living justly) and the common good (the collective good which individuals communally desire and work toward). According to this systematic argument, we existentially belong to each other in the common human community bound together by familial friendship, through which alone we realize our individual good in helping others achieve their good as they also do for us (Aristotle 1984, 2012). Thus, autonomy is fulfilled in well-being. And freedom is fulfilled when it is freedom *for* choosing the good life (giving to others what they deserve as they do for us), rather than simply remaining as freedom *from* constraint (afraid of others getting too much from oneself). This historical trajectory reinforces our modern understanding from the societal and strategic dimensions of the power and justice struggle which help define the relationship between AI and global public health (and thus our future). In this line of reasoning, power without justice can devolve into tyranny (elitist or autocratic), while justice without power can devolve into irrelevance (unable to substantively advance individual flourishing at scale, i.e., societal development). For AI-empowered global public health to help define a future that can be a common home we collectively desire, it needs just power driving and directing it—a common home built on the foundation of the common good, from which we build a sustainable framework with common tools (which otherwise devolve into destructive weapons).

1.2 Why this book matters for you

So if we need health to survive (and global public health is the most effective societal tool for that, which we will seek to establish below shortly), and we need AI to make it work (as its most efficient technical tool, which we will also demonstrate), then this book matters for you as it is the first to comprehensively demonstrate the above, and how to make these trends work better for our shared tomorrow with a breadth, depth, scale, and practicality to make that vision a reality. The COVID-19 pandemic, the 2022 Russo-Ukrainian war, African debt crises, growing global economic slowdowns and inequities, and rising US–China tensions have highlighted our world's surging global political, economic, and related health crises that are crashing against the reality of our governments, institutions, healthcare systems, and public health agencies that are often seen as insufficient to meet this historic moment. There is widespread consensus that we need effective, efficient, and equitable solutions to these challenges, in addition to guardrails on their overarching global cooperative competition (without the collateral damage of catastrophic conflict), amid rising fears of these trends' related risks of disruptive AI technology, nuclear war, climate change, and pandemics. Otherwise, as the UN Secretary-General in 2022 warned, "humanity is just one misunderstanding, one miscalculation away from...annihilation" (UN 2022). From the UN to the WHO to leaders and populations at the national and local levels, there is broad agreement that modern healthcare is falling short of patients and populations' needs (without any clear solutions in sight to fixing the practical and structural issues) at scale and at speed. It appears that we may only be able to face our shared existential crises when we generate new shared, effective, and fair global solutions.

This book thus provides the first known comprehensive global analysis of how AI can revolutionize the decolonized global public health ecosystem to equitably empower the world to solve our era's defining crises, by detailing the diagnosis (of inadequate global public health) and treatment (the responsible ecosystem AI and governance transforming the above change). Written by the world's first triple doctorate-trained physician−data scientist and AI ethicist (and the author of the first three integrated AI books on healthcare systems, bioethics, and multicultural metaphysics), this critical resource shows practically and technologically how our different political economics, belief systems, and cultures can unite in cooperative competition, without sacrificing our identity, rights, or sustainable (and fair) development. This book makes global public health accessible and actionable by integrating global health, public health, medicine, data science, political economics, ethics, and related emerging technologies and strategies (including deep learning [DL], AGI, quantum computing, global disease surveillance, adaptive value supply chains, demographic shifts, integral development, network science, health financing, healthcare system design, and multicultural global ethics underlying diverse political economic systems) for a clear and concrete way forward together in a divided but digitized and globalized world. This work, therefore, is meant to be a compelling and coherent guide to help empower and equip students, practitioners, policymakers, researchers, and leaders in digital technology, public health, healthcare, health policy, public policy, political science, economics, and ethics to generate the solutions that will define humanity's next era—while recovering what that humanity means and why it is worth saving.

As such, this book provides the first known unifying strategic vision (and principles and examples operationalizing it) for the AI-accelerated effective, efficient, and equitable global public health ecosystem of the future. Prior books provide partial answers. This book seeks to detail the complete ones, by defining the first ecosystem-based approach to understand how AI is transforming and globalizing public health (and thus our underlying political economics, contextualized in our diverse values and cultures). The book's broad audience of students, practitioners, and leaders noted earlier can therefore understand how their sector fits with others in a cooperative global digital health ecosystem, both at a conceptual level and practical level. The strategic problems that this book helps solve include clarifying the structure and content of this global public health ecosystem, its decentralized and organic evolution (with elements of centralized planning and coordination), its suprastructure of global institutions, its structure of political economics (bridging decentralized democratic and more centralized autocratic capitalist and socialist systems), and the substructure of its moral foundation (uniting diverse belief systems through the UN-based approach of modern human rights theory). The operational problems this book helps solve include describing how AI is both now and in the foreseeable future being deployed through emerging models of private–public partnerships among technology companies, healthcare systems, global health and public health agencies, and governments, at the local, national, and international levels (addressing both current challenges and emerging solutions to the productivity and equity of these force-multiplying partnerships). This approach attempts to balance the breadth and depth needed to make this vision actionable, by giving enough theoretical depth to understand key concepts and principles without sacrificing the range of diverse disciplines and actors constituting the AI-enabled global public health ecosystem (as explained through concrete examples). The daily challenges the book addresses are how to understand the major barriers faced by you, the broad audience in your diverse sectors and regions, and how disruptive AI technologies along with the strategic vision or conceptual framework of Personalist Liberalism (integrating data science, global public health, and political economics) can unite sectors to solve our shared problems. This book has three features that may be the most valuable to modern readers: (a) a comprehensive and cross-sector strategic vision, (b) clear and practical explanations of complicated technological and societal trends, and (c) a novel formula generating agile shared solutions to our era's most urgent existential health challenges. Pairing AI and global political economics (explained through Personalist Liberalism) shaping the global public health ecosystem serve as a simplifying conceptual and narrative framework that may allow the book to be sufficiently broad and deep (while still remaining as coherent and concise as possible for a wide audience), and so relevant and actionable for you.

In addition, this book grounds its approach with particular emphasis on inclusion and diversity. It utilizes a similar approach to my first three AI books which pioneered the first known inclusive, multicultural, pluralistic, and global AI ethics comprehensive framework (recognized in the world's top doctoral dissertation award by the 2020 international expert symposium from the UN, Microsoft, and IBM, which provided the first multisector global consensus standard for AI ethics, which in turn informed the 2021 WHO's similar standard; Monlezun 2023, 2022). This fourth book applies this novel approach to global public health specifically to champion previously underrepresented voices in this field, and so facilitating more just, united, and effective global solutions to our modern health challenges.

This book is meant to complement and advance the important contributions from a number of excellent earlier books by other authors that hopefully will further equip you according to your particular interests, passions, and purpose (including to disagree with and improve upon yourself). While this book attempts to provide you novel value as the first known comprehensive book on the AI-enabled global public health ecosystem (and thus also the first scholarly book on this topic, the first written for a broad audience, and the first from the integrated perspective of a physician−data scientist and ethicist), the following competing works also deserve particular mention (with which I have no prior or current relationship): Jain et al. 2022 (*Artificial Intelligence, Machine Learning, and Mental Health in Pandemics*), Santosh and Gaur 2021 (*Artificial Intelligence and Machine Learning in Public Healthcare*), Detels et al. 2021 (*Oxford: Oxford Textbook of Global Public Health*), and Murth and Ansehl 2020 (*Technology and Global Public Health*). The major strengths of each include their academic rigor, attempted real-world utility, and novelty. Their primary weaknesses (which allow this book to potentially build upon theirs in novelty and utility for readers) include excessive superficiality, narrow focus, and real-world application. This work differentiates itself from such competitors by allowing accessible depth of content, integrated cross-sector approach, and a coherent real world−supportive narrative demonstrating my novel conceptual approach to explain the modern trends driving the emerging model of the next era of the AI-enabled global public health ecosystem. The future of healthcare is this ecosystem (which this book will argue links communities, global and public health agencies, healthcare systems, businesses, and governments). But to defend this bold claim and make it an actionable formula for how to realize a future that the world wants and needs, this book uniquely balances the above-noted breadth and depth with firsthand multidisciplinary expertise, made accessible for a broad audience to show how we can reach this commonly desired destination strategically, operationally, and technologically.

1.3 Book's structure as the blueprint for the artificial intelligence−empowered global public health ecosystem: humanity's common home

To accomplish the above, the book is structured like a home. Each chapter describes a critical element of the AI-empowered global public health ecosystem, building sequentially to the unified vision of how today's such ecosystem is giving way to the ecosystem of tomorrow, along with how to accelerate that reality: design (financing and integral development), framework (data architecture and political economics), inhabitants (culture and demographics), and foundation (security and ethics). Each chapter begins with the basic terms and concepts (including those for AI in the next chapter), considers their larger global and strategic contexts, and then zooms in to related concrete AI use cases. We will consider each of the abovementioned aspects in their dual dimensions of operational means and strategic ends. We will then conclude with an analysis of the emerging future of the AI transformed global public health ecosystem by constructing the adaptive building materials which enable this home to grow and respond to emerging and future challenges and opportunities. The chapters therefore are as follows:

1. Chapter 1. Power and AI: transformation of the global public health ecosystem
2. Chapter 2. Design part I: AI + financing
3. Chapter 3. Design part II: AI I(integral) + S(sustainable) development

4. Chapter 4. Framework part I: AI + data architecture
5. Chapter 5. Framework part II: AI + political economics
6. Chapter 6. Foundations and families: AI ethics of demographic, multicultural, and security shifts
7. Chapter 7. Our common home: AI + global public health ecosystem
   a. History: public health to global public health to its ecosystem

1.3.1 Public health's early days: quarantines to vaccines

Public health essentially consisted of politically imposed and socially accepted measures to control infections from our earliest records up to the 1900s, often as part of larger cultural and religious customs predicated upon individual duties to the common good (Monlezun 2023). If you were sick with a mysterious disease, you often were exiled from the community until the danger seemed to pass, as the cause behind it was often unclear and its treatment largely ineffective. Additional documented measures date back to approximately 2000 BCE with European sanitation efforts, including installing home water supplies along with toilets and drainage (Juuti Katko and Vuorinen 2007). By the 5th century BCE, the Torah or Jewish sacred scriptures specified within individual religious duties such daily practices as healthy diets and personal hygiene, like the later 2nd century BCE Buddhist and traditional Chinese medicine instructions for disease prevention and well-being (Chattopadhyay 1968). Contemporaneously, the ancient Greeks appeared to develop the first scientific or systematic reason-based cause−effect approach to understand, prevent, and treat diseases (Bryant and Rhodes 2021). The "father of medicine," Hippocrates developed this tradition further with his 4th-century book (*Airs, Waters, and Places*), generally recognized as the first methodical account of the causal relationship between diseases and the environment. This milestone cast a millennia-long shadow by enabling the eventual 16th-century germ theory of disease (describing how environmental and infectious germs or microorganism pathogens cause diseases), after informing the premodern public health measures attempting to mitigate local clusters of infectious diseases (endemics), particularly when they first emerged to impact a specific population in its initial time frame (epidemics).

By the late 17th century, such theories and research became increasingly formalized and translated into public policies and government action as seen with Europe directing public officials to record plague cases (individuals meeting defined criteria for a particular disease or condition) and enforce quarantines (mandatory isolation for individuals exposed to or who contracted diseases to reduce further transmission; Goudsblom 1986). By the 1800s, the British-born Industrial Revolution triggered pervasive social upheaval that in turn precipitated the widely acknowledged birth of early modern public health as its own social enterprise and scientific discipline (Wohl 1983). Machine manufacturing increasingly began to replace products traditionally made by hand, giving way to the commercial incorporation of more powerful energy methods including steam and water and eventually commercial electricity−driven mass production. Precipitating this technological revolution was the Catholic and then Protestant-informed 17th-century Western Enlightenment and its focus on human dignity and derivative individual rights, which influenced strong property laws in what is today the United Kingdom, allowing private individuals to retain the rights to their intellectual property and capital. This facilitated the resultant innovation surge that drove the technological breakthroughs required for their economic commercial upheavals, which in turn drove their political upheavals (shifting the global power balance to these industrialized empire states) and societal upheavals (in the structures and content of their social networks, cultures, and values). Britain externally expanded its global empire to bring in more raw materials and export more finished products, concurrent with its internal swell in the standard of living for its general population. This in turn increased its birth rate, life expectancy, workforce productivity, and related political economic and military hegemonic or dominant world power. Its industrialization spread to the rest of Europe and North America before peaking around World War I (WWI), after which it was eclipsed by the United States that preserved that global dominance into the early 21st century at least (more on this in Chapter 5 on political economics). But the rapid technological-driven industrialization and political economic power explosion of Britain—and that of the emergent "West"—came at a massive societal cost. Factories ravenously consumed workers, catalyzing a plummeting in workplace safety, urban sanitation, and living conditions. Contagious diseases ripped through these increasingly densely packed cities, inflicting a deadly disproportionate disease burden on vulnerable communities, including racial minorities, immigrants, and the poor. As more workers were sick more often, economic productivity dropped and political pressure mounted on governments to improve such societal conditions through the new field of early modern public health, in which science and technology moved not only into political economics but also into health.

Then the 1838 Chadwick Report changed it all. Bowing to popular and elite demand, the English social reformer, Edwin Chadwick, was tapped to lead the British Poor Law Commission and its publication of the first statistical analysis of societywide life expectancy (Hanlon and Pickett 1984). It detailed the hard evidence for a 20-year difference between when rich elites and poor workers, with the latter making it to only 16 years of age on average. These results informed Chadwick's subsequent wide-ranging public health recommendations, including waste and sewage removal. They ultimately ushered in the landmark 1848 Public Health Act and the new age of modern scientific public health at societal scale. Progressively spreading to the rest of Europe and North America along with the rest of the industrialized Western world, systematic studies on the causes and spread of diseases guided the creation of civil engineering, social countermeasures, and public education (about disease prevention and treatment) that governments funded and enforced in the name of public health, justified by appeals to the common good. The next major leap forward in public health came from France with Louis Pasteur's discovery in 1877 that the *Bacillus anthracis* bacteria caused anthrax disease, enabling his 1884 creation of the first effective vaccine by training the human body's immune system to successfully fight a pathogen and so prevent its disease manifestation (Winslow 1923). This kicked off the surge in European and American vaccines for tuberculosis, diphtheria, typhoid, and yellow fever. The early 1900s solidified public health's transition from its ancient and early modern paradigm (cultural and religious directives for individual health behaviors and quarantines, with questionable impact at best) to its late modern form: scientific, targeted, coordinated, and increasingly effective measures prioritizing low-cost attempts to boost well-being, with particular focus on vulnerable communities. Riding this historical wave, the American bacteriologist, Charles-Edward Winslow, became a modern public health pioneer, pushing the field forward while providing its widely accepted definition that outlined its field-defining priorities for the ensuing century as a professional discipline, progressively recognized as a necessary pillar of modern societies to grow and thrive (Winkelstein 2022; Winslow 1923):

The science and the art of preventing disease, prolonging life, and promoting physical health and efficiency through organized community efforts for the sanitation of the environment, the control of community infections, the education of the individual in principles of personal hygiene, the organization of medical and nursing service for the early diagnosis and preventive treatment of disease, and the development of the social machinery [civil engineering] which will ensure to every individual in the community a standard of living adequate for the maintenance of health; organizing these benefits in such fashion as to enable every citizen to realize his birthright of health and longevity.

1.3.2 Modernization and globalization of public health

In the 1940s ashes of World War II (WWII), the United States emerged with its victorious allies set on remaking the old world order in their new image to prevent what many feared would be a world-ending, nuclear war–powered World War III. The postwar hyperglobalization led by the United States increasingly replaced the power vacuum left by decolonization. The early modern empires were succeeded by the emergent US-led global network of nations, bound by a minimum set of common values supporting the suprastructure of institutions generated by and advancing liberal democratic capitalist political economics (Slobodian 2018). Recognizing the rise of the communist Soviet Union as its main peer competitor, the United States integrated public health with its diplomatic efforts (i.e. "global health diplomacy"), along with its humanitarian, cultural, and economic efforts to build a global network of allies built on a pragmatic proposition backed up by the integration of hard power (military) power and soft power (everything else): we guarantee your security and prosperity, and you join our alliance (Katz et al. 2011; Sachs 2020; Mearsheimer 2018). The United States deployed its enormous navy and middle-class demand for cheap goods to catalyze what became the later 20th century marked by increasingly rapid industrialization, capitalization, globalization, digitalization, and (though with notable autocratic exceptions) even liberalization and democratization. As introduced earlier, Deaton demonstrated how this historic revolution in population well-being—the product of health and wealth in his account—was accelerated by the historic success of public health measures, enacted at scale by adequate institutional and political economic support at both the national and international levels (Deaton 2022; Bondarenko 2021). The flip side though was that insufficient public health institutionalization and investment particularly in healthcare systems became the primary cause of societies' worsening inequalities. In this analysis, poor people generally remain sicker and less able to become rich in a negative reinforcing cycle: they bear the heavier burden of diseases (that sufficient public health could begin reversing), which in turn undermines their productivity capacities that then limits their opportunities to more equally benefit from economic and health progress. But sufficient public health (including its boost for vulnerable populations benefiting from greater public education) unleashes their capacity to benefit from the diffusion of technological innovations through enhanced productivity in a positive reinforcement cycle, resulting in complementary improvements to wealth and health for them and their subsequent generations. Public health thus grew not only across borders but more densely within them, taking on increasingly central roles for integrating and force multiplying synergistic networking and capacities across international, government, business, academic, and community organizations. The more equitable the public health, the healthier the workforce, the wealthier the society, the safer the state, and the more peaceful the international community of nations.

In this historical account, by 1991 the Soviet Union's fall hastened what was largely characterized in retrospect as 20 years of overoptimism of the "liberal international order" under the unchallenged global hegemon of the United States and its global alliance. It created many winners—including the rise of China's "state capitalism" and developed nations, especially their upper middle class and upper class—and also many losers (especially in developing nations). The proliferation of increasingly powerful global institutions in this order, including the UN (which the United States remains the largest funder), WHO, and World Trade Organization (WTO), manifested and furthered much of America's values and political economic model that integrated public health as soft power to the point that the UN's 2008 General Assembly declared the "interdependence" of such "foreign policy...and global public health" (UN 2008). But the structural shocks of the UN 2008 Great Recession and China-born 2020 COVID-19 pandemic accelerated the popular and even a popularist backlash (on the left and right of the political spectrum) against the supposed threats of such a hyperglobalized world order. Claiming it undermined national sovereignty, self-determination, and identity, such a backlash generally asserted that this world order gave away too much power to international institutions that failed to deliver sufficient prosperity, stability, and well-being equally to the locals. (And that leaves out the colonization and COVID critique as well as the AI disruptive shocks, which we will get to shortly).

1.3.3 Strategic and organic ecosystem transition into global public health

Broadly, the rise and peak of the liberal world order correlated with the rise and potential peak of the international power of public health, leading up to the 2008 Recession and ultimately the 2020 pandemic (Brown et al. 2006; Monlezun 2023). The US-led alliance of WWII victors and the non-Axis countries who created the UN in 1945 at the same time voted to create a new international health organization, eventually giving back in 1948 to the WHO and the adoption of its Constitution the same year (during which the UN's own *Universal*

Declaration of Human Rights or *UDHR* was ratified by the representative nations). Echoing the Western liberal values etched into the *UDHR*, the WHO's Constitution held the consensus that it would "in conformity with the Charter of the United Nations" protect humanity's health, which is "basic to the happiness, harmonious relations and security of all peoples" (WHO 1948, p. 1). The Constitution defined health as a "state of complete physical, mental, and social well-being and not merely the absence of disease or infirmity," which is not only "one of the fundamental rights of every human being," but also "is fundamental to the attainment of peace and security." When the Communist Soviet Union and its allies left the UN a year later, the West increasingly exercised outsized influence laying its foundation and trajectory. By 1955 (a year before the Soviets rejoined) the Brazilian WHO Director-General oversaw the global malaria eradication program which the United States and its allies backed to increase international economic growth, facilitating increased markets for their goods and boosting America's soft power appeal to the world's nations to move further from the communist Soviets. Public health was again hyperpoliticized in 1959. But this time, it was done by the Soviets who pushed a global smallpox eradication program for similar reasons (which the United States later coopted in 1967 under the American Donald Henderson to deploy new US scientific and technological innovations mass producing and distributing more effective, affordable, and convenient vaccines). The WHO shifted focus from the 1960s to 1990s to additionally embrace primary healthcare amid the growing cultural and political economic influence of decolonized African nations and socialist movements. A major milestone occurred in 1978 as such developing nations led the push to enact the Alma Ata Declaration, asserting primary healthcare care as a human right, and so an essential socioeconomic good and means to achieve "Health for All" (Hameiri 2020). It succeeded in building a historic bridge between public health, healthcare, and public and foreign policy. It also triggered retaliatory measures by the developed world. Reportedly worried about the risk of subsequent redistributive pressures, the WHO's main funders, the United States and western Europe, slashed their funding and shunted the majority of international health aid through the World Bank's structural adjustment budget for developing nations.

The WHO attempted to ease such growing tensions in the 1980s (including with its "Essential Drug Program," which the US pharmaceutical companies protested), while the World Bank increasingly appropriated domains of international health that were traditionally recognized as the WHO territory (i.e., as the World Bank promoted Western-style liberal capitalist "structural adjustments" integrated with family planning and health education requirements as part of national development loans; Brown et al. 2006; Monlezun 2023). These trends collided in 1990 when the World Bank's health loans exceeded the WHO's total budget and the WHO's own budget was progressively dominated by wealthy multinational organizations (including the UN Development Program, Western public health academic institutions, and UNICEF). Donor nations earmarked their preferred international health projects aligned with their interests, further undermining the comparative effectiveness and influence of the WHO in international health. The WHO's May 1993 working group report therefore strongly pushed for the WHO to pivot to what would become the formal language and framework of "global public health" in which it attempted to regain its former undisputed role in public health on the international stage (but now by positioning itself as a streamlined strategic coordinator, leader, and technical experts of such programs). This pivot manifested in the Harvard-educated former Norwegian prime minister, Gro Harlem Brundtland, who became the WHO's Director-General in 1998 and subsequently pioneered the WHO's rapid reframing of the competitive public-health domain through its enhanced partnerships and funding schemes. Brundtland's WHO thus accelerated the evolution of global public health as an ecosystem of partnerships. The WHO, for instance, launched the Commission on Macroeconomics and Health, uniting globally recognized public health leaders with academics including from Harvard University and the UN with its derivative and related intergovernmental agencies, including the World Bank, the UN Development Program, the WTO, and the International Monetary Fund [IMF]). The 2001 commission report ultimately asserted that developing nations had to improve their populations' health if they were to improve their economic development, while developing and developed nations should deepen the interdependence of the international structures and values of public health and political economics that notably reflected the then-dominant Western liberal world order (that underlay and shaped its political economic dominance). Brundtland's WHO pushed this ecosystem to produce robust deliverables in related public health initiatives through streamlined and globalized funding schemes. The global public health ecosystem therefore generated a growing list of "global health partnerships" of governments, intergovernmental organizations, and private donors linking overlapping interests and funding programs, including the Bill & Melinda Gates Foundation's vaccine programs, the 2001 Stop TB, and the 1998 Roll Back Malaria initiatives.

Concurrently, the semantic and conceptual developments in public health continued with these major strategic and structural trends as 20th-century public health transitioned into early 21st-century global public health (particularly as it operated increasingly as the emergent global public health ecosystem; Brown et al. 2006; Monlezun 2023). The growing public health successes during this time (and the international optimism for it) surged even faster from the 1990s to early 2000s as hyperglobalization brought greater health coordination, investment, and technological innovations across the Western-driven institutions in the Global East and South. During this time, the term "international health" and its primary leading institution, the WHO, dominated the public health agenda, discussion, and vocabulary. The term principally referred to the attempted prevention and mitigation of epidemics spreading across national borders, as public health practiced at an international level prioritized this dimension. The WHO appeared to introduce the term "global" in relation to international (public) health even earlier in their 1950s "global malarial eradication program" to denote the increasing recognition and importance of the worldwide dimension of health challenges (that do not recognize state borders) and involved actors (expanding to not just governments as in the early 20th-century model of public health but also to powerful transnational private funders, corporations, academic institutions, nongovernmental organizations, and media by the late 20th century). Throughout the US–Soviet geopolitical competition and proxy conflicts in the Cold War, public health was tugged back and forth as its main drivers sought to navigate global public health initiatives, priorities, and influence in a divided world. The political economic toll noted earlier in the 1960s and particularly in the 1980s were replaced following the Soviet Union's fall with the infighting of international agencies (particularly with the WHO and World Bank). This was until Brundtland helped position the WHO strategically and structurally as a complementary technical public health leader that again dominated public health into the 21st century, while defining the field's technical pivot into global public health.

This conceptual pivot was articulated at the time by the influential 1998 publications by the WHO's Derek Yach and Douglas Bettcher, who provided a high-profile formalization of this transition to "global public health" with their two-part publication in the *American Journal of Public Health* (AJPH, the official publication for the American Public Health Association and one of the world's oldest and most influential journals in public health) on "The Globalization of Public Health" (Yach and Bettcher 1998). They defined this globalization as "the process of increasing economic, political, and social interdependence and integration as capital, goods, persons, concepts, images, ideas and values cross state boundaries." When applied to public health, it accelerated its positive aspects (values such as human rights and technological innovations as vaccines and sanitation systems) and negative aspects (enhanced consumption of tobacco, infectious disease spread, and environmental harm). The WHO authors invoked such challenges from the political economic inflexion point of hyperglobalization to argue for the unique importance of the WHO to champion global public health solutions, including with "global early warning systems" (i.e., for infectious disease surveillance through volunteer collaboration and data sharing by government and nongovernment actors for the mutual benefit of the world's peoples and leaders). As an aside to illustrate this interdependency of global actors on global health problems—and how they are largely driven by the West and specifically the United States—Yach moved on from the WHO as the Cabinet Director for its Director-General to also fill roles in business (as the Senior Vice President of Global Health for the US beverage company, PepsiCo), academics (as a Professor of Global Health for Yale University), and nongovernment organizations (including leadership and senior advisory roles for the Rockefeller Foundation and the Clinton Global Initiative). By then, the WHO appeared to be back on top leading public health on the world stage (with its early 1900s modern public health transition to the mid-1900s international health into the latter post-1990s global [public] health).

1.3.4 Global public health as (competitive) foreign policy

The early 2000s witnessed the WHO taking the lead role technically crafting global public health initiatives (complementing local healthcare system and national public health agencies) and then coordinating their funding and deliverables with UN development agencies, the World Bank, and the WHO's globalized ecosystem of governments and nongovernment organizational partners. The optimism of the Western liberal world order bled into the related optimism of this ecosystem that generally believed its globally coordinated, technologically enabled programs would continue their linear march toward greater health, wealth, and thus peace the world over. This optimism progressively translated into greater acceptance and then pressure from not just the West but also the Global South and East to promote the greater institutionalization of global public health within and among countries, national public health agencies, and local healthcare systems. By 2007, the Ministers of Foreign Affairs for Indonesia, Thailand, Brazil, Senegal, South Africa, and Norway (4 years after Brundtland left the WHO and eventually moved to PepsiCo) published the Oslo Ministerial Declaration advocating for "broaden[ing] the scope of foreign policy [to include] health" (Ministers of Foreign Affairs 2007). They justified this move as "today's era of globalization and interdependence" underlines how poor health "may compromise a country's stability and security" by undermining "economic growth" within countries (echoing again the 1998 *Lancet* paper and 2001 WHO commission report) and our "common vulnerability" across nations. Thus "multilateral cooperation for global health security" is a modern necessity. By 2008, the UN General Assembly adopted Resolution 63/33 that recognized the "contribution...of the Oslo Ministerial Declaration" pushing for the expanded role of global public health in the international agenda among nations, while declaring (boldly) the seemingly successful reclaiming by the WHO (following Brundtland's strategic pivot) of its original "leading role...as the primary specialized agency for health" (UN 2008). This resolution approved by the world's nations followed the now well-worn US-born post-WWII formula justifying public health investments for national and international political economic net benefits. But it did so now under the formalized banner of "global public health" to advance the MDGs as its political economic operationalization on the world stage through "enhanced coordination," given the "interdependence" "between foreign policy and global health." It appeared the WHO had won the later 20th-century semantic and strategic battle for the soul and future of public health—it would be structurally global, accelerated technologically (through the internet and then AI), driven economically (by capitalism), navigated politically (by liberal democracies), and coordinated institutionally (including with agenda setting) primarily by the UN's WHO.

The practical operationalization within nations of this ambitious vision was (a) manifested with the 2008 Consortium of Universities for Global Health (CUGH) and the 2009 US Global Health Initiative, (b) articulated by the 2013 *Lancet* Commission, and (c) debated extensively in the academic literature and in real-world practice.

The US-based Bill & Melinda Gates Foundation and Rockefeller Foundation launched the CUGH the same year as the abovementioned UN Resolution to facilitate the pipeline of global public health trainees, professionals, and leaders to staff the health programs by the WHO and similar intergovernmental organizations in parallel with governments (Koplan et al. 2009; CUGH 2023). The CUGH has since significantly expanded internationally to over 170 institutions, while codifying and propagating the agenda, frameworks, content, and standards of global public health (translating the modern scientific discipline of public health increasingly into our era's globalized political economic structures and programs at the international, national, and local levels). Within this development, the CUGH asserted the formal definition of the increasingly dominant iteration of public health as a development of the WHO's 1998 strategic pivot, overshadowed by the contemporaneous liberal world (political economic) order:

Global [public] health is an area of study, research and practice that places a priority on achieving equity in health for all people…[while it] emphasizes transnational health issues, determinants and solutions; involves many disciplines within and beyond the health sciences and promotes interdisciplinary collaboration; and is a synthesis of population-based prevention with individual-level clinical care (Koplan et al. 2009).

The ultimate strategic end or objective of global public health is equitable well-being or health for all people, achieved through the primary means of WHO-coordinated prevention and treatment (uniting traditional public health, medicine, and political economics). Building on this growing historical momentum, the US President, Barak Obama, in 2009 launched the US Global Health Initiative (GHI) as the country's signature global health program and among the highest profile and funded programs in this new iteration of a globalized public health, catalyzing technology-enabled strategic and structural reform of earlier attempts to scale and coordinate public health worldwide (Alcorn 2012; Chen et al. 2023). Like the 1950s US-dominated efforts through the UN and WHO in international health, the GHI framed global health within globalization as a vehicle of the larger US national security strategy: peace purportedly through shared prosperity, accelerated through streamlined technical and funding "expertise" and "capacity building" in care delivery, education, research, and policy. Yet similar to the infighting within the international health community in the later 20th century, tensions over territory, authority, agency, and funding undermined GHI, until it was closed before the decade did.

1. By 2013 the *Lancet* Commission on Investing in Health provided a further articulation and application of this formula with its "Global Health 2035" framework (Jamison et al. 2013). It espoused an almost exuberant confidence in the "'grand convergence' in health [that] would be achievable within our lifetimes" in which the unprecedented 20th-century twin health and wealth explosions could be followed by their equitable diffusion internationally. LMICs could catch up with HICs by 2035 as global public health efforts controlling NCDs (in the more traditional public health domain) and improving healthcare system performance (by public health extending their affordable accessibility to vulnerable populations through universal health coverage). Similar to the 2001 WHO commission, the 2013 *Lancet* commission justified this evolution on health grounds (i.e., 10 million lives saved particularly among children and mothers) and economic grounds (generating net benefits 20-fold).

2. Yet throughout the 2010s, successes in global public health (and larger political economic successes in globalization-related interdependencies and cooperation among the world's nations) were accompanied by persistent disagreements among influential public health circles about what are the distinctions, if any, among global public health, international health, global health, and public health (and if they actually matter), in addition to their critiques (but mostly on the margin of mainstream discourse; Fried et al. 2010). By the end of the decade (and 6 months prior to the emergence of COVID-19 in Wuhan) (Chen et al., 2020), the Editorial Board Meeting of the China-based academic journal, *Global*

Health Research and Policy, met in Wuhan to further codify the articulated framework of global health from a non-Western perspective that still largely echoed the abovementioned Western-dominated historical narrative, including the assertion that "we will continue to learn global health from the WHO" that "established [its] knowledge base [and] methodologies" (Chen et al. 2023). Like the Western efforts implicitly or explicitly meant to expand its power reach (politically, economically, culturally, and even arguably militarily in certain contexts) through global public health, this high-level emblematic Chinese Board "recommend[s] to take advantage of [China's] Belt and Road Initiative" (BRI) to "advance global health science" and "to share China's lessons and successful experience with other countries." Proponents of the BRI note how China's President Xi Jinping launched BRI in 2013 and since then grew to be among history's largest infrastructure programs, covering up to 100 nations, 60% of the global population, and $4 trillion of roads, railways, trade, transportation, cultural, and digital exchange in a modern Silk Road stretching from Asia to Europe; opponents counter it is a debt trap preying on LMICs, emboldened by Russian and Iranian autocratic leaders, and enabling Chinese military and economic power expansion that benefits China at the expense of neo-colonized states (Chatzky and McBride 2020). Regardless the march continued toward developing and practically implementing global public health—as the intersection of the traditional scientific discipline with globalized foreign policy—through the accelerated proliferation of its institutions and conceptual frameworks, all within its increasingly dense ecosystem of partners, funding, and political economic influence on the wider global society. So historically, public health emerged as religious-informed cultural practices in ancient times, developed for two millennia as political mandates for societal security, leapt forward into scientific-based and economically motivated national policy in early modern times, and crossed the threshold of the 21st century as a global public health ecosystem where health, wealth, and equity were meant to synergistically power each other (framed and furthered by powerful political economic blocs, particularly in the West). It became difficult to therefore distinguish between global public health and power by another name.

By 2021, a systematic review and thematic analysis by Salm et al. of 1363 publications in the academic literature from the preceding decade reflected the debate and disagreements about what "global health" actually is and thus how it should be conducted (reflecting the broader underlying ideological-informed foreign policy campaigns of political economic competitions for power, and thus the historical competing forces in the development of the global public health ecosystem encompassing these factions; Salm et al. 2021). This comprehensive study demonstrated how there is no clear consensus distinguishing "global health" (or "global public health" from "public health" nor "international health"). It did illustrate how differing conceptions of "global health" generally do express a multidisciplinary approach to solving health problems spanning the world in an academic dimension (through research organizations like universities and think tanks) and practical dimension (through governmental, intergovernmental, and international organizations collaborating on health programs, often intertwined with political economic and human development investments).

Ultimately, the systematic review concluded that defining global health can be better accomplished by answering "who" is seeking to define (and enforce) it, rather than "what" is being defined. So as global (public) health became increasingly in the 2000s an ecosystem overlapping national and supra-national blocs' foreign policy powered by their political economic systems, the 2010s grappled with where does global public health go from there (including how to fix its inherent problems and beginning with deciding what needs to be fixed and by whom). This conceptual ambiguity set it up for the anticolonial critique that built up in that decade and the practical shortcomings painfully demonstrated following the WHO's 2020 COVID-19 pandemic declaration.

1.4 Anticolonial and COVID critiques

To better understand how and why AI is transforming the future of the global public health ecosystem, we will wrap up its historical analysis by understanding how the anticolonial and COVID critiques are pressuring it to more rapidly and fundamentally embrace the responsible AI shaping its future.

1.4.1 Anticolonial backlash

The 2010s witnessed a growing push in the academic and practical sectors of global health for its "decolonization" (King and Koski 2020). In this trajectory, the abovesaid Canadian anthropologist and epidemiologist team built on the conceptual ambiguity of global health to influentially (and provocatively) argue essentially that "global health is public health somewhere else": self-identified experts and practitioners of public health do such work in regions outside of where they live, "imposing" on others their own conceptions of health and the means of achieving it. Although there have been resultant disagreements on this sharp distinction within the public and global health academic literature, such critics have not up to this point articulated a robust alternative; nonetheless, they do share their concern for colonial aspects of global health programs (Turcotte-Tremblay et al. 2020). Regardless, King and Koski's bold definition highlighted the (1) academic observation that there are no clear methodologies or ends (ultimate strategic objectives) distinguishing global and public health, in addition to the (2) practical observation that global health interventions often have embedded problematic assumptions limiting their moral and social defensibility and stated technical objectives. Such assumptions include the "expertise gradient" (assuming typically Global North "experts" know better how to direct Southern health programs and policies), the "accountability gap" (downplaying local community agency and program sustainability), and unnecessary inefficiency (in potentially excessive academic training to become an "expert" and then transporting and deploying such human and capital resources often at great distances, increasing program costs that may negatively impact local communities where the programs are deployed). While King and Koski explicitly reject the notion that "all global health efforts are inherently flawed or unjustifiable," they do encourage a "more widespread and transparent discussion of the unexamined normative dimensions of global health." They explicitly link this anticolonial critique, following global health's historical development from the 19th-century West-born modern public health, with the wider critique of the Global North and particularly Western international aid, as articulated by Angus Deaton:

> *The aid endeavor [in general and global health in particular] is inspired by the question of what we should do, or by its imperative version that we must do something. Yet. . .Why is it is we who have to do something? Who put us in charge?. . .We often have such a poor understanding of what they need or want, of how their societies work, that our clumsy attempts to help on our terms do more harm than good. . .Negative unintended consequences are pretty much guaranteed when we try. And when we fail, we continue on because our interests are now at stake—it is our aid industry, staffed largely by our professionals, and generating kudos and votes for our politicians—and because, after all, we must do something (Deaton 2022).*

A sharper line of critique of global health (especially as it gained international influence and integration with foreign policy of Northern geopolitical blocs) questioned if global health must account for its "inherent colonialism, uncritical faith in Western expertise and technology, [and a] lack of accountability and inefficient use of resources" (Packard 2016; Horton 2013; Deaton 2022). Such research flowed from the earlier work of John-Paul Sartre, the French philosopher who articulated the term "neo-colonialism" to describe the larger supposed societal trend in which a stronger state that was historically a former colonial power (typically in the Global West or East) continued or reimposed imperialist control or influence economically, politically, and/or culturally over a weaker state (Sartre 1956; Stanard 2018, p. 5). From the 17th to 20th centuries, European nations translated the Industrial Revolutions' technological innovations into more powerful economies and militaries. They then used them to dominate African, Middle Eastern, Asian, and American peoples to extract their raw resources for (or stimulate their consumption of) their manufactured refined products. The long colonial shadow during the 21st-century decolonization period often meant the stronger states retained over the weaker states' residual political economic influence (often in the form of perpetuating political systems of local leaders sympathetic to the stronger states or North-run global health programs as foreign policy, economic arrangements with often unsustainable debts, and influential foreign cultural practices); these often conflicted with or even overpowered the weaker states' historical or preferred societal, political economic, and cultural arrangements (Prashad 2007, pp. 231−3). The anticolonial critique responded progressively in the first three decades of the 21st century against not only Western international aid but increasingly also Chinese infrastructure investments (Chatzky and McBride 2020).

In parallel with Deaton's anticolonial critique against international aid mentioned earlier (and King and Koski's emphasizing its global health applications), Eugene Richardson extends it even to global and public health's methodologies. Richardson, the Rwanda and Harvard-based University of Global Health Equity physician−anthropologist, followed the French Michel Foucault by arguing that the new techniques of AI, Big Data, and causal inference statistics alongside the older techniques of infectious disease containment and epidemiological modeling "play an essential role in perpetuating a range of global inequities" (Richardson 2020). Even the essential public health tool of disease causation modeling supposedly "serve protected affluence" by "setting epistemic limits" on healthy versus sick populations, and so ultimately unleashes the world's "biggest epidemic": "an epidemic of illusions," "propagated by the coloniality of knowledge production" to "achieve monopolies on truth" (p. 5). According to this argument, modern global health following its early modern public health progenitor creates problems it then professes to solve with an authority it invents for and enforces itself.

Such 21st-century anticolonial critique from within the North echoes the earlier lesser known 20th-century critique from within the South. Kwame Nkrumah, the philosopher—politician who served as Ghana's first Prime Minister, argued that public health was essentially colonial power under the guise of compassionate care with questionable at best practical benefit for the South's communities. He highlighted in 1965 how the March Bulletin of the US-based American Federation of Labor and Congress of Industrial Organizations (physically neighboring the UN's headquarters) stated "In mobilizing capital resources for investment...[including in] Health Clinics and Housing...we will encourage labor-management co-operation to expand American capital investment in the African nations" (p. 245). He noted how this period featured both Western democratic and Eastern communist nations (particularly the Soviet Union and China) competing with each other in the explosion of politically tied economic investment especially in Africa to expand their influence over it. This critique argues therefore that Northern nations extended international "aid" (encompassing public health) to the South with the central imperial pitch of "We make you wealthy and healthy, and you play on our team by our rules to beat the other guy." Such neo-imperialism according to Nkrumah gives the weaker colonized modern state the illusion of "international sovereignty," while "[i]n reality its economic system and thus its political policy is directed from outside" (p. ix). This long-standing anticolonial questioning of public and now global health is only intensifying especially as AI is transforming it. The most advanced AI—including its governance and intellectual and technical capital—is based in America, China, and the larger North which "extracts" data globally, particularly from weaker states and communities in the South, without providing mutual benefit or honoring sufficient consent in this growing global digital ecosystem. Such critics question if the 21st-century data in the South (used to refine the global health algorithms of the North and its derivative products and programs) have replaced the colonized people's 17th- to 20th-century raw natural resources (refined into colonial power's manufactured products principally for their benefit).

It should be finally noted that the more immediate and intense anticolonial pressure on global public health (with its emphasis on disruptive technologies like AI) is the highly polarizing political event ongoing as of the early 2023 writing of the book, namely, the Russo-Ukrainian war mentioned earlier. It has been widely heralded as an emblematic conflict embodying a new era of technologically accelerated great power conflict dividing the world (along with different supranational blocs' global health, economic, and foreign policies that are deeply intertwined). The UN and WHO noted in March 2023b, a year following Russia's "full-scale invasion of Ukraine," that Ukraine provides an unprecedented case example not only of modern local conflicts with globalized repercussions, including threatening food and energy shortages capable of undermining healthcare systems and public health agencies globally (WHO 2023c; Nchasi et al. 2022). But it also accentuates the public health lessons for how a "country's health system [can] remain resilient"—particularly with enhanced WHO-coordinated support to maintain healthcare systems' vital operations and access—in a new era of unpredictable and unprecedented national, health, and human security threats. Russia's government and affiliates defended their invasion by asserting "'the West is literally rotting' yet becoming more expansionist while only Eastern civilization has a future," with the Russian Foreign Minister declared that "Russia's military operation in Ukraine contributes to liberating the world from the neo-colonial oppression of the West" (Kirillova 2022). The UN responded on the war's 1-year anniversary with 141 member nations voting to condemn Russia and repeated "its demand that the Russian Federation immediately...withdraw all of its military forces from...Ukraine" (UN 2023a). This was followed by the International Criminal Court, with jurisdiction in 123 countries, issuing an arrest warrant in March 2023 for Russia's President, Vladimir Putin, for "the war crime of unlawful deportation of [a] population" by separating nearly a million Ukrainian children from their parents in the first year and sending them to Russia (ICC 2023). Aligned critiques argue rather it is Russia which is the most significant and immediate neo-colonial threat to global, health, and human security with its "imperial aggression," including over its post-Soviet colonies in Eastern Europe and Asia, particularly with their main interstate institutions spanning Belarus, Armenia, and Kazakhstan still remaining "dominated by Russia and [which still] largely serve as vessels for the Kremlin's strategic agenda" (Couch 2023). The Yale University genocide historian, Timothy Snyder, similarly argues that like the darkest premodern period of European empires treating weaker colonized "tribes" as being unable to govern themselves, Putin publicly and repeatedly denied Ukrainian exists as a sovereign nation: "we see in the [modern] ruins of Ukrainian cities, and in the Russian practice of mass killing, rape, and deportation, the claim that a nation does not exist is the rhetorical preparation for destroying it" (Snyder 2022). This includes upward of 200 000 Russian conscript casualties within only the first year of the full-scale war, the majority of which were drawn from Russian peripheral ethnic minorities and former colonies rather than the higher income central Russian region (Snyder 2022; Ivanova et al. 2022).

A parallel analytic consensus notes that the self-identified Putin ally, friend, and autocratic Chinese leader, Xi Jinping, has declared that China will use force if necessary to achieve "reunification" of its supposed breakaway province, the decades-long self-governing island democracy of Taiwan (Blanchette and DiPippo 2022). Chinese and Russian proponents generally assert that the postcolonial West needs to make room for a more multipolar world. Yet their critics counter that Putin and Xi actually mean they want a world they dominate through greater global influence and domestic control by their autocratic regimes, threatened by supposedly peaceful and prosperous democratic neighbors (particularly in Ukraine and Taiwan, which must therefore be eliminated as separate states and subjugated as neo-colonialized weaker powers). Such analysts worry that while Russia's Ukrainian invasion still threatens to trigger worsening global food, energy, and health crises at least as of 2023. But a Chinese invasion of Taiwan—with the expected resultant defensive support by the United States, Japan, and the larger West—would bring the entire global digital economy to a halt. Taiwan produces the vast bulk of the semiconductors it runs on, along with the global public health ecosystem it enables. AI cannot run without data and analytics, nor can its digitally enabled global public health (or even its international coordination, communication, and supply chains). Such colonial critique thus argues that the 21st-century AI-enabled and de-colonized global public health must finally take seriously not only such structural threats to its resilience, but also the sovereignty and security of all nations—including post-colonial states—which constitute it.

1.4.2 Great COVID Reset

As this decolonial global debate was ramping up amid worsening geopolitical shocks, COVID-19 struck. The AI-based Canadian firm, BlueDot, released on December 31, 2019, the first known warning about a novel cluster of pneumonia cases in China's Wuhan Hubei Province (over a week before the WHO released its public warning) using its natural language processing algorithms scanning publicly available news reports, airline tickets, and disease networks continuously every 15 minutes year-round (Stieg 2020). The day before China even locked down Wuhan, within just 2 weeks of the WHO reporting this cluster was caused by a novel coronavirus, and 3 months before it declared this "COVID-19" virus was a pandemic, BlueDot submitted a manuscript that would become the first published peer-reviewed scientific paper on the virus, and the first known of any public report to accurately predict the initial international spread of the virus from China to "support public health planning and readiness" (AP 2021; WHO 2020; Bogoch et al. 2020). Within the pandemic's subsequent 2 years, the WHO estimated that the pandemic caused 14.83 million excess deaths internationally (with the highest mortality in LMICs), while costing the global economy $12.5 trillion over its first 5 years (or 1 of every 10 dollars the world makes; Msemburi et al. 2023; Wang and COVID-19 Excess Mortality Collaborators 2022; IMF 2022). Vaccine nationalism may heap on an additional $9.2 trillion, as HICs hoarded 84% of COVID-19 vaccines in the pandemic's first year compared to 1% being available in LICs—despite the global health and economic cost of more dangerous viral variants generated and supply chains further disrupted by inadequate global vaccination (Çakmaklı et al. 2021). Aside from interstate inequities, intra-state inequities were further exposed by the global health response to COVID-19. Low-income peoples shouldered the disproportionately higher health and financial burden of the pandemic, revealing not only the "hollowness of the global health rhetoric of equity, the weaknesses of a health security-driven global health agenda, and the negative health impacts of power differentials not only globally, but also regionally and locally," which therefore highlighted the urgent need to "reimagine and repair the broken systems of global health" (Shamasunder et al. 2020). Such critics questioned if COVID-19 laid bare how we are "failing another…stress test on health disparities (Owen Carmona and Pomeroy 2020). COVID-19 thus ultimately demonstrated the "collapse of global cooperation and solidarity," according to the 2016−22 Director of the African Centers for Disease Control and Prevention (CDC), Dr. John Nkengasong (Myers 2022). And without cooperation, it is unclear how global health can survive. The modern global health ecosystem boasts the most advanced and globalized science, technology, and political economic cooperation for societal well-being in history. And yet there is no substantive agreement that its pandemic interventions (one of its primary objectives) equitably worked at the scale and cost the world needed, to the point that even within the highest profile and influential public health agencies on the planet, its own internal critics even questioned if "public health...failed" (Varma 2022).

The anticolonial critique (centered on the alleged problematic abstract and structural features) of the global public health ecosystem assumed new urgency with the COVID-19 critique (centered on the concrete and ineffective features of the ecosystem). A decade after the world's countries proclaimed the WHO was the "leading...specialized agency for health," the WHO's Independent Panel concluded its "failure to enact fundamental change...has left the world dangerously exposed" to global health risks "as the Covid-19 pandemic proves" (UN 2008; Clark et al. 2021; AP 2021). Two pandemics propagating from China in just the first two decades of the 21st century showed according to the Panel how global public health came up short leading the world "in our collective capacity to come together in solidarity to create a protective web of human security." Beginning with the WHO down to national governments and local healthcare systems and public health agencies, the Panel found there was inadequate preparedness for the pandemic, early warning of it, response to the warning, efficient and equitable creation and distribution of effective countermeasures, and substantive change to better respond to the next global health crises (as China initially withheld the viral genome while urging the WHO and other nations against emergency declaration, followed by other nations being slow to respond to the eventual WHO warnings and guidance). Strategic, operational, coordination, and equitable failures painfully exposed how the WHO seemed to have made no substantive course corrections or structural improvements after the COVID-19 pandemic emerged in 2020 (or even after similar problems were identified in 2015 following the Ebola epidemic) to better respond to current or future threats (Kupperschmidt 2021; Hameiri 2020). If the WHO is the face of the modern global public health ecosystem, such criticism alleges it hides its history of international power struggles and current political and funding constraints (with approximately 85% of its $5.6 billion annual budget by the 2000s controlled by donors' earmarked projects), leaving little capacity for generating and sustaining true and equitable global health progress. Such critics argue that it is simply an expensive source of declarations and documents, with limited demonstrated success or concrete development. Nonetheless, even high-profile critics of global health in general and the WHO in particular (including the Independent Panel) argue the WHO may still be the best positioned force to lead effective and equitable global public health (as an attainable strategic means for global peace, prosperity, and thus justice). Yet it lacks the necessary power politically (to enforce health measures, including mandatory reporting by nations for disease surveillance and internal health investment) and economically (to move efficiently enough to create, distribute, and coordinate health interventions). The World Economic Forum thus proposed "The Great COVID Reset" in 2020 to highlight how the health crisis showcased not only the failings in the global public health ecosystem—and those in its underlying political economic and even deeper societal ecosystems—but also how it can transform this failure into the historic opportunity reclaiming our common values and revolutionize the informed institutional relations, governance structures, and finance models. This Great COVID Reset is ambitiously described by its proponents as the critical chance "to build a new social contract that honours the dignity of every human being" (WEF 2023). According to this critique, the pandemic thus allows global health to not only confront its own existential crisis of identity and practical operations, but it also can catalyze our larger global human society to rethink, retool, and reform according to a renewed vision of our humanity and the future worthy of it.

1.5 Part II: Future

1.5.1 Emerging trends shaping artificial intelligence's global public health ecosystem

The abovementioned history of the global public health ecosystem now allows us to consider its future. In this section, we will consider an overview of three emerging trends shaping AI in this ecosystem, setting up the next section introducing how they frame three primary domains in which global health is developing. We will then conclude this introductory chapter with an overview of how the book will delve deeper into those domains driven by those trends using an interpretative key to understand and even shape them.

AI is at the center of the (1) digitalization, (2) deglobalization, and (3) demographic trends shaping the trajectory of the global public health ecosystem by accelerating how technology is changing our national and international societies and political economic structures impacting health.

1.5.2 Digitalization

The earlier sections introduced how early modern public health developed alongside its concurrent Industrial Revolutions: rapid technological changes produced seismic societal changes within nations (particularly in populations' health) and in turn fueled cooperation, competition, and conflict among nations which culminated in the US-led international liberal world order of the 1990s and early 2000s (McKinsey 2022; Monlezun 2023; Schwab 2016; Allison and Schmidt 2020). The First, Second, and Third Industrial Revolutions. Respectively, centered on steam-driven mechanization, electricity-driven mass production, and digital-driven computation and automation. They progressively enabled more rapid, numerous, affordable, and valuable products until a critical mass of the world's nations became industrialized, globalized, and then digitalized in the Fourth Industrial Revolution since the 2010s. The US-accelerated economic expansion of capitalism in the later 20th century (along with its liberal democratic dominated institutions including the UN, WHO, World Bank, and WTO) increasingly connected the world in global supply and value chains for this global capitalist economy. Cyber-physical systems linked customers, producers, organizations, and governments to a degree and depth previously unseen in near real-time feedback about what individuals demand and how suppliers can respond. Technology progressively rewrote the lines between health, society, politics, and economics and rearranged them into the single dimension of digits.

By the end of that decade, digitalization had reached the heights of global health. Its projects and their creation, funding, and management had up to that point followed the larger 2000s−10s societal changes of digitalization-driven globalization. Health projects were devised, deployed, and managed with teams typically relying on internet connectivity, remote telecommunications, and digital data collection and analysis. All this occurred in a self-reinforcing feedback loop of increasingly interconnected and interdependent cooperation across multiple sectors of societies, states, and organizations. The WHO followed by the rest of the global health community in turn formulated guidance and instruments to further the fundamental digital makeover of global health. In July 2019, the Chinese businessman, Jack Ma, and the American philanthropist−computer scientist, Melinda Gates, chaired the UN High-Level Panel on Digital Cooperation that released its report on "The age of digital interdependence" (UN 2020). This informed the UN Secretary-General's June 2020 "Roadmap for Digital Cooperation" to implement those recommendations for the government, academic, business, and technology sectors (UN 2020). The panel and roadmap identified the current transition into a new human era of digital interconnectedness that they argued can accelerate greater peace and prosperity for our planet—or war and devastation —while detailing a practical vision for how to make digital technologies safe, equitable, and just for the global society (not just for profit or power of a local few). To make this AI-driven digitalization therefore good for humanity, the Panel recommended we together "build an inclusive digital economy and society" that nourishes "human and institutional capacity" through "protecting[ing] human rights and human agency," beginning with "promot[ing] digital trust, security, and stability" and "foster[ing] global digital cooperation" (p. 4). The UN Secretary-General therefore called for "an inclusive digital ecosystem" in which "technology is harnessed for good," achieved by the roadmap's plan to implement these recommendations that were essentially aimed at realizing the health-focused sustainable development goals (SDGs; with an urgency accelerated by the "global health crisis" of COVID-19; p. 12, 17, 20).

The WHO adapted the UN roadmap's eight action items for its eight "principles to reflect the imperatives of the Digital Transformation" for global health: universal connectivity, digital goods, inclusive digital health, interoperability, human rights, AI, information security, and public health architecture (García Saisó and D'Agostino 2021, p. 5; Saisó et al. 2022). We previously considered how the WHO as the UN's chief health body had recognized 20 years prior its need to strategically pivot to the roles of expert and coordinator of global health cooperative projects (spanning traditional public health, medicine, and political economics). And at the dawn of the 2020s, the WHO recognized its next needed pivot to AI-accelerated digitalization. The new "globalized, interconnected reality that is now part of the human condition" requires "global participation in artificial intelligence" that "should be part of public health policies" (p. 5). Speaking reportedly as our collective global health voice, the WHO essentially was saying our modern lives are digitalized because they are globalized, interconnected, and increasingly AI augmented. Health is multifaceted (individually, collectively, and structurally) and contextualized in progressively digitalized societies (interchangeable with the AI they progressively run on). Thus the WHO argued that health AI should promote "equity…and diversity" through "secure, reliable and open algorithms" (p. 5). And as done in the twilight of the 20th century, the WHO specifically and global health generally (according to this line of argument) should take a lead role in ensuring this new reality gives rise to our emergent future that works for our common good, "grounded in the globally-agreed ethical principles of human dignity, beneficence, non-maleficence and justice" (p. 2). The WHO sees such ethical principles as critical since the major technical drivers of AI development and deployment cannot be assumed to do so without assistance, pressure, and even compulsion to put ethical parameters on their supposed primary focus of expanding their power economically and/or politically). The WHO's AI principles therefore highlighted equitable expansion of safe, reliable, and affordable access to the global digital ecosystem as basic public digital goods, characterized as individual rights, and necessary for individual and collective flourishing in our digital world. This would make the ecosystem therefore more inclusive and so an effective means to improve global health.

The first year of the COVID-19 pandemic accelerated the global push for greater digitalization and thus connectivity, speed, and complexity of data sharing as our interconnected world sought to rewrite in real-time basic rules for our societies, economies, and governance. Tracking the viral spread, managing limited hospital resources, advising updated public health guidance (from masking to quarantines to treatments to recovery), rerouting global supply chains—it all ran (and runs) on data that we used (and use) to guide our decisions, undermined by uncertainty and challenged by massive negative consequences if we got those decisions wrong. By 2021, the WHO buffeted by the supposed opposing forces of financial concerns (to "reopen economies") and health concerns (to "control the virus" often through quarantine and lockdowns) published its "Global strategy on digital health," following its history of rebranding international health as global health and then as digital health in response to overarching global societal changes. The report refined its strategic pivot in this new era of global health's digitalization by detailing a unifying conceptual framework with derivative principles, strategies, objectives, and stepwise implementation. Hearkening back to Alma Ata and the 1970s decolonization push for more equitable health, the report sought to bolster global health by "strengthen[ing] health systems through the application of digital health technologies for consumers, health professionals, health care providers and industry" as a means to "empowering patients and achieving the vision of health for all" (WHO 2021). To achieve global health (that is global and health), it must become digital. And to be maximally useful, it must be supercharged by AI. The WHO according to this argument advocated for "artificial intelligence solutions and big data analyses" as the primary means to "improve the quality of health care and research effectiveness," which are the primary strategic objectives of global health (p. 12, 15). But to make AI-fueled digitalized global health happen, it needs "principles for...[their] ethical use," "sharing of learning," "sustainable financing models," and appropriate "governance structures" (pp. 23−24).

By February 2022, a WHO-coordinated international multisector consortium emphasized how the "weaknesses in global health care delivery systems and public health responses" revealed by the COVID-19 pandemic could and should be addressed by effectively deploying digital health in the global public health system (Al Knawy et al. 2022). In line with the WHO's report, the G20's related 2020 Riyadh Global Digital Health Summit assembled a panel spanning representatives from governments (including Saudi Arabia and the United Kingdom), businesses (including IBM and CVS), and academics (including universities from Finland, Scotland, Australia, Singapore, South Korea, and the United States). They then published their consensus blueprint for implementing such a vision of digitalized global health. The consortium highlighted how the 21st century's digital advances were dizzyingly advanced in notable areas, though the pandemic showed how they were generally still fragmented, inefficient, and underfunded, and so failed to deliver on international needs in the major stress test that COVID-19 posed to the global public health ecosystem. The lack of sufficient data interoperability (sharing, using, and understanding information across different stakeholders), integrity (the quality, accuracy, and precision of information making it trustworthy), effectiveness (fit-for-purpose architecture), scale (expanding or shrinking capacities and their applications based on user needs and timeframes), maturity (the degree of embeddedness and usability within groups enabling digital operations), and equity (disparate capacities across stakeholders) across states and within them (including governments, academics, business, organizations, and communities) blunted the potential of global health's digital promise for us. Their recommendations therefore outlined concretely how to optimize AI-powered digital transformation, teamwork, transparency (and related trust), technology, and "techuity" (technology-accelerated health equities). Moving on, we will spend the remaining chapters filling out the practical details how such responsible AI-accelerated digitalization continues to frame and fuel global public health in its various domains noted in the above section's introduction of the book's structure. Specifically, we will analyze the explosive technological development of various AI forms and their wide variations in deployment especially for health in our digitalized world.

1.5.3 Deglobalization

Late modernity's "deglobalization" snowballed with the 2008 Great Recession, 2010s populist movements (including the 2016 Brexit referendum and Donald Trump's US presidential election), the 2020 declaration of the COVID-19 pandemic, Russia's 2022 full-scale invasion of Ukraine (with resultant Western decoupling from Russia), and China's increasing AI technological competition and military aggression in the South China Sea along with threats of force against Taiwan (prompting further Western "de-risking" from China in key technologies and Western strengthening of defensive alliances; Irwin 2020; Oxford 2022; Monlezun 2023). Globalization describes the degree of international exchange and interdependence of trade, investment, ideas, technology, data, and people (as students, workers, and tourists). It can be measured empirically as global trade, or the international exports and imports over world gross domestic product (GDP), which is the monetary value of services and goods measuring a nation's total yearly output. In the 1800s, European colonial powers leveraged their Industrial Revolutions to integrate the peoples and resources populating their spheres of influence through supply chains that produced final refined goods and services for their domestic and international markets. Global trade initially measured at 17.6% in 1870 and stayed largely stable through 1914. It then plummeted by nearly half to its lowest levels in recorded history during the interwar era of WWI and WWII amid hostilities, conflicts, and protectionist policies (promoting domestic industries while limiting foreign ones). The United States largely drove the postwar rebound of global trade up to 1980 when it reached 39.5%, as its global navy facilitated more open borders and markets (particularly with American reconstruction investments enabling the economic surge of a Japan-led Asia and Germany-led Europe). As Soviet power progressively faltered, US-driven digitalization surged, along with its parallel decolonization process of democratic liberalization in the 1980s–2000s which facilitated an explosive increase of global trade to its 2008 peak of 61.1% (with most of the global economic output coming from generating goods nationally for exchange internationally). Digital technologies accelerated health, wealth, and security, while also more deeply intertwining them into global value supply chains, making nations increasingly economically interdependent in a densely interconnected global ecosystem. But in the 2010s, the party was over (or at least toned down). When the Great Recession hit, economic damage in the US housing market raged outward throughout the globalized economic markets (followed by COVID-19 at the end of the decade when the health damage of COVID-19 poured outward from China through our globalized travel networks). Although, the more extreme interpretation of these trends as "deglobalization" may rather be more a period of "slowbalization." Global trade appears to actually be stabilizing at around 53.5% going into the 2020s, such that our globalized society may be restructuring rather than unraveling, or pulling back the reins of "runaway" hyperglobalization rather than abandoning the model.

This interpretation argues the world is entering a more stable period of slower growth and interdependence from the intense rate seen in the hyperglobalization of the 1990s–2000s (with the unchallenged dominance of the US-led liberal world order). The IMF describes this slowbalization phenomenon as a more gradual pace of globalization, or what I term "secure globalization," referring to how this slower rate comes specifically from trade bounded by reportedly necessary national security concerns (Aiyar and Illyina 2023; Irwin 2020; Oxford 2022; Monlezun 2023). Consider the latest "hot" tech business in which everyone who can seem to be rapidly buying stocks (or shares of public ownership) believing it will become the next Apple or Microsoft, becoming worth much more tomorrow than it is today (generating a greater return on that investment). Yet it can be overhyped and overvalued, leading to its value bubble to burst. This market correction (in which prices for such shares shift back to a more accurate value now and likely value for the near term at least) occurs for companies and economic sectors cyclically and predictably. Such secure globalization emerging from the 2020s onward may thus be the new normal for the foreseeable digital future as this political economic reality frames businesses and nations—particularly their public health and even global public health stakeholders. Hyperglobalization accentuated globalization's benefits: cheaper and easier products for consumers (through global value supply chains), greater equality across nations (through developing nations growing richer through their cheaper labor force in those global chains), more peaceful international relations (through greater economic interdependence tamping down occasional political tensions), reduced military conflicts (with a nearly 50% reduction in defense spending globally in the last 50 years up to 2022), and enhanced green energy investments (through cheaper credit or cost of borrowing enabling technological breakthroughs that make renewable or nonfossil fuel energy sources more affordable and effective; Bokat-Lindell, 2022; Hayashi and DeBarros 2023). But the Great Recession and the COVID-19 pandemic finally may have broken this model. After benefiting from the American global liberalization efforts including its 2001 WTO entrance into more frictionless global trade, China became the main manufacturing nation for the world, such that most if not all global value chains moved through it by 2019—until President Xi Jinping's Chinese Communist Party (CCP) locked down the country from 2020 to 2022. Unless countries rapidly diversified and reshored their supply chains, their lockdown may have locked down the global economy. For public health resources like masks and vaccines to economic resources like raw materials and digital technology components, the world's countries increasingly moved to diversity, shorten, and overlap their supply chains to avoid single points of failure that were unintended hallmarks of hyperglobalization. When Russia launched a full-scale invasion of Ukraine in 2022, hundreds of Western companies pulled out of Russia (along with billions of dollars and thousands of jobs), while dozens of states weaned themselves off energy dependence on it. The capitalist liberal democracies of the West (Europe, North America, and its Pacific allies including Japan, South Korea, and Australia) and the more illiberal democracies or autocracies of the East (including China, Russia, and Iran) sharpened the borders of their political economic blocs at least rhetorically (like China and Russia) and if not also materially (with deepening North Korean, Iranian, and Russian military cooperation skirting Western sanctions; Lemco et al. 2021, p. 8).

In the most substantive and intense geopolitical rivalry during this period, secure globalization therefore seems increasingly manifested by the US business community arguing for instance that "the US should be de-risking from China, not decoupling" (Hayashi and DeBarros 2023). So, while US good imports to China dropped in 2022 to their lowest level since 2005, its trade deficit with China remained near record levels. This occurred even as China escalated its threats to seize Taiwan (with their advanced semiconductors), despite the specter of Western interference, while America implemented export controls to block China from accessing advanced semiconductors that power the most advanced AI-driven digital technologies (including for military purposes) that run our modern global economy. This microchip war is driving the de-risking deglobalization aspect of our current larger secure globalization era that has particular global health implications (Miller 2022). Consider a transistor, the basic building block of the digital age that controls an electric current's flow between two terminals, allowing a machine to compute or generate output based on preprogrammed rules. Transistors make up "semiconductors" or microchips that are the brains of modern digital technologies. The chip industry every year creates more transistors than all other goods made by all other businesses in all other economic sectors in all of human history—combined. From being nonexistent less than a century ago, semiconductors now dominate the devices that generate the majority of the global GDP. Arguably, the United States beat the Soviet Union in the Cold War and remains the sole global military superpower because it designed and manufactured the best chips that produced the smartest and so most powerful computers. And now, China spends more on chips every year than oil. For this vital lifeblood of the global economy, the United States and its allies are increasingly in an explicit strategic competition with China to secure it (progressively forcing countries to "pick a side"), while more generally the world's countries are seeking to shorten and duplicate global supply chains to make them more resilient and thus reliable.

Secure globalization is dominated by its two primary strategic competitors in AI technology, economics, international relations, and thus global health: China and the United States. According to Anthony Saich (the Chinese Tsinghua University and American Harvard University Professor of International Affairs), President Xi defends China's more assertive strategic pivot as necessary for the "rejuvenation of the Chinese nation" by making it not only *a* "global leader in terms of composite strength and international influence" but *the* leader (Saich 2022). To purportedly preserve its national security (as the survivability of its autocratic government regime), it seeks to displace the United States at the center of the current global order (with its societal values of individual rights and freedom and political economic structure of liberal democratic capitalism). It then seeks to replace them with China's own values of collective security and sovereignty, along with its political economic structure of increasingly illiberal autocratic socialism with key capitalist features. This grand strategy requires such ultimate objectives even if it requires China prioritizing political control over economic growth (maximizing state control while minimizing business innovation and citizen rights) as Xi supposedly sees the survival of the CCP as indispensable for the survival of China and its global destiny (Doshi 2021). In contrast, the US President Joe Biden continued Trump's push to accelerate "more secure and resilient supply chains" for the United States that are "essential for our national security, our economic security, and our technology leadership" (Sullivan and Deese 2021, p. 6). A central "deglobalization" strategy for this is "friend-shoring," restructuring supply chains with countries who share compatible or comparable values and related political economic structural features. And interestingly, the United States uses public health to at least in part defend this strategic pivot to enhanced national security within global commerce: "the COVID-19 pandemic highlighted the critical importance of a resilient U.S. public health industrial base" preserved by a "supply chain resilience strategy" as one of the "six critical industrial base sectors that underpin America's economic and national security" (p. 4, 8–9). AI runs on data and computing, and both run on semiconductors, as does our modern global societal and so health ecosystems. Thus the story of AI's digitalization and deglobalization of global public health cannot escape the basic reality of these intertwined societal trends, which shape the lives of a rapidly changing global demographic.

1.5.4 Demographics

Demographics societally drive digitalization and deglobalization (which synergistically feedback to it), as before we can have technology and economics, we need to first have people to build and use them. The different values of populations and their structural manifestations in political economics domestically and internationally—including in public and global health—order the rate and magnitude of the oscillation between competition and cooperation. Demographics, as the statistical description of a population and its constitutive aspects, help us to begin to frame and eventually answer the questions that our shared existence on a common planetary home pose to us. We have limited resources and yet seemingly unlimited desires (particularly for health as a necessary good for all other pursuits). "Health" is after all always health *for* someone rather than an abstract isolated concept. The global public health ecosystem must therefore understand who health is for if it is to generate the products and services to optimize it. And as the seismic societal trends mentioned earlier are advancing, so are similar changes in global demographics.

We are approaching a demographic challenge humanity has never faced before: there are globally more old people than young, which will likely stay like this indefinitely (Dobriansky et al. 2017, p. 3; Weng 2010). Using global data including from the UN, the US National Institutes of Health, and the WHO's World Bank—commissioned Global Burden of Disease Study (GBDS), consensus demographic studies demonstrate how the global population is aging faster than at any time in history. By 2020, we crossed the unprecedented threshold of having more people over 65 years of age than under 5. By 2050, 78% of the world's countries are expected to fall below replacement levels (total fertility rate [TFR], or the average number of children born per women, less than 2.1; Vollset et al. 2020). By 2064, our species is projected to peak at 9.73 billion (95% uncertainty interval 8.84–10.90) and by 2010, 95% of nations will likely fail to reach replacement levels with a TFR of only 1.66 billion. By then, India is expected to be the most populous country—exceeding China likely by 2023—followed by Nigeria, as China's population is expected to collapse by nearly 50% (accentuating questions not only if it will remain among the top global economies, but also if it will even be able to overtake the United States). While women experience higher levels of education and contraception rates and societywide mortality rates decline (particularly with continued global health investments), developed nations have led the way in demographic decline over developing nations in early modernity. Yet fertility and thus demographic decline has progressively accelerated for developing nations (as France took 115 years for over 65 year olds to double in population size compared to China's 26 years), generating rapid shifts in "age structure" as increasingly more "countries may grow old before they grow rich" (Dobriansky et al. 2017, p. 7).

The IMF describes the related "middle-income trap." Poor developing nations rapidly grow (with globalization shifting manufacturing supply chains initially to their low-cost worker population), but this growth into middle-income levels (as growth boosts wages) stagnates before they can transition into a high-income service-based domestic economy (as their advantage of low-cost labor for the global economy fades and thus their hopes of escaping this "trap"; Aiyar et al. 2013; p. 3). China may be the quintessential example of this. It generated what may be humanity's fastest surge in health and wealth from the 1990s to 2000s, increasing life expectancy through public health and antipoverty policies along with free market-orientated reforms driving explosive GDP growth (CSIS, 2020). But by the 2010s (after decades of its one-child policy of state-mandated caps including through contraception, abortion, and sterilization), China began facing one of history's fastest aging demographics. Digitalization and globalization (and their related public health advances) seem to power LICs into rapid growth, but unsustainable demographics (without sufficient societal adaptations) slam on the brakes as they get bogged down in the middle-income level. As more countries fall into the trap, more spotlight is placed on the remaining nations with healthy demographics to avoid it (for their sake and that of the global public health ecosystem and economy). As the more developed Global North rapidly ages, there is a growing reliance on the South to sustain the needed global value supply chains (particularly in digital technologies) and growth in healthy and wealthier populations. Although Nigeria is set to surpass China over the next few decades in demographics, Africa significantly trails the rest of the world in health improvements and life expectancy (Kuate Defo 2014). There have been significant advances in child health and HIV/AIDS treatments with the last 50 years of global public health investments. But continued conflicts, epidemics, and poverty-related complications (especially in NCDs) along with public health underinvestment hampers health and economic growth (and the capacity to achieve sustainable growth that avoids the middle-income trap, which Ghana and Cote d'Ivoire manifest unlike the more sustained growth of India and Vietnam; Aiyar et al. 2013; p. 5). As digitalization and globalization catalyze structural transformations of societies especially among developing countries, it appears that healthy growth is key to both global health and its interrelated equitable economic prosperity (highlighting how political economic considerations can be indispensable in effective AI-driven global public health programs and policies in this digital era).

Population aging in a sense is a historic victory for global public health: more and more of us generally live longer and healthier lives. But it also is a historic challenge, as concurrent declining fertility rates mean less workers must pay to support more retirees who are living longer with more NCD, which in turn push up their demand for more resources from public health and healthcare systems (as the COVID-19 pandemic demonstrated systems worldwide already are generally plagued by a fundamental strain delivering and financing care, even at current demographic levels; Monlezun 2023). Social safety nets (of government financial and material assistance to vulnerable populations) and welfare states (especially nationally financed or discounted healthcare) over the last century generated massive health gains. And developed nations (which are already generally facing demographic decline if not collapse) drive most of AI-accelerated technologies. Yet the needed capital investments and workforce is undercut by demographic changes which threaten the technological innovations needed to support the global economy, thus pressuring it to be more labor and capital efficient. With less taxpayers and workers and more patients, how can global public health keep pace with these seismic societal trends, let alone the need for AI-driven technological innovation to which global health is increasingly dependent? And how do changes in the number and makeup of nations' peoples affect global public health? (Especially as international challenges and crises require coordinated international responses, which can be undermined if national security is cited as reasons to, i.e., withhold local health data from the global health community at the onset of a new infection cluster with high potential to become a pandemic). Digitalization and deglobalization (sharpening countries' competition on the global stage for technological superiority in the name of national security) is thus indirectly strengthening the global health movement for "human security" to ensure the collective focus of national security is balanced with protection for individual security (inside and outside of one's national borders).

The concept of the "security of person" was introduced in what was likely the first global consensus description in the UN's 1948 *UDHR*, the global moral charter and foundation for the modern UN, WHO, rights, international law, and the West-driven liberal world order (Monlezun 2023). The *UDHR* defined the most fundamental intrinsic rights of each human individual as "life, liberty and security of person." This was distinct from "national security" which describes sufficient defense from external and internal threats to the collective sovereignty, identity, and territorial integrity of the state (particularly through military force to protect its domestic political economic structures, social institutions, [and for some critics even] cultural values). The UN Development Programme (UNDP) popularized this concept especially with its 1994 "Human Development Report," which provided the first widely accepted definition of "human security" as derived from individual human dignity (articulated by the *UDHR*), central to global public health, critical for domestic and international political stability and economic prosperity, and manifested as safety from acute and chronic threats to sustainable development of the individual (and thus of the global human society in which human security is scaled globally; UNDP 1994). The concept and its operationalization particularly in global public health was subsequently refined to describe essentially each person's "freedom from fear and want" (quoting and elaborating on the *UDHR*'s definition; Takemi et al. 2008; Anand, 2012).

"Human security" articulates how this freedom is required to "protect the vital core [well-being] of all human lives in ways that enhance human freedoms and human fulfilment," consisting of the pursuit of one's goals needed for one's good, unhindered by the internal threat of poor health and the external threats of poverty, disaster, war, and pandemics. To formalize, develop, and apply this concept further, the UN in 2000 launched the Commission for Human Security which was coordinated by Japan's government and funded by Sweden, the World Bank, and the Rockefeller Foundation. It produced its landmark 2003 report that cited how liberalization and globalization accelerated the new reality of global interdependence across state borders (at the individual and collective levels), while highlighting the need for human security to "balance" national security concerns (at both levels). Set during the height of the liberal world order, the Commission justified its positioning of human security as a central component of global public health (that itself is central for political stability and economic prosperity within and across developed and developing countries) by the "political liberalization." This global process spurred "movements towards democracy" as an assumed linear trend toward greater interdependence in a Western-weighted world view (privileging a dignity-based capitalist liberal democracy model of culturally conditioned political economics). Notably, the UN

Commission framed the WHO's "core functions of public health" as "primary prevention and care for major health threats" that directly advance the dual necessities of human security: "empowerment" and "protection" (p. 107). Global public health therefore becomes a critical means of "mobilizing social action" to facilitate personal development of individual capacities essential for lifelong well-being (including preventing NCDs and its complications through healthy behaviors), in addition to stimulating individual resiliency (responding to acute threats like wars and epidemics). Conceptually global public health and human security are distinguishable by their primary means (health vs larger political economics and social institutional efforts). But they are not clearly distinct in their primary practice or ultimate end. Both seek to integrate different partners and efforts from the larger global human ecosystem—encompassing the health, political economic, and technological subecosystems—to leverage their synergies for the ultimate end of individual well-being at scale, which produces global well-being that is manifested as "peace and [sustainable and integral] development."

Concurrent with the Commission, the WHO by 2002 joined global public health with human security, whose "essential determinants" are "justice and equity" (WHO 2002). Throughout the transition into the third millennium, continued demographic changes riding the societal waves of digitalization and globalization deepened the institutional model to more coordinated multisector approaches within the global public health ecosystem, particularly as decolonization accelerated the previously underrepresented voices in the increasingly populous Global South (which notably like the West and East are *not* monolithic value blocs, but richly diverse peoples, cultures, and histories; accordingly, this book seeks to balance the utility of the popular use of this general language to discuss overarching global trends with the respect due to those peoples by invoking their local communities with as great specificity as the high number of topics in this book permit). By 2012, the world's nations adopted the General Assembly Resolution 64/291 formalizing the equitable human security–driven approach to "improving global health" (UN 2012, p. 13). They went so far as to assert that global health requires the "human security approach" which enables "multidimensional analysis" and thus "comprehensive strategies" (UN 2012, p. 13). The UN consensus was that global public health cannot achieve its needed dual objectives of effectiveness or equity optimizing humanity's well-being (concretely in the context of the MDGs) without the "bigger picture view" that human security facilitates (to see how health is "shaped by social, economic and environmental conditions" in which individual and global health is contextualized and largely shaped). According to the UN, security-driven global health therefore should equitably focus on empowerment ("improving health-care systems," educating health professionals and their societies, and strengthening health financing) and protection ("preventing, monitoring and anticipating health-related threats" particularly epidemic early warning systems, preparedness plans, and action plans) within and across nations.

1.6 Emerging artificial intelligence categories of applications

These trends of digitalization, deglobalization (or secure globalization), and demographics (especially with their security) shape how AI is being developed and deployed in the global public health ecosystem in three primary domains: (a) population health, (b) precision public health, and (c) system optimization (Monlezun 2023). This grouping echoes that which was used by the milestone 2019 report by the USAID (United States Agency for International Development), Rockefeller Foundation, and Bill & Melinda Gates Foundation on global health AI (USAID 2019, p. 8). It additionally enables us to see how they differentiate the major categories of global health AI applications (and how they interrelate, which will allow us to dive deeper to understand specific applications in their different contexts and angles in the following chapters).

To begin with a high-level view, global health AI can be generally grouped into population health (including risk management, surveillance, and intervention selection and targeting), precision public health (population health, multiomics, and infectious disease surveillance integrated with data analytics to accelerate culturally sensitive integral sustainable development), and system optimization (enhancing health systems and ecosystem's clinical, organizational, and supply-chain performance; USAID 2019, p. 8; Monlezun 2023).

1.6.1 Population health

According to the high-profile distinction by the AJPH and the *New England Journal of Medicine* (respectively, the leading public health and medicine journals internationally), "public health is about what we're doing as a society and population health is about what a system is doing for its community" (Roux 2016; Bharel and Mohta 2020). The US National Academy of Medicine clarifies how what we are doing collectively as a society in public health programs is to "to assure the conditions in which people can be healthy," echoing the abovementioned UN's emphasis on the protection and empowerment dimensions of human security-based global public health (IoM 2002). The CDC details how population health in contrast practically focuses on the activities of healthcare systems (accelerated by their ecosystem partners) enhancing "the health outcomes of the communities they serve." In order words, population health is the practical interface or bridge between public health and healthcare together seeking to optimize societal well-being, top-down and bottom-up. Healthcare systems go out from their traditional physical and digital borders through population health into their communities to improve their well-being. Over the last century, public health has facilitated healthcare's expansion into population health to broaden its primary focus on disease (diagnosing and treating individuals one at a time) to the larger ecosystem vision (understanding the social determinants of health and how they affect not only disease but also how the community affects the individual and vice versa). Notably, this strategic broadening of healthcare systems follows the consensus in the abovementioned UN General Assembly Resolution 64/291 to also feature a human security–based approach to global health, rather than simply the traditional disease-only approach. This expanded vision is both communal (treating the person as a member of the community and thus treating the community also) and conceptual (treating diseases and their determinants). Responsibility to one's local community—improving care and costs for communities and systems—propels this strategic push (Bharel and Mohta 2020; Jha 2019; Kelley et al. 2020). Conversely, public health assumes and relies more on the "principle of social justice" as responsibility to the larger society, including globally. Within the AI-powered global public health ecosystem, there are growing coordinated investments and institutional support to accelerate AI-enabled population health as a means to improving local healthcare systems' performance optimizing their acute medical treatments concurrently with the chronic integral well-being of their communities.

This new wave of population health includes increasing AI use cases embedded in or in parallel with electronic health records (EHRs) that focus on interconnected phases of well-being and healthcare delivery: (1) data integration (of clinical, behavioral, environmental, socioeconomic, and financial especially claims data) to (2) inform dynamic risk stratification (identifying the patients within a population who will likely get sick and the time window in which that will occur), (3) resource allocation (enhancing healthcare professional resilience and time management while prioritizing higher risk patients, especially those more likely to benefit from greater resources through improved prevention and chronic comorbidity management and reduced preventable hospital admissions and readmissions), and (4) improved experience (of the abovementioned life cycle of well-being and healthcare delivery for patients and clinicians) through actionable data-driven health insights (CardinalHealth 2023; Kennedy 2022; Monlezun 2023). The surge in AI use cases parallels and complements the surge in healthcare ecosystem partners, including health and health-complementary businesses offering AI-based digital capacities for traditional healthcare systems (like hospitals and clinics), including in concert with universities and local governments (especially those focused on low-income populations). Recent higher profile AI-enabled and cloud computing–based population health measures include early epidemic modeling and prediction to guide local containment and mitigation measures, like with COVID early warning systems for inpatient clinical worsening, for or against targeted versus blanket societal lockdowns, and mRNA-based vaccines (Bogoch et al. 2020; Tuli et al. 2020; Allen 2021; Ball 2020).

1.6.2 Precision public health

In the previous section, we considered an overview of how public health is helping expand traditional healthcare systems' focus from individual-based medicine to also include population health (treating *both* the individual *and* their community rather than *either* the individual *or* the community). Similarly, the 20th-century rise of precision medicine within healthcare is spurring the developing of precision public health within global public health (Velmovitsky et al. 2021; Monlezun 2023). The former refers to more targeted Big Data–driven approaches to treat diseases for individuals based on applying population-level clinical, multiomics, socioeconomic, and environmental data to the individual level (integrated with individuals' own unique data) to match the best treatment and intervention time with the most accurate diagnosis. The latter refers to using Big Data for a similar process, but at scale across multiple individuals until it begins to approximate the population level (with a greater emphasis on low-cost prevention and societal wide interventions such as maternal and childcare in addition to vaccines). Precision public health therefore is the bridge between precision medicine and public health (using AI to quickly analyze and inform policy and program decisions based on large, diverse, continuous, and real-time data streams). "Multi-omics" refers to combining multiple data dimensions or layers of interconnected biological data to more completely understand causal mechanisms underlying health and disease states, including proteomics (for proteins), transciptomics (how RNA makes copies of DNA, which details the genetics defining the biological makeup of organisms), epigenetics (how DNA's genetic expression is modified by processes outside the genetic code), and genomics (the structure and function of an organisms' genes acting together). When paired with clinical data, AI case uses suggest that multiomics within precision public health can increasingly help tailor public health measures to boost their effectiveness and efficiency for the populations on which they focus (by addressing macro- and micro-level factors to improve the match between person and intervention).

Emerging examples of AI-enabled precision public health including real-time analytics, modeling, and insights for designing and deploying health programs and policies. Consider the modern public health pioneer, John Snow, the British physician who eventually had enough of seeing more and more patients die from cholera in the early 1800s. He left the confines of the hospital to go door to door carefully mapping cases until he traced it to what he became convinced was the contaminated source of the Broad Street public water pump (Snow 2008). The skeptical government officials closed the pump, the cases plummeted, and Snow accidentally helped found what became the modern public health subdiscipline of epidemiology (the study of diseases' determinants and distribution). A modern precision public health example is SaTScan, the "hyper-local public health" program that is an open-source (freely available online) data analytics platform (Arnold 2022). SaTScan generates digital maps of infectious disease clusters like COVID-19 that are near real-time, high-resolution, and actionable. It crunches rapid and diverse data streams from hospitals, laboratories, and social media networks cross-checked off census data to detail how cases are spreading now and likely in the future. This in turn allows more precise and prompt management of resources for healthcare systems working in tandem with each other to ensure they have the testing, protective equipment, treatments, and staffing to respond to their communities' needs.

Aside from such spatial–temporal applications, AI-driven precision public health is broadening into policymaking through causal inference analytics (statistics on nonrandomized observational data that may reasonably allow one to infer certain risk factors like smoking on cancer or protective factors like smoking cessation support; Flaxman and Vos 2018). In healthcare, physicians like me in the hospital often have to make our best educated guess as to what treatment will likely effect the patient's recovery. And then by closely checking their exams, vitals like blood pressure, laboratory tests, and images, we can adjust the treatment by what is showing signs of helping or not helping as quickly as possible. But in public health, the most effective and efficient policy is rarely known in advance, its rollout is slow, and its revision (if it does not work) is even slower and more costly. Precision public health provides what appears to be early examples of successful causal inference AI: different policies can be simulated early, tested precisely, and expanded quickly with greater safety, efficiency, and cost compared to the historic model. The COVID pandemic spotlighted not only how public health policies can be costly blunders and politically polarizing within and across states, but also how such causal inference AI can give leaders the best chance of putting the best programs forward (and fixing what does not work quickly), along with the case uses advancing their practical impact. In the theoretical or methodological front, there are advances for instance with a newer ML approach that appears to outperform older traditional non-AI causal inference statistics (Schuler and Rose 2017). It seems to especially supersede targeted maximum likelihood estimation, which is a popular regression method to generate doubly robust estimates of an intervention's average treatment effect (the difference in the average outcome between an intervention and a control). More recent methodological advances show how pairing AI with statistical causal inference techniques like propensity scores may produce more accurate, reliable, and efficient results, particularly when coupling the above with real-time EHR integration to provide timely clinical decision support at the bedside (Monlezun et al. 2022b).

1.6.3 System optimization

The previous section surveys how AI-enabled public health is deepening its operational and institutional collaboration with healthcare systems through population health and precision public health between their two domains. But it is also expanding to overall system optimization (Monlezun 2023). It particularly focuses in the clinical realm on process improvements in prevention, diagnosis, treatment, and rehabilitation of diseases in parallel with traditional healthcare systems. Organizationally, it is deployed to improve staffing (predicting and matching staffing with patient population's changing utilization patterns of healthcare) and charge capture (coding, billing, processing claims, preventing fraud, and ensuring quality). In supply chains, global health AI generally is concentrated in boosting efficient clinical trials (in their design, recruitment, analysis, and adaptation often embedded in current clinical care) and drug research and design or research and development (R&D; notably in pharmaceutical, medical, and digital technology companies for compound selection, testing, safety, pharmacovigilance, data storage, analysis, and adaptive supply chains predicting and responding to healthcare ecosystems' dynamic needs).

To clarify terms, a system generally is a network of parts (and their relationships) that operate in relation to each other to achieve a larger purpose they cannot do alone. Historically, "healthcare systems" from the 1990s onward described the network of hospitals and clinics that work together to deliver clinical care to patients. This especially applied to managed care organizations and then later accountable care organizations (ACOs) in the 2000s onward, which operationally and financially tied hospitals and clinics together to provide more coordinated and cost-efficient care. Public health and global public health were differentiated from such clinical care by their institutional context (in government and inter-government agencies outside of hospitals) and strategic focus (increasingly on equitable societywide well-being through prevention and mitigation, rather than just local communities' disease management through acute medical care, medications, and procedures for chronic diseases). But by 2022, the largest professional services and consulting firm, the UK-based Deloitte, articulated the substantive cross-sector consensus across academics, governments, and businesses about how AI is pushing our world to the "brink of large-scale disruption" through the Fourth Industrial Revolution (Dhar et al. 2022). AI is not only accelerating productivity within economic sectors but also the deepening relationships among them in an increasingly dense and interdependent relationships. Unlike "two-dimensional" systems, these networks more resemble three-dimensional "ecosystems" we find in nature, like in forests or deserts. Within them, individual organisms from plants to insects to birds to large predators seek to maximize their survival. The collective decentralized effect is the enhanced survival of these complex adaptive networks of life. Such ecosystems seem to take on a life of their own as they operate according to predictable mechanisms or laws of cause and effect, supply and demand, prey and predator, incentives and disincentives, and specialization and adaptation.

Similarly, Deloitte sees how this process is overtaking the health sector as progressively mature and networkwide AI-driven digital technologies are generating an increasingly dynamic network, joining both value-based healthcare systems (hospitals and clinics) and public health agencies (government and academic agencies), along with their complementary partners (pharmaceutical, medical technology, and digital technology companies). This AI transformation is collectively generating the "health ecosystem" technically characterized by "radically interoperable data, open yet secure platforms, and consumer-driven care." This "interoperable" term refers to the technical ability for different computer systems often from different organizations to communicate with each other by exchanging data often in a common data language, platform, and architecture (the digital structure of defined rules determining how data is collected, processed, stored, analyzed, and reported). Comprehensive integration of data (digitally uniting diverse members of the ecosystem in and outside traditional silos of healthcare systems and public health agencies) and well-being focus (not simply healthy functioning of organs but the more integral flourishing of the person and communities) structurally characterize this future's emerging health ecosystem achieved through efficiency and equity (Monlezun 2023). Existentially and practically, no person exists in or as an empty island, but is rather understood and differentiated through their relationships in a densely interdependent global village. And AI is helping accelerate our technical understanding of how we exist in a global human ecosystem that encompasses the AI-driven digital ecosystem (integrating our economic sectors and political networks) and its underlying health ecosystem generally and global public health ecosystem specifically (which emphasizes the partners structurally and strategically seeking solutions to health and well-being with international scope).

This technical system optimization with AI also extends to and presupposes its embedded and foundational moral optimization. The ecosystem is widely and multiculturally understood as an outcome, end, or teleologically ordered hierarchy in classical Aristotelian terms as a vertical network orientated toward the "common good" (WHO 2023a). This is the ecosystem's ultimate strategic aim, according to the WHO as articulated with the UN's health-focused SDGs (WHO 2023a). It describes global health as "public policy" that is meant to "strengthen the benefits" of modern "digital transformation." It does this through the "design

[of] an equitable economic that serves human development," ecological stewardship that "preserve[s] the planet," and responsible financial governance that "achieve[s] universal health coverage." The WHO specifies that well-being is a "positive state" for "individuals and societies," characterized by "quality of life and the ability…to contribute to the world with a sense of meaning and purpose," as individual lives lived relationally in local communities find their flourishing in caring for their communities which in turn care for them. It is "determined by social, economic and environmental conditions" and produces "resilient and sustainable communities," adapted to "current and emerging health threats" to empower this "overall thriving" for persons and their local and global communities. The AI digitalization of global public health technically supports and is supported by this expansive vision of well-being in a global context (informed by the convergence of our metaphysical and moral pluralism) as a systemic optimization in the metaphysical sense (Monlezun 2023).

In these institutional, technical, and metaphysical (or personal) dimensions, AI is generally strengthening the global human ecosystem while advancing its system optimization specifically (improving how the parts work together), including at the global public health level. Within it, emergent case uses typically focus on (1) design, (2) governance, and (3) financing, given how practical experience and empirical research highlight how inefficiency and inequity in modern global public health often flow from its structural weaknesses in these areas (Birn 2014; Monlezun 2023). Excessive fixation on disease (rather than larger individual and societal well-being), postcolonial and great power governance (dominated by richer Global North nations particularly the United States and China), and its related donor-controlled financing (imposing programs from foreign players on poorer countries with limited input, while the "brain drain" pulls young talented professionals from the South to the North with better pay) persist in undermining sustained improvements in global public health.

1. Design: ML applications are allowing local health bodies to more comprehensively model health and sickness states to better create, simulate, deploy, and improve local interventions more quickly and precisely (relying less on external and foreign global health bodies to provide more generic programs; Mhasawade Zhao and Chunara et al. 2021). These AI models enable enhanced mapping of complex factors and causal inferences. They thus empower more complete interventions from a socio-ecological standpoint (understanding individuals as members of a community that shapes them as they shape the community). To improve the burden of cardiovascular disease in a poor community, a global public health agency can simply provide nutritious meals (that can temporarily improve diets). Or they can provide improved education in schools about healthy diet, nutritious food assistance for the poorest families, hands-on cooking lessons for families about healthy and appetizing foods, and training for medical professionals to reinforce dietary counseling (that can allow more sustainable diet and subsequently health improvements) as a multisector, cost-effective, capacity building ecological approach spanning complementary interventions, as has been demonstrated through the world's first randomized controlled trial and multisite prospective cohort study in this area (Monlezun et al. 2015, 2022a). The smarter the intervention, the better the chance of

success usually. Such sophisticated ML-driven modeling of system dynamics has been expanded outside of nutrition to address smoking cessation, pandemic resource allocation, depression treatment, mobile phone data, tax codes, and ACO programs (Birn 2014).

2. Governance: As introduced earlier, most of global public health and AI are created, governed, and deployed by the North (which principally benefits the people there; Owoyemi et al. 2020; Monlezun 2023). So how can a health program or algorithm designed in New York or Shanghai have the same effectiveness or equity in Kinshasa or Lagos as it does in those power centers? (Who do not first-hand see, understand, [and vocal critics also suggest] even belong to the reality on the ground as those who live and work there do). The COVID-19 pandemic this century following the decolonization movement at the end of the last century are accelerating the global push for greater representation, collaboration, and shared benefit in the South and other historically underrepresented groups through more inclusive governance structures in both global public health and AI. Accordingly, Dr. Tedros Adhanom Ghebreyesus transitioned from his early career as an Ethiopian public health researcher and practitioner to become the first African to lead the WHO in 2017 as its Director-General (WHO 2023b). He initiated what the WHO describes as its "most significant transformation in the Organization's history" through an agile "data-driven strategy" built on efficiency, equity, and the global human ecosystem. These structural changes sought to provide a global public health governance model that was inclusive, impactful, and innovative, setting the stage for its COVID-accelerated AI transformation to catalyze digital capacity in lower income and resource countries by fundamental and operational readiness in AI (Ghebreyesus and Swaminathan 2021). Fundamental readiness refers to the WHO's initiatives to assist countries technically and organizationally to develop their own health AI through improved high-quality universal internet access (including for data collection and analysis, digital communication, EHRs, and telemedicine), data infrastructure (coordinating the diverse data sources and types across diverse health ecosystem partners), and "intelligent connectivity" (digitally plugging LMICs into the global digital and public health ecosystems which HICs already run on to allow greater shared utilization of AI-accelerated Internet of Things data running on 5G [fifth generation mobile network]). More inclusive data governance examples include the WHO Hub for Pandemic and Epidemic Intelligence, created in 2021 amid COVID as a publicly available global public health version of the private BlueDot (UN 2021). It is meant to allow secure data sharing, early warnings, and emergent best practices for LMICs and HICs using AI-augmented supercomputing to inform more precisely tailored local rollouts of public health interventions. Operational readiness indicates the ability to draw on fundamental capacities to responsibly and sustainably coordinate public health AI applications, especially through a sufficiently trained workforce and trustworthy governance models. The WHO's Digital Health Leadership Training Programme and WHO-G7 regulatory and ethical standards for health AI created jointly by LMICs and HICs provide examples of such readiness advancing fairer governance in global public health AI.

3. Financing: Direct fund transfers are increasingly replacing at least part of the donor-directed public health and health AI funding to allow local public health agencies and healthcare systems to create and obtain funding for their programs (Shamasunder et al. 2020). UNICEF with the Bill & Melinda Gates Foundation through their Global Grand Challenges for example utilize a public—private finance model to fund more collaborative, precise, and local health programs across over 55 African countries and 110 equity-free investments (Akogo 2021). The Vietnamese Ministry of Health, Novartis (Swiss pharmaceutical company), and Harvard University provide a partnership-based finance model leveraging diverse ecosystem partners' capacities to better integrate public health with healthcare systems' primary care and population health (Shaaban 2020).

Such system optimization particularly in design, governance, and financing of global public health illustrate emblematic examples of the major emerging AI use cases. The general trend is that particularly in the wake of perceived COVID-19 failures by global public health authorities and agencies, decentralized technical solutions to local health problems are having an ecosystemwide impact on these structural challenges by making "global" health more intelligent, agile, and local. Yet there is still significant progress required for more efficient, equitable, and mature global public health AI through a more effective leveraging of its ecosystem reality, as evidenced by the influential USAID report mentioned earlier that defines "global [public] health" as healthcare narrowly for LMICs (USAID 2019, p. 5). There are potentially problematic neo-colonial undertones and framing (doing public health "somewhere else"), conceptual ambiguity (excluding the data and institutional interconnectedness of LMICs and HICs that constitute the global public health ecosystem), and potentially excessive dependence on the outdated simplistic disease-based approach to health. (This book therefore returns to its central argument about a more ecosystem and so comprehensive approach to the responsible AI reengineering of the global public health ecosystem, including foundational, metaphysical, personal, structural, and strategic considerations spanning political economic, multicultural, and ethical dimensions, rather than solely technical considerations to advance the power of one's region and sector in which those technical advances are deployed).

1.7 Just power: artificial intelligence reengineering the global public health ecosystem

1.7.1 Aims and angle: an ethical ecosystem

Now that we have set the scene, we are ready to get into the substance of what is new and needed in this book for your unique interests and purposes. The central question we are asking in this work is the central question of our era: how can we make just power reengineer (or regenerate) the world we want? (In our modern digital age increasingly dominated by AI and its transformation of our health, which is critical for enabling or limiting all other social structures from our politics to economics to cultures that flow from the health of individuals and our communities). But a book about everything is a book really about nothing, and so we will focus on specific concrete aims and a transparent angle to reach them. As introduced earlier, this work seeks to provide you the first comprehensive, rigorous, accessible, and actionable book on how AI is reengineering the global public health ecosystem—and thus our larger global society it sustains and is shaped by—by translating the on-the-ground perspective of a physician−data scientist and AI ethicist into a shared formula for a better future for us all. It is meant to be broad enough to be defensible (by understanding how our global public health exists within our global digital ecosystem with its underlying political economics, generated by our underlying diverse cultures, manifesting our common values and beliefs about who we are as individuals and members of a human community). But it must also be narrow enough to be effective (using a broad theoretical base to inform targeted and detailed explanations of how AI is changing global public health in trends and use cases illuminating where this ecosystem is likely going and what it will look like in our emergent future). This chapter therefore introduced the metaphorical (and thus conceptual) methodological angle of an ecosystem as a home. We surveyed generally the trends shaping the AI-enabled global public health ecosystem that we will unpack in the subsequent chapters: digitalization, deglobalization, and demographics. We considered a high-level first look at its major categories of use cases within those trends of population health, precision public health, and system optimization. Our dual assessment of the above will focus on what they are now and what they can be (if we optimize a just future together, seeing the AI-driven global public health ecosystem as a common home for all of humanity). And so we will analyze them from the specific AI domains or perspectives broken down by chapters like the various dimensions of a home's architectural plan: financing and development as its design, data architecture and political economics as its framework, culture and demographics as its inhabitants, and security and ethics as its foundation (before putting it all together by doing a "walk-through" of the home with you in the final chapter that explores its emergent future in concrete terms to make this vision one of sovereignty, solidarity, and success; Monlezun 2023).

The angle by which we will frame these topics is therefore an "ethical ecosystem," or a comprehensive 360-degree perspective on how to mobilize collective societal action fairly to realize the aim of AI-enabled global public health (namely health for all in a way that helps ensure power is orientated toward justice, or giving to each what is owed to them as members of the global human family). Healthcare typically focuses on individual agency, but public health (and its latest development phase of global public health) focuses on societal agency, or how soft power through societal influence and hard power through force, laws, and penalties are leveraged to achieve its aims of collective well-being (as the prerequisite for the healthy functioning of any society or state). Power is essentially an idea endowed with practical force. Its end or objective and its guard rails (avoiding undue harm or use of others) determines if it is used rightly. Public will wielding it can be easily swayed for different ends either good or bad (i.e., care for the underserved or racist abuse of minorities)—which only gets more complicated on an international level with more people and factors involved. Global public health therefore must contend with this societal context if it is to be effective and trustworthy. We will include a chapter not only on political economics but also ethics for the AI global public health ecosystem because of fundamental and practical reasons. For power to be just, we have to know its right end (common conception of the good) and means (good ways) to reaching it. And it takes a common metaphysical and derivative moral vision spanning our diverse belief systems to anchor and sustain these common values and vision. Consider how the Allied powers responded to Hitler's genocidal power gab with their collective reorientation of power (militarily) as a means to the end of justice (national sovereignty and international peace). This concrete plan was justified ethically by individual rights and global security (which became individual security at scale by the 1990s), articulated by the WHO's Constitution (as derived from the UN Charter), and more fully elaborated by the *UDHR* (WHO 1948; UN 1948, 1945). If power is our age-old ground on which society is established, then justice must be the new floor of the modern home for our global human family. Since the creation of the UN, global public health was a central and fundamental strategic focus to ensure more bandages and less bullets in a world made more just (respecting rights and security), interdependent (through collaborative aid and globalized capitalist economics), and thus peaceful and prosperous. As this ethical ecosystem angle became increasingly manifest by the 21st century, the UN in its 2008 Resolution 63/33 asserted the WHO was "*the* [emphasis added] primary specialized agency for health" promotion and protection globally, "leading that effort within the UN system" as the "global guardian of public health" (UN 2008, 2023b). But critics will ask who gave it that power? Supporters respond that the power from the supra-democratic consensus of the world's nations (both democratic and autocratic) make it so, to preserve global health by preventing power's descent into self-serving violence of the strong against the weak, and instead setting power's strategic end ethically on dignity and security-based justice. By its 2021 "Global strategy on digital health," the WHO recognized that global public health had become "the health ecosystem" digitally transformed, and through effective collaboration, had to be made "ethical, safe, secure, reliable, equitable, and sustainable" (WHO 2021, p. 8). To be so, this ethical ecosystem specifically requires "international solidarity" in collaborative progress toward "justice and equity as essential determinants of human security," as the world's countries' jointly asserted in the UN General Resolution 64/291, noting that "improving global health" requires the "human security approach" (WHO 2002; UN 2012, p. 13). At this intersection of ethics and pragmatism, justice and power, health and security, lies this human security concept on which our ethical ecosystem angle is based. We will thus use it to help us frame how we understand, influence, and to some degree even direct the complex and often competing forces shaping the various dimensions of the AI-powered global public health ecosystem.

1.8 Personalist Liberalism: health spanning global divisions

To use this angle to achieve the abovementioned aims, this book adopts the particular approach of Personalist Liberalism (with as honest and clear description as possible of its influences and biases, in addition to its defensibility elaborated progressively throughout the book). This novel political economic theoretical framework bridges democracies' personal defense of dignity (and thus rights decentralizing power through the societal network) and autocracies' reported national defense of sovereignty (and thus security centralizing power in a hierarchy, often with socialist or oligarchical management of a society's resources—but with Personalist Liberalism not sacrificing the good of the individual in the hierarchy to achieve the overall good of the hierarchy). The political dimension of this framework is paired with the economic one, a science and technology—driven capitalist-free market dominating our modern world. The strategic justification for the use of this framework is that in the political dimension it bridges the dominant power players, as the world's primary AI and global public health influencers are the democratic United States and the autocratic China, with their respective value blocs they lead (in the West and East seeking to "win" over the South). The justification in the economic dimension is that it articulates and sustains the durable ethical guardrails for our era's dominant economic paradigm. Empirically speaking, the world generally became capitalist by the 1990s with the vast majority of nations (including Russia and China, along with South American and African countries) adopting the fundamentals of the free markets (Sachs 1999). The historical justification is that it is the political economic translation of the Personalist Social Contract, the first global ethical framework comprehensively articulating and metaphysically defending modernity's dominant ethics (human dignity—based rights and duties detailed by the *UDHR* as the basis for modern international law and institutions), facilitating substantive pluralistic convergence of diverse belief systems, and embedded in real-time AI analytics (AI-driven Computational Ethics and policy analysis or AiCE; Monlezun 2023; Monlezun et al. 2022b). The substantive justification for Personalist Liberalism is that it argues for the fundamental (metaphysical) reality of the dignity of each person as a member of the global human family, and thus the (practical) necessity to guide how AI reengineers a global public health ecosystem that is efficient and equitable, enabling just AI to empower an ecosystem we commonly desire and depend on (more on this in the ethics chapter). And finally, its technical justification is that it is compatible with and facilitates the AI transformation of the global public health ecosystem in (1) scope, (2) scale, and (3) speed.

1. *Scope*: "Economies of scope" refers to the economic principle explaining how large organizations can reduce their average costs per product by increasing the *variety* of their complementary products (to maximize outputs from shared inputs). An example is when a public health agency can use the same input i.e., a single mRNA-based vaccine manufacturer to reduce costs to produce a wider range of complementary vaccines to multiple diseases, rather than using more manufacturers for each disease individually, each with their own negotiated contracts. Personalist Liberalism helps unpack the aggregate advances in a net forward vector direction through economies of scope for the AI global public health ecosystem, but through the lens of seeing the competing divergent vectors in the dynamic power struggle between the more decentralized democratic and more hierarchical autocracies central to both AI and global health (Ferguson 2018). Consider how the US-based research laboratory, OpenAI, triggered in

November 2022 what has been hailed as AI's "iPhone moment" that "kicked off a. . .[new phase of the] AI arms race" when it publicly and freely published ChatGPT, a generative AI chatbot (Forman 2023; Roose 2023). This large language model, drawing from the internet's vast data and optimized by reinforcement and supervised learning, became one of the most rapidly growing software products in history with over 30 million users in its first 2 months alone. Elon Musk (founder−CEO of the Tesla and SpaceX companies in addition to the CEO of X, formerly known as Twitter), described ChatGPT's articulate and detailed responses ranging from poetry to apps to human user questions as so "scary good" that it can fool many users trying to differentiate whether it is human or AI, while garnering a $10 billion acquisition from Microsoft and catalyzing a frenzied race among competitors from Google to China's Baidu, Alibaba, and JD.com to respond with their alternatives (Forman 2023; Iyengar and Scott 2023). Personalist Liberalism can illustrate the driving forces underlying the spectrum of relationships of power versus values, networks versus hierarchies, democracies versus autocracies, and AI versus health, to help generate and guide the AI global public health ecosystem by expanding the scope of its partners, services, and communities served.

2. *Scale*: "Economies of scale" is the economic principle showing how large firms can decrease their averages costs per product by increasing the *volume* of those products. An example is how it is cheaper for a healthcare system to offer new population health preventive services in enhanced child health by spreading medical specialists among newly acquired hospitals, rather than trying to create a new healthcare system to offer traditional specialties. Personalist Liberalism helps illustrate the collaboration, organizational, and technical steps required (and their benefit) of the above and related efforts like with the WHO building fundamental and operational health AI readiness, particularly in LMICs to accelerate the effectiveness of the AI global public health ecosystem. By setting up more data collection, processing, and analytic centers including with edge computing, the ecosystem builds better economies of scale. It lowers the computing costs and thus the output of data-driven efficient and equitable programs, rather than sending the bulk of data from developing to developed nations (more on this later). Yet scale requires cooperation, which requires stewarding power throughout often competing networks within the ecosystem—cooperation that Personalist Liberalism can defend and facilitate. The dean of Boston University School of Public Health, Dr. Sandro Galea, captures this dynamic of public health and power in its three forms: overt power (i.e., political leaders over populations), covert power (i.e., institutional leaders shaping agendas), and societal power (i.e., persuasion through common values such as with smoking cessation to improve health, or propaganda through disinformation such as excessive politicization of COVID policies):

Given that the promotion of the health of populations depends on improving the social, economic, and cultural conditions that shape well-being, we have little choice but to grapple with how we can engage with the three dimensions of power, with special emphasis on influencing values to promote health (Galea 2018).

1 *Speed*: In our modern digital economy, innovation can longitudinally lower costs by increasing the value of goods and services by boosting the rate of the above volume and variety of those goods and services. There is growing separation in the top- and low-performing public health agencies and healthcare systems, driven by the high versus low speed of AI transformation particularly when it breaks into the level of enterprise-wide or mature AI (Chebrolu et al., 2023; Monlezun 2023). Typically, organizations begin with piloting discrete AI projects or applications, scale them up to span the organization for process applications, and then finally embed them fundamentally in the governance, organizational, and data structure of the organization to achieve its vital strategic objectives. AI then informs and drives the firm by better strategic and operational decision-making across and within the organization. The greater the data capture, AI penetration, and embeddedness of the iterative cycle (of programing, data capture from it, and AI analytics identifying growth areas which subsequently guide better programming), the greater the organization's speed leveraging its ecosystem to achieve its strategic ends. Personalist Liberalism helps map the organizational elements of the health value chain (from digitalization of organizational operations to consumer engagement to clinical and public health delivery to financial and compliance performance to smart workforce and back to operations). It then applies it to the AI global public health ecosystem that bridges diverse health, political economic, and value paradigms and structures. Unlike in healthcare systems typically restricted to a narrow range of the above, the global public health ecosystem to be efficient and equitable must engage the full spectrum of the abovementioned domains while lowering collaboration barriers among them to ensure the needed speed of AI transformation. Personalist Liberalism in the subsequent chapters will help us map out how to actualize this. Therefore, this approach will allow us to understand how to grow the partners and their size as appropriate in the AI global public health ecosystem for scale, the quality and sustainability of their partnerships for scope, and the maturity of the end-to-end integrated AI capacities for speed and thus agility adapting in real-time to dynamic health challenges and preemptively for foreseeable ones.

1.8.1 Why the global public health ecosystem?

Now let us finalize this chapter's framing why we are applying Personalist Liberalism to the AI-transformed "global public health ecosystem" rather than "global health," "public health," or those domains without an ecosystem view. Modern reality, not simply rhetoric, supports this nuance shift. As this chapter has progressively built up to this point, the ecosystem perspective allows a novelty and thus value for this book addressing global public health that is unique among its predecessors, enabling a more comprehensive, agile, and actionable approach for optimizing AI-accelerated health and thus humanity's future. Aside from the abovementioned pragmatic reasons, the historical and structural ones below specify how our modern global society came to, operates, and likely will go from here. Earlier we introduced how Deloitte articulates the international thought leader consensus about how the future of health is the "health ecosystem" integrating our globalized society, digital ecosystem, public health agencies, traditional brick-and-mortar healthcare systems, governments, academics, businesses, institutions, and community groups focused on the equitable well-being of all individuals and thus of our world (Dhar et al. 2022). The UN Secretary General echoed this vision in the above-noted 2020 Roadmap for Digital Cooperation with the multisector push to "accelerate…an inclusive digital ecosystem," which entails "digital public goods in the form of actionable real-time and predictive insights" for efficient and equitable global public health, from West Africa's 2014 Ebola to the 2020 COVID-19 pandemic outbreaks (UN 2020; para. 81, 22).

The specific modifier for this ecosystem is "global public health" for further structural reasons. The UN's 2008 General Assembly 63/33 Resolution enshrined the term "global public health" at the intersection of "global health and foreign policy" of states, regardless if they are democratic or autocratic, for "achieving the health-related Millennium Development Goals" (being replaced by the SDGs; UN 2008). It justified such health objectives as necessary for "socio-economic development" explicitly within the UN's explicit ultimate end of global peace through just political stability, especially among the competing value blocs of nations. The resolution referenced the UN's Economic and Social Council's 2009 annual review that focused on further developing, implementing, and so "achieving the global public health agenda" (DESA 2009). This echoes Dr. Sandro Galeo's emphasis of overt power (political leaders advancing the concept and realization of global public health through the resolution), covert power (setting its agenda), and societal or soft power (persuading its personalization and adoption by local communities). We previously analyzed how we arrived at this point after the 20th century's historical and structural shifts in global power alliances that pressured the WHO as the UN's primary health agency to shift its strategy, brand, and operations from international to "global public health" to retain relevance and survival (while simultaneously exerting significant covert and soft power on the field itself which shifted its strategy, brand, and operations accordingly; Brown et al. 2006). Yet importantly, this is still in line with the original 1940s modernization and globalization of the science-based public health of the 1800s when the representative countries through the UN assigned the WHO its constitutional mission advancing the "health of all peoples," not simply "public health," as the former is "fundamental to the attainment of peace and security" for "all peoples" (WHO 1948). Such historical and structural evidence supports how the "global public health" framework is the pragmatic refinement of the initial vision of a world seeking to avoid the horrors and apocalyptic risk of another global conflict by anchoring a stable political economic structure (with its various subtypes of more free market democracies and more centralized capitalist or socialist autocracies) in a common moral and health foundation of a common existential home for humanity.

Finally, such a framework within the structure of our digitalizing modern society is already being operationalized with growing influence. New York University rebranded and reorganized its top ranked public health program in 2015 as the "School of Global Public Health" for the "next generation of public health pioneers" to "reinvent the public health paradigm" (NYU 2023). Yet in this digital generation opening up to a new AI age, there is still no clear consensus for defining "digital public health" on the international stage nor the "digital transformation" of global health (Iyamu et al. 2021). In this open conceptual frontier, "global public health" may help provide the needed differentiation and direction through what the WHO terms the "multisectoral and interdisciplinary networks" defining our new "human condition," constituted by the AI-driven health ecosystem through which the needed "global cooperation" can be nourished to achieve health for all (García Saisó and D'Agostino 2021). Proponents note that such a pivot may avoid the above-discussed critique of "global health as public health somewhere else" by retaining the local agency of public health accelerated by the international resources of global health (King and Koski 2020; Monlezun 2023). We noted earlier how the world's AI technical experts are pessimistic or at least guarded about the prospect of ethical AI breaking out from its current trajectory in a political economic power race to be an effective, responsible, and moral force for global good (Rainie Anderson and Vogels 2021). Framing such dynamics within the larger understanding of AI's transformation of the global public health ecosystem helps to shift this trajectory from arbitrary to just (not sole) power, from one of simple zero-sum competition for national security alone to one positive sum cooperative competition for "human security" (underlying, anchoring, and justifying the global public health ecosystem; UN 2012; Monlezun 2023). It is the later trajectory that is reorientated to a human horizon fixed on our shared common good, what the world's nations in the 2012 UN General Assembly's 64/291 resolution described as our end realized through the means of safeguarding "human security [which] aims at ensuring the survival, livelihood and dignity of people…where the protection and empowerment of individuals form the basis for achieving stability, development and human progress" (p. 5). This ecosystem approach to global public health can thus help balance the spectrum relationship rather than imposing a false choice for the world between collectivism and individualism (underlying our competing political economic systems) by orientating them to the common good *via* human security (existentially and structurally deeper than even these world views, by recovering the person inherent in both ideologies). We do not know if we should turn left or right on our current road unless we know the desired destination. The fixed metaphysical and moral summit of the common good therefore can help us navigate this new AI era by being that destination for our shared ascent up modernity's mountain. Thus, this book will use this operational approach in its two interchangeable mathematical formulations:

$$\text{Global} \quad \text{public health ecosystem}_{\text{structurally}} = \left(\frac{\text{Global health} + \text{Healthcare}}{\text{Digital ecosystem}} \right)^{\text{Human security} \times \text{AI}}$$

$$\text{Global public health ecosystem}_{\text{principally}} = \text{Personalist Liberalism}^{\text{Health AI}}$$

We will explicate these formulations by examining the different dimensions of the global public health ecosystem in the subsequent chapters. But suffice it for now to summarize them as an approach to understanding the different supra-domains (with their major components) of the global (or technological) public (cultural, political economic, and ethical) health (public health, global health, and healthcare) ecosystem (existentially as the global level with its derivative layer of the global digital and subderivative layer of the global public health ecosystem).

1.9 Artificial intelligence × global public health ecosystem: AI × *Equity*^{2}

Following Hurricane Katrina's 2005 devastation of New Orleans costing the lives of over 1392 and \$161 billion (NOAA 2023), I gathered with a team of physicians, public health professionals, biomedical researchers, data scientists, statisticians, students, and community members to build what became the world's first medical school-based teaching kitchen, united with the simple mission of feeding and so healing a shared city through our diverse backgrounds (Monlezun et al. 2022a). Housed in a low-income community's abandoned grocery store complex renovated into a community health hub, we steadily built public health programs with low-income families, students, and medical professionals. We then translated them through a community-based participatory research study I designed, led, and analyzed —Cooking for Health Optimization with Patients (CHOP; US National Institutes of Health ClinicalTrials.gov ID number NCT03443635)—that scientifically established the field of culinary medicine. It was the field's first and remains the largest AI-driven multisite cohort study with nested Bayesian adaptive randomized trials scaled to over 60 academic centers and 10,000 participants. CHOP sought to rapidly innovate the science, adapt for local community needs, and improve health outcomes and inequities through low cost, sustainable, and workforce-multiplying public health programming led by the local community leveraging global resources.

And I propose a similar process here. Now that we have a common theoretical foundation, conceptual framework, and technical vocabulary in this chapter, we can embark on a shared discussion, deliberation, and decisions based on the concrete details of the various domains of the AI global public health ecosystem, remaking humanity's health the world over. As this requires reuniting the typically conflicting camps (and so reordering them to their original relationships on a shared spectrum) of AI and health, science and ethics, democracies and autocracies, rights and security, efficiency and equity, we will use this novel approach of the AI-empowered global health ecosystem in which they operate through the interpretive key of Personalist Liberalism. In a natural ecosystem, networks of synergistic relationships allow growth through shared attempts at self-survival. At scale, this enables ecosystem survival in a hierarchy orientated to the common goal of preserving life. In the AI-enabled global public health ecosystem, we will thus analyze how the network relationships in their various domains can be made more human through more deliberate, sustained, and institutionalized efforts to orientate them to the common good, constituting the good of each individual in our global human family—science at the service of human dignity and security. But unlike in nature in which ecosystems evolve, such an AI ecosystem requires deliberately cooperative reengineering or regenerating toward this shared strategy and ultimate end. And in this common ecosystem home, we will unpack the domains of its design (financing and integral development), framework (data architecture and political economics), inhabitants (culture and demographics), and foundation (security and ethics) with an overarching strategic approach of the ultimate relationship of AI and equity ordering all other derivative ones.

As introduced in *The Thinking Healthcare System: Artificial Intelligence and Human Equity* (Monlezun 2023), the organic formula or system DNA of the future's thinking healthcare system (bridging AI-enabled public health and traditional healthcare systems in the health ecosystem) represents health (H) as the product of AI (A) and equity (E) squared:

$$H = AE^2$$

Einstein's landmark equation described energy as the product of mass and the speed of light squared ($E = MC^2$). This physics formula describes how energy is power put into motion to produce change. Our formula on the other hand in this emerging AI era describes how humanity's power can be translated into progress as "human health and artificial intelligence" become interchangeable (under the right conditions that are generated rather than happen accidentally). When the ecosystem partnership of global public health and healthcare generate efficient AI at scale, it signals individual well-being is optimized to the point that it becomes global (unhindered by inequities which produce system inefficiencies by dragging down aggregate ecosystem growth, as sickness and debility for enough people produce political instability and economic stagnation forces on the global human ecosystem). And health "travels" (or advances at a global level) at the speed of equity. The "kinetic energy" or speed of health's motion is proportional to this effective AI. The richer the AI collaboration in the global public health ecosystem, the faster it propagates, embeds, and maturates itself and its ecosystem as edge partners (in LMICs) and more central partners (HICs) generate more interconnected, interchangeable, and informative data in the ecosystem's digital architecture.

The significance of this similitude between energy and health deepens with their similar strategic and structural problems that are particularly illuminative in global public health. The World Energy Council's 2011 report described the "Energy Trilemma" as the modern trade-off of three seemingly mutually exclusive options in which governments and businesses are pressured to balance the competing goods of security, affordability, and sustainability (WEC 2011). As Russia's 2022 full-scale invasion of Ukraine accentuated amid the ongoing climate and debt crises, the fundamental challenges accessing affordable energy without worsening planetary health for subsequent generations affects every aspect of our states and global society as modernity materially runs on energy. Similarly, humanity existentially runs on health as without equitable well-being the overarching political stability and economic prosperity is compromised. Sick individuals (with the lack of healthy functioning in our network of organs internally and social network externally) at scale produce a sick humanity. Our strategic approach of equitable AI at global scale (and the book's derivative approach of the AI-empowered global public health ecosystem) is meant to help us appropriately balance health's security, affordability, and sustainability needs in the following formula interchangeable with the above:

$$\text{Global public health ecosystem}_{\text{strategically}} = \left(\frac{\text{AI} \times \text{Equity}^2}{\text{Global public health}} \right)$$

This approach does not force false choices between power or justice, global or public health, AI or health, and efficient or equity. It chooses them all. But it orders their proper relationship (and dynamic emphasis on one end of the spectrum periodically compared to the other) by reenvisioning them rather as two-dimensional partnerships orientated to a third dimension. To break out the false dichotomy or flat earth tension of *A* versus *B*, or us versus them, it orientates and so orders both ends of each spectrum to the ultimate destination of the common good. This approach is thus meant to enable us to advance toward the responsible AI transformation of the global public health ecosystem operating through just power. We began this chapter facing the personal trilemma of a monster storm and pandemic bearing down on an underserved hospital. And we launch into this book with the shared proposed solution of the just AI-engineered global public health ecosystem in which effectiveness, efficiency, and equity face off against security, affordability, and sustainability challenges. Saving some will not save the system, and vice versa. Saving a common and real vision of who we are as unique members of the common human family may thus be key to ensuring we can build and preserve a new AI ecosystem in which we all can call home.

References

Agrawal, A., Gans, J., and A. Goldfarb. 2018. *Prediction Machines: The Simple Economics of Artificial Intelligence*. Boston, MA: Harvard Business Review Press.

Aiyar, S., R. Duval, D. Puy, Y. Wu, and L. Zhang. 2013. "Growth Slowdowns and the Middle-Income Trap." IMF Working paper 13/71. International Monetary Fund. Accessed February 14, 2023. imf.org/external/pubs/ft/wp/2013/wp1371.pdf.

Aiyar, S., and A. Illyina. 2023. "Charting Globalization's Turn to Slowbalization After Global Financial Crisis." International Monetary Fund. Accessed February 9, 2023. https://www.imf.org/en/Blogs/Articles/2023/02/08/charting-globalizations-turn-to-slowbalization-after-global-financial-crisis.

Akogo, D. 2021. "Five Ways AI Can Democratise African Healthcare." *Financial Times*. Accessed June 20, 2022. https://www.ft.com/content/8649e35f-29d2-4da0-a1cd-7eece48b7152.

Al Knawy, B., McKillop, M.M., Abduljawad, J., Tarkoma, S., Adil, M., Schaper, L., and A. Chee, et al., 2022. "Successfully Implementing Digital Health to Ensure Future Global Health Security During Pandemics: A consensus statement." *JAMA Network Open* 5 (2): e220214.

Alcorn, T. 2012. "What Has the US Global Health Initiative Achieved? ." *Lancet* 380 (9849): P1215–P1216.

Allen, D.W. 2021. "Covid-19 Lockdown Cost/Benefits: A Critical Assessment of the Literature." *International Journal of the Economics of Business* 29 (1): 1–32.

Allison, G., and E. Schmidt. 2020. "Is China Beating the U.S. to AI Supremacy?" Harvard University Kennedy School Belfer Center. Accessed January 8, 2023. https://www.belfercenter.org/publication/china-beating-us-ai-supremacy.

AP. 2021. "Timeline: China's COVID-19 Outbreak and Lockdown of Wuhan." Associated Press. Accessed February 5, 2023. https://apnews.com/article/pandemics-wuhan-china-coronavirus-pandemic-e6147ec0ff88affb99c811149424239d.

Aristotle. 1984. *Politics*. Chicago: University of Chicago Press, Translated by C. Lord.

Aristotle. 2012. *Nicomachean Ethics*. Chicago: University of Chicago Press, Translated by R. C. Bartlett, and S. D. Collin.

Arnold, C. 2022. "Is Precision Public Health the Future—or a Contradiction?" *Nature*. Accessed February 22, 2023. https://www.nature.com/articles/d41586-021-03819-2.

Ball, P. 2020. "The Lightning-Fast Quest for COVID Vaccines—and What It Means for Other Diseases." *Nature*. Accessed February 22, 2023. https://www.nature.com/articles/d41586-020-03626-1.

Barrat, J. 2013. *Our Final Invention: Artificial Intelligence and the End of the Human Era.* New York: Macmillan Publishers Thomas Dunne Books.

Bharel, M., and N.S. Mohta. 2020. "Defining Distinctions Between Public and Population Health to Knock Down Barriers that Impede Care." New England Journal of Medicine Catalyst. Accessed February 18, 2023. https://catalyst.nejm.org/doi/full/10.1056/CAT.20.0432.

Birn, A.E. 2014. "Philanthrocapitalism, Past and Present: The Rockefeller Foundation, the Gates Foundation, and the Setting(s) of the International/Global Health Agenda." *Hypothesis* 12 (1): e8.

Blanchette, J. and G. DiPippo. 2022. "'Reunification' with Taiwan through Force Would Be a Pyrrhic Victory for China." Center for Strategic and International Studies. Accessed March 22, 2023. https://www.csis.org/analysis/reunification-taiwan-through-force-would-be-pyrrhic-victory-china.

Bogoch, I.I, Watts, A., Thomas-Bachli, A., Huber, C., Kraemer, M.U.G., and K. Khan. 2020. "Potential for Global Spread of a Novel Coronavirus from China." *Journal of Travel Medicine* 27 (2): taaa011.

Bokat-Lindell, S. 2022. *Will the Ukraine War Spell the End of Globalization?* The New York Times. https://www.nytimes.com/2022/03/30/opinion/ukrainne-russia-globalization-end.html (accessed 30.03.23).

Bondarenko, P. 2021. Angus Deaton. Encyclopedia Britannica. Accessed June 13, 2022. https://www.britannica.com/biography/Angus-S-Deaton.

Bostrom, N. 2014. *Superintelligence: Paths, Dangers, Strategies.* Oxford: Oxford University Press.

Boyd, M., and N. Wilson. 2020. "Existential Risks to Humanity Should Concern International Policymakers and More Could Be Done in Considering Them at the International Governance Level." *Risk Analysis* 40 (11): 2303−2312.

Bremmer, I. 2022. *The Power of Crisis: How Three Threats—and Our Response—Will Change The World.* New York: Simon & Schuster.

Brown, T.M., Cueto, M., and E. Fee. 2006. "The World Health Organization and the Transition From "International" to "Global" Public Health." *American Journal of Public Health* 96 (1): 62−72.

Bryant, J.H., and P. Rhodes. 2021. "Public Health." Encyclopedia Britannica. Accessed June 7, 2022. https://www.britannica.com/topic/public-health.

Buckley, C., A. Stevenson, and K. Bradsher. 2022. "From Zero Covid to No Plan: Behind China's Pandemic U-Turn." *New York Times*. Accessed January 12, 2023. https://www.nytimes.com/2022/12/19/world/asia/china-zero-covid-xi-jinping.html.

Çakmaklı, C., S. Demiralp, Kalemli-Özcan, S. Yeşiltaş, and M.A. Yıldırım. 2021. "The Economic Case for Global Vaccinations." National Bureau of Economic Research. Accessed February 20, 2023. https://www.nber.org/papers/w28395.

CardinalHealth. 2023. "AI-Enabled Population Health." CardinalHealth. Accessed February 21, 2023. https://www.cardinalhealth.com/en/services/specialty-physician-practice/solutions/navista/ai-enabled-population-health.html.

Chattopadhyay, A. 1968. "Hygienic Principles in the Regulations of Food Habits in the Dharma Sūtras." *Nagarjun* 11, 194−199.

Chatzky, A., and J. McBride. 2020. "China's Massive Belt and Road Initiative." Council on Foreign Relations. Accessed January 31, 2023. https://www.cfr.org/backgrounder/chinas-massive-belt-and-road-initiative.

Chen, X., Li, H., Lucero-Prisno, D.E., Abdullah, A.S., Huang, J., and C. Laurence, et al., 2020. "What is global health? Key concepts and clarification of misperceptions." *Global Health Research and Policy* 5 (14). https://doi.org/10.1186/s41256-020-00142-7.

Chen, X., H. Li, D.E. Lucero-Prisno, K. AChebrolu, K. Cherco, M. Shukla, and H. Varia. 2023. "Health Care's Quest For An Enterprisewide AI Strategy." Deloitte. Accessed March 9, 2023. https://www2.deloitte.com/us/en/insights/industry/health-care/ai-led-transformations-in-health-care.html.

Clark, H., E.J. Sirleaf, M. Cárdenas, A. Chebbi, M. Dybul, M. Kazatchkine, J. Liu, P. Matsoso, D. Miliband et al. 2021. "COVID-19: Make It the Last Pandemic." World Health Organization Independent Panel for Pandemic Preparedness and Response. Accessed February 5, 2023. https://theindependentpanel.org/mainreport.

Couch, E. 2023. "Is the Ukraine War an Anti-Colonial Struggle?" *Foreign Policy*. Accessed March 22, 2023. https://foreignpolicy.com/2023/03/07/russia-colonialism-imperialism-solidarity-ukraine/.

CSIS. 2020. "Developing or Developed? Assessing Chinese Life Expectancy." Center for Strategic and International Studies: China Power Team. Accessed February 15, 2023. https://chinapower.csis.org/life-expectancy.

CUGH. 2023. "Mission and Vision." Consortium of Universities for Global Health. Accessed January 22, 2023. https://www.cugh.org/about/mission-vision.

Deaton, A. 2022. *The Great Escape: Health, Wealth, and the Origins of Inequality*. Princeton, NJ: Princeton University Press.

Deci, E.L., and M. Vansteenkiste. 2004. "Self-Determination Theory and Basic Need Satisfaction: Understanding Human Development in Positive Psychology." *Ricerche di Psicologia* 27 (1): 23–40.

DESA (Department of Economic and Social Affairs). 2009. "Achieving the Global Public Health Agenda." United Nations Department of Economic and Social Affairs. Accessed January 22, 2023. https://www.un.org/en/ecosoc/docs/pdfs/achieving_global_public_health_agenda.pdf.

Detels, R., Karim, Q.A., Baum, F., Li, L., A.H. Leyland, eds. 2021. *Oxford Textbook of Global Public Health*. Oxford: Oxford University Press.

Dhar, A., N. Batra, D. Betts, R. Judah, L. Sterrett, and S. Thomas. 2022. "The Future of Health." Deloitte. Accessed February 25, 2023. https://www2.deloitte.com/us/en/pages/life-sciences-and-health-care/articles/future-of-health.html.

Dobriansky, P.J., R.M. Suzman, and R.J. Hodes. 2017. "Why Population Aging Matters: A Global Perspective." Accessed February 10, 2023. United States National Institutes of Health and Department of State. https://www.nia.nih.gov/sites/default/files/2017-06/WPAM.pdf.

Doshi, R. 2021. *The Long Game: China's Grand Strategy to Displace American Order*. Oxford: Oxford University Press.

Eurasia. 2023. "Top Risks for 2023." Eurasia Group. Accessed February 13, 2023. https://www.eurasiagroup.net/issues/top-risks-2023.

Ferguson, N. 2018. *The Square and the Tower: Networks and Power, from the Freemasons to Facebook*. New York: Penguin Press.

Flaxman, A.D., and T. Vos. 2018. "Machine Learning in Population Health: Opportunities and Threats." *PLoS Medicine* 15 (11): e1002702.

Forman, L. 2023. "AI Has Its 'iPhone Moment'." *The Wall Street Journal*. Accessed March 9, 2023. https://www.wsj.com/articles/ai-has-its-iphone-moment-d9b47f4e.

Fried, L.P., Bentley, M.E., Buekens, P., Burke, D.S., Frenk, J.J., Klag, M.J., and H.C. Spencer. 2010. "Global Health is Public Health." *Lancet* 375 (9714): 535–537.

Galea, S. 2018. "Power and Public Health." Boston University School of Public Health Dean's Note. Accessed January 22, 2023. https://www.bu.edu/sph/news/articles/2018/power-and-public-health.

Galea, S., Tracy, M., Hoggatt, K.J., Dimaggio, C., and A. Karpati. 2011. "Estimated Deaths Attributable to Social Factors in the United States." *American Journal of Public Health* 101 (8): 1456–1465.

García Saisó, S., and M. D'Agostino. 2021. "Artificial Intelligence in Public Health." World Health Organization. Accessed February 8, 2023. https://iris.paho.org/bitstream/handle/10665.2/53732/PAHOEIHIS21011_eng.pdf?sequence = 5.

García Saisó, S., Marti, M.C., Medina, F.M., Pascha, V.M., Nelson, J., Tejerina, L., Bagolle, A., and M. D'Agostino. 2022. "Digital Transformation for More Equitable and Sustainable Public Health in the Age of Digital Interdependence." *American Journal of Public Health* 112 (S6): S621−S624.

GBD 2017 Diet Collaborators. 2019. "Health Effects of Dietary Risks in 195 Countries, 1990−2017: A Systematic Analysis for the Global Burden of Disease Study 2017." *Lancet* 393 (10184): 1958−1972.

Ghebreyesus, T.A., and S. Swaminathan. 2021. "Get Ready for AI in Pandemic Response and Healthcare." *BMJ (Clinical Research Ed.)*. Accessed February 28, 2023. https://blogs.bmj.com/bmj/2021/10/28/get-ready-for-ai-in-pandemic-response-and-healthcare.

Goudsblom, J. 1986. "Public Health and the Civilizing Process." *The Milbank Quarterly* 64 (2): 161−188.

Groseclose, S.L. 1999. "Ten Great Public Health Achievements: United States, 1900−1999. Centers for Disease Control and Prevention." *MMWR* 48 (12): 241−242Accessed June 7, 2022. https://www.cdc.gov/mmwr/PDF/wk/mm4812.pdf.

Hameiri, S. 2020. "COVID-19: Why Did Global Health Governance Fail?" The Lowy Institute. Accessed February 5, 2023. https://www.lowyinstitute.org/the-interpreter/covid-19-why-did-global-health-governance-fail.

Hanlon, G., and J. Pickett. 1984. *Public Health: Administration and Practice.* St. Louis, MO: C.V. Mosby.

Hayashi, Y., and A. DeBarros 2023. "U.S.−China Trade Grows as Spy Balloon Raises Tensions." *The Wall Street Journal*. Accessed February 9, 2023. https://www.wsj.com/articles/u-s-china-tensions-are-high-so-is-commerce-between-the-nations-11675920444.

Himmelstein, D.U., and S. Woolhandler. 2016. "Public Health's Falling Share of US Health Spending." *American Journal of Public Health* 106 (1): 56−57.

Horton, R. 2013. "Offline: Is Global Health Neocolonialist? ." *Lancet* 382 (9906): 1690.

Huang, Y. 2022. "The COVID-19 Pandemic and China's Global Health Leadership." Council on Foreign Relations. Accessed January 11, 2023. https://cdn.cfr.org/sites/default/files/report_pdf/Huang_CSR-92.pdf.

ICC. 2023. "Situation in Ukraine: ICC Judges Issue Arrest Warrants Against Vladimir Vladimirovich Putin and Maria Alekseyevna Lvova-Belova." International Criminal Court. Accessed March 22, 2023. https://www.icc-cpi.int/news/situation-ukraine-icc-judges-issue-arrest-warrants-against-vladimir-vladimirovich-putin-and.

IMF. 2022. "World Economic Outlook Update: Rising Caseloads, a Disrupted Recovery, and Higher Inflation." International Monetary Fund. Accessed February 5, 2023. https://www.imf.org/en/Publications/WEO/Issues/2022/01/25/world-economic-outlook-update-january-2022.

IoM. 2002. *Institute of Medicine's Future of the Public's Health in the 21st Century.* Washington, DC: National Academies Press.

Irwin, D.A. 2020. "The Pandemic Adds Momentum to the Deglobalization Trend." Peterson Institute for International Economics. Accessed February 9, 2023. https://www.piie.com/blogs/realtime-economic-issues-watch/pandemic-adds-momentum-deglobalization-trend.

Ivanova, P., M. Seddon, and B. Hall. 2022. "'We're Minor Losses': Russia's Mobilisation Targets Ethnic Minorities." *Financial Times*. Accessed March 22, 2023. https://www.ft.com/content/ae06c532-e1ff-488a-b77c-cb93422d3dd7.

Iyengar, R., and L. Scott. 2023. "What the ChatGPT Moment Means for U.S.−China Tech Competition." *Foreign Policy*. Accessed March 9, 2023. https://foreignpolicy.com/2023/03/03/chatgpt-us-china-tech-competition/.

Jain, S., Pandey, K., Jain, P., and K.P. Seng. 2022. *Artificial Intelligence, Machine Learning, and Mental Health in Pandemics.* New York: Elsevier.

Jamison, D.T., Summers, L.H., Alleyne, G., Arrow, K.J., Berkley, S., Binagwaho, A., and F. Bustreo, et al., 2013. "Global Health 2035: A World Converging Within a Generation." *Lancet* 382 (9908): 1898−1955.

Jha, A.K. 2019. "Population Health Management: Saving Lives and Saving Money? ." *JAMA: The Journal of the American Medical Association* 322 (5): 390−391.

Juuti, P.S., Katko, T.S., and H.S. Vuorinen. 2007. *Environmental History of Water*. London: International Water Association Publishing.

Katz, R., Kornblet, S., Arnold, G., Lief, E., and J.E. Fischer. 2011. "Defining Health Diplomacy: Changing Demands in the Era of Globalization." *The Milbank Quarterly* 89 (3): 503−523.

Kelley, M., Ferrand, R.A., Muraya, K., Chigudu, S., Molyneux, S., Pai, M., and E. Barasa. 2020. "An Appeal for Practical Social Justice in the COVID-19 Global Response in Low-Income and Middle-Income Countries." *The Lancet Global Health* 8 (7): e888−e889.

Kennedy, S. 2022. "Coalition Will Use Health Computing, AI for Population Health." Health IT Analytics. Accessed February 2, 2023. https://healthitanalytics.com/news/coalition-will-use-health-computing-ai-for-population-health.

Khalil, L. 2020. "Digital Authoritarianism, China and COVID." Lowry Institute. Accessed January 11, 2023. https://www.lowyinstitute.org/publications/digital-authoritarianism-china-covid.

Kifer, Y., Heller, D., Perunovic, W.Q.E., and A.D. Galinsky. 2013. "The Good Life of the Powerful: The Experience of Power and Authenticity Enhances Subjective Well-Being." *Psychological Science* 24 (3). https://doi.org/10.1177/0956797612450891.

King, N.B., and A. Koski. 2020. "Defining Global Health as Public Health Somewhere Else." *BMJ Global Health* 5 (1): e002172.

Kirillova, K. 2022. "Imperial Russia Declares War on Colonialism." Center for European Policy Analysis. Accessed March 22, 2023. https://cepa.org/article/imperial-russia-declares-war-on-colonialism/.

Koplan, J.P., Bond, T.C., Merson, M.H., Reddy, K.S., Rodriguez, M.H., Sewankambo, N.K., and J.N. Wasserheit. 2009. "Consortium of Universities for Global Health Executive Board: Towards a Common Definition of Global Health." *Lancet* 373 (9679): 1993−1995.

Kuate Defo, B. 2014. "Demographic, Epidemiological, and Health Transitions: Are They Relevant to Population Health Patterns in Africa? ." *Global Health Action* 7, 22443.

Kupperschmidt, K. 2021. 'A Toxic Cocktail': Panel Delivers Harsh Verdict on the World's Failure to Prepare for Pandemic. Science (New York, N.Y.). Accessed February 5, 2023. https://www.science.org/content/article/toxic-cocktail-panel-delivers-harsh-verdict-world-s-failure-prepare-pandemic.

Lammers, J., Stoker, J.I., Rink, F., and A.D. Galinsky. 2016. "To Have Control Over or to Be Free From Others? The Desire for Power Reflects a Need for Autonomy." *Personality and Social Psychology Bulletin* 42 (4). https://doi.org/10.1177/0146167216634064.

Lemco, J., A. Sathe, A.J. Schickling, M. Weiland, B. Yeo. 2021. "The Deglobalization Myth(s)." Vanguard. Accessed February 10, 2023. https://corporate.vanguard.com/content/dam/corp/research/pdf/Megatrends-The-deglobalization-myths-ISG052021%20(1).pdf.

Lusigi, A. 2022. "Shaping Our Future in a World of Transformation." United Nations Development Programme. Accessed January 13, 2023. https://www.undp.org/ghana/blog/shaping-our-future-world-transformation.

McArthur, J.W., and Rasmussen, K. 2017. "How Successful Were the Millennium Development Goals?" Brookings Institute. Accessed January 8, 2023. https://www.brookings.edu/blog/future-development/2017/01/11/how-successful-were-the-millennium-development-goals.

McKinsey. 2022. "What are Industry 4.0, the Fourth Industrial Revolution, and 4IR?" McKinsey & Company. Accessed February 6, 2023. https://www.mckinsey.com/featured-insights/mckinsey-explainers/what-are-industry-4-0-the-fourth-industrial-revolution-and-4ir.

Mearsheimer, J. 2018. *The Great Delusion. New Haven, CT.* Yale University Press.

Mecklin, J. 2022. "At Doom's Doorstep: It is 100 Seconds to Midnight." *Bulletin of the Atomic Scientists.* Accessed January 9, 2023. https://thebulletin.org/doomsday-clock/current-time.

Mhasawade, V., Zhao, Y., and R. Chunara. 2021. "Machine Learning and Algorithmic Fairness in Public and Population Health." *Nature Machine Intelligence* 3, 659−666.

Miller, C. 2022. *Chip War: The Fight for the World's Most Critical Technology.* New York: Simon & Schuster (Scribner Books).

Ministers of Foreign Affairs. 2007. "Oslo Ministerial Declaration—Global Health: A Pressing Foreign Policy Issue of Our Time." *Lancet* 369 (9570): 1373−1378.

Monlezun, D.J. 2022. *Personalist Social Contract: Saving Multiculturalism, Artificial Intelligence, and Civilization.* Newcastle upon Tyne: Cambridge Scholars Press.

Monlezun, D.J. 2023. *The Thinking Healthcare System: Artificial Intelligence and Human Equity.* New York: Elsevier.

Monlezun, D.J., Carr, C., Niu, T., Nordio, F., DeValle, N., Sarris, L., and T. Harlan. 2022a. "Meta-Analysis and Machine Learning-Augmented Mixed Effects Cohort Analysis of Improved Diets Among 5847 Medical Trainees, Providers and Patients." *Public Health Nutrition* 25 (2): 281−289.

Monlezun, D.J., Kasprowicz, E., Tosh, K.W., Nix, J., Urday, P., Tice, D., Sarris, L., and T. Harlan. 2015. "Medical School-Based Teaching Kitchen Improves HbA1c, Blood Pressure, and Cholesterol For Patients With Type 2 Diabetes: Results From a Novel Randomized Controlled Trial." *Diabetes Research and Clinical Practice* 109 (2): 420−426.

Monlezun, D.J., Sinyavskiy, O., Sotomayor, C., Peters, N., Steigner, L., Girault, M., Garcia, A., et al., Gallagher, C., et al., and C. Iliescu 2022b. "Artificial Intelligence-Augmented Propensity Score, Cost Effectiveness, and Computational Ethical Analysis of Cardiac Arrest and Active Cancer With Novel Mortality Predictive Score." *Medicina (CardioOncology)* 58 (8): 1039.

Msemburi, W., Karlinsky, A., Knutson, V., Aleshin-Guendel, S., Chatterji, S., and J. Wakefield. 2023. "The WHO Estimates of Excess Mortality Associated With the COVID-19 Pandemic." *Nature* 613 (7942): 130−137.

Murth, P., and A. Ansehl. 2020. *Technology and Global Public Health.* New York: Springer.

Myers, J. 2022. "From Pandemic to Endemic." World Economic Forum. Accessed February 4, 2023. https://www.weforum.org/agenda/2022/01/covid-19-pandemic-2022-what-next-expert-voices-from-davos.

Nchasi, G., Mwasha, C., Shaban, M.M., Rwegasira, R., Mallilah, B., Chesco, J., Volkova, A., and A. Mahmoud. 2022. "Ukraine's Triple Emergency: Food Crisis Amid Conflicts and COVID-19 Pandemic." *Health Science Reports* 5 (6): e862.

Nkrumah, K. 1965. *Neo-Colonialism, the Last Stage of Imperialism.* London: Thomas Nelson & Sons.

NOAA. 2023. "Hurricane Costs." National Oceanic and Atmospheric Administration. Accessed March 11, 2023. https://coast.noaa.gov/states/fast-facts/hurricane-costs.html.

NYU. 2023. "Reinventing the Public Health Paradigm." New York University. Accessed March 8, 2023. https://publichealth.nyu.edu/.

OECD. 2011. "Education at a Glance: OECD Indicators." Organisation for Economic Co-operation and Development. Paris, France: OECD Press.

Owen Jr., W.F., Carmona, R., and C. Pomeroy. 2020. "Failing Another National Stress Test on Health Disparities." *JAMA: the Journal of the American Medical Association* 323 (19): 1905−1906.

Owens, D., and J. Parry. 2022. "COVID-19: What Can China Learn From Hong Kong and Singapore About Exiting Zero COVID? ." *BMJ (Clinical Research Ed.)* 379, o3043.

Owoyemi, A., Owoyemi, J., Osiyemi, A., and A. Boyd. 2020. "Artificial Intelligence for Healthcare in Africa." *Frontiers in Digital Health* 2, 6.

Oxford. 2022. "Deglobalization and Russia's War on Ukraine." Oxford Economics Group. Accessed February 9, 2023. https://www.oxfordeconomics.com/resource/deglobalisation-and-russias-war-on-ukraine.

Packard, R.M. 2016. *A History of Global Health: Interventions Into the Lives of Other Peoples.* Baltimore, MD: Johns Hopkins University Press.

Plato. 1991. Translated by B. Jowett *The Republic.* New York: Vintage Books (375 B.C.).

Prashad, V. 2007. *The Darker Nations: A People's History of the Third World.* New York: The New Press.

Rainie, L., Anderson, J., and Vogels, E.A. 2021. "Experts Doubt Ethical AI Design Will Be Broadly Adopted As the Norm Within the Next Decade." Pew Research Center. Accessed October 15, 2022. https://www.pewresearch.org/internet/2021/06/16/experts-doubt-ethical-ai-design-will-be-broadly-adopted-as-the-norm-within-the-next-decade.

Richardson, E. 2020. *Epidemic Illusions: On the Coloniality of Global Public Health.* Cambridge, MA: MIT Press.

Roose, K. 2023. "How ChatGPT Kicked Off an A.I. Arms Race." *The New York Times.* Accessed March 9, 2023. https://www.nytimes.com/2023/02/03/technology/chatgpt-openai-artificial-intelligence.html.

Roux, A.V. 2016. "On the Distinction—or Lack of Distinction—Between Population Health and Public Health." *American Journal of Public Health* 106 (4): 619−620.

Sachs, J. 1999. "Twentieth-Century Political Economy: A brief History of Global Capitalism." *Oxford University Review of Economic Policy* 15 (4): 90−101.

Sachs, J. 2020. *The Ages of Globalization: Geography, Technology, and Institutions.* New York: Columbia University Press.

Saich, T. 2022. "What Kind of World Does Xi Jinping Want?" Harvard University Kennedy School of Government Policy Topics. Accessed February 10, 2023. https://www.hks.harvard.edu/faculty-research/policy-topics/international-relations-security/what-kind-world-does-xi-jinping.

Salm, M., Ali, M., Minihane, M., and P. Conrad. 2021. "Defining Global Health: Findings From a Systematic Review and Thematic Analysis of the Literature." *BMJ Global Health* 6 (6): e005292.

Santosh, K.C., and L. Gaur. 2021. *Artificial Intelligence and Machine Learning in Public Healthcare.* New York: Springer.

Sartre, J.P. 1956. "La Mystification Néo-Colonialiste." *Les Temps Modernes* 123, 125.

Schuler, M.S., and S. Rose. 2017. "Targeted Maximum Likelihood Estimation for Causal Inference in Observational Studies." *American Journal of Epidemiology* 185 (1): 65−73.

Schwab, K. 2016. "The Fourth Industrial Revolution: What it Means, How to Respond." World Economic Forum. Accessed January 8, 2023. https://www.weforum.org/agenda/2016/01/the-fourth-industrial-revolution-what-it-means-and-how-to-respond.

Shaaban, N. 2020. "Digital Health Entrepreneurship in Vietnam." Massachusetts Institute of Technology. Accessed February 28, 2023. https://legatum.mit.edu/wp-content/uploads/2020/07/Digital-Health-Vietnam-MIT-Legatum-Center.pdf.

Shamasunder, S., Holmes, S.M., Goronga, T., Carrasco, H., Katz, E., Frankfurter, R., and S. Keshavjee. 2020. "COVID-19 Reveals Weak Health Systems by Design: Why We Must Re-Make Global Health in This Historic Moment." *Global Public Health* 15 (7): 1083−1089.

Slobodian, Q. 2018. *Globalists: The End of Empire and the Birth of Neoliberalism.* Cambridge, MA: Harvard University Press.

Snow, S. 2008. "John Snow: The Making of a Hero? ." *The Art of Medicine* 372 (9632): P22−P23.

Snyder, T. 2022. The War in Ukraine is a Colonial War. New Yorker. Accessed March 22, 2023. https://www.newyorker.com/news/essay/the-war-in-ukraine-is-a-colonial-war.

Stanard, M.G. 2018. *European Overseas Empire, 1879–1999: A Short History*. Hoboken, NJ: John Wiley & Sons.

Stieg, C. 2020. "How This Canadian Start-Up Spotted Coronavirus Before Everyone Else Knew About It." CNBC. Accessed February 5, 2023. https://www.cnbc.com/2020/03/03/bluedot-used-artificial-intelligence-to-predict-coronavirus-spread.html.

Sullivan, J., and B. Deese. 2021. "Building Resilient Supply Chains, Revitalizing American Manufacturing, and Fostering Broad-Based Growth." The US White House. Accessed February 10, 2023. https://www.whitehouse.gov/wp-content/uploads/2021/06/100-day-supply-chain-review-report.pdf.

Takemi, K., Jimba, M., Ishii, S., Katsuma, Y., Nakamura, Y., Working Group on Challenges in Global Health and Japan's Contribution. 2008. "Human Security Approach for Global Health." *Lancet* 372 (9632): 13–14.

Thucydides. 1972. *History of the Peloponnesian War*. New York: Penguin Classics, Edited by M. I. Finley. Translated by R. Warner.

Tuli, S., Tuli, S., Tuli, R., and S.S. Gill. 2020. "Predicting the Growth and Trend of COVID-19 Pandemic Using Machine Learning and Cloud Computing." *Internet of Things* 11, 100222.

Turcotte-Tremblay, A.M., Fregonese, F., Kadio, K., Alam, N., and L. Merry. 2020. "Global Health is More Than Just 'Public Health Somewhere Else." *BMJ Global Health* 5 (5): e002545.

UN. 1945. "Charter." United Nations. Accessed January 13, 2023. https://www.un.org/en/about-us/un-charter/full-text.

UN. 1948. "Universal Declaration of Human Rights." United Nations. Accessed January 16, 2023. https://www.un.org/en/about-us/universal-declaration-of-human-rights.

UN. 2008. "Global Health and Foreign Policy: Resolution 63/33 Adopted by the General Assembly." United Nations. Accessed March 8, 2023. https://digitallibrary.un.org/record/642456?ln = en.

UN. 2012. "Follow-Up to General Assembly Resolution 64/291 on Human Security: Report of the Secretary-General." United Nations. Accessed March 8, 2023. https://digitallibrary.un.org/record/726045?ln = en.

UN. 2020. "Road Map for Digital Cooperation: Implementation of the Recommendations of the High-level Panel on Digital Cooperation. United Nations 74th General Assembly." United Nations. Accessed June 11, 2022. https://www.un.org/en/content/digital-cooperation-roadmap/.

UN. 2021. "Early-Warning 'Pandemic Hub' Plan Unveiled by WHO's Tedros and Germany's Merkel." United Nations News. Accessed February 28, 2023. https://news.un.org/en/story/2021/05/1091332.

UN. 2022. "Humanity's Just One Misunderstanding Away From 'Nuclear Annihilation' Warns UN Chief." United Nation News. Accessed January 13, 2023. https://news.un.org/en/story/2022/08/1123752.

UN. 2023a. "UN General Assembly Calls for Immediate End to War in Ukraine." United Nations. Accessed February 23, 2023. https://news.un.org/en/story/2023/02/1133847.

UN. 2023b. "Global Issues on Health." United Nations. Accessed January 22, 2023. https://www.un.org/en/global-issues/health.

UNDP. 1994. "Human Development Report 1994: New Dimensions of Human Security." United Nations Development Programme. Accessed February 15, 2023. https://hdr.undp.org/content/human-development-report-1994.

USAID. 2019. "Artificial Intelligence in Global Health: Defining a Collective Path Forward." United States Agency for International Development. Accessed February 18, 2023. https://www.usaid.gov/cii/ai-in-global-health.

Varma, J. 2022. "How Public Health Failed America." *The Atlantic*. Accessed February 2023. https://www.theatlantic.com/ideas/archive/2022/05/how-public-health-failed-america/629869.

Veenhoven, R. 2010. "Life is Getting Better: Societal Evolution and Fit With Human Nature." *Social Indicators Research* 97 (1): 105–122.

Velmovitsky, P.E., Bevilacqua, T., Alencar, P., Cowan, D., and P.P. Morita. 2021. "Convergence of Precision Medicine and Public Health Into Precision Public Health: Toward a Big Data Perspective." *Frontiers in Public Health* 9, 561873.

Vollset, S.E., Goren, E., Yuan, C.W., Cao, J., Smith, A.E., Hsiao, T., and C. Bisignano, et al., 2020. "Fertility, Mortality, Migration, and Population Scenarios for 195 Countries and Territories from 2017 to 2100: A Forecasting Analysis For the Global Burden of Disease Study." *Lancet* 396 (10258): 1285–1306.

Wang, H., COVID-19 Excess Mortality Collaborators. 2022. "Estimating Excess Mortality Due to the COVID-19 Pandemic: A Systematic Analysis of COVID-19-Related Mortality, 2020–21." *Lancet* 399 (10334): 1513–1536.

WEC (World Energy Council). 2011. "Policies For the Future: 2011 Assessment of Country Energy and Climate Policies." World Energy Council. Accessed March 11, 2023. https://www.worldenergy.org/assets/downloads/PUB_wec_2011_assessment_of_energy_and_climate_policies_2011_WEC.pdf.

WEF. 2023. "The Great Reset." World Economic Forum. Accessed February 5, 2023. https://www.weforum.org/great-reset.

Weng, F. 2010. "China's Population Destiny: The Looming Crisis." Brookings Institute. Accessed June 12, 2023. https://www.brookings.edu/articles/chinas-population-destiny-the-looming-crisis.

WHO. 1948. "Constitution." World Health Organization. Accessed January 16, 2023. https://apps.who.int/gb/bd/PDF/bd47/EN/constitution-en.pdf?ua = 1.

WHO. 2002. "Health and Human Security." World Health Organization. Accessed January 16, 2023. https://apps.who.int/iris/handle/10665/122074.

WHO. 2010. Global Status Report on Noncommunicable Diseases. Geneva, Switzerland: World Health Organization Press. https://apps.who.int/iris/bitstream/handle/10665/44579/9789240686458_eng.pdf.

WHO. 2020. "Listings of WHO's Response to COVID-19." World Health Organization. Accessed February 5, 2023. https://www.who.int/news/item/29-06-2020-covidtimeline.

WHO. 2021. "Global Strategy on Digital Health 2020–2025." World Health Organization. Accessed June 11. 2023. https://www.who.int/docs/default-source/documents/gs4dhdaa2a9f352b0445bafbc79ca799dce4d.pdf.

WHO. 2023a. "Promoting Wellbeing." World Health Organization. Accessed February 25, 2023. https://www.who.int/activities/promoting-well-being

WHO. 2023b. "Biography: Dr. Tedros Adhanom Ghebreyesus." World Health Organization. Accessed February 25, 2023. https://www.who.int/director-general/biography.

WHO. 2023c. "Ukraine's Health System Shows Resilience, But Barriers Remain." World Health Organization. Accessed March 22, 2023. https://www.who.int/europe/news/item/17-03-2023-ukraine-s-health-system-shows-resilience--but-barriers-remain.

Winkelstein, W. 2022. "History of Public Health." *Encyclopedia of Public Health*. Accessed March 25, 2023. https://www.encyclopedia.com/education/encyclopedias-almanacs-transcripts-and-maps/history-public-health.

Winslow, C.E. 1923. *The Evolution and Significance of The Modern Public Health Campaign*. New Haven, CT: Yale University Press.

Woetzel, J., J. Mischke, A. Madgavkar, E. Windhagen, S. Smit, M. Birshan, S. Kemeny, and R.J. Anderson. 2021. "The Rise and Rise of the Global Balance Sheet: How Productively Are We Using Our Wealth?" McKinsey & Company. Accessed January 13, 2023. https://www.mckinsey.com/industries/financial-services/our-insights/the-rise-and-rise-of-the-global-balance-sheet-how-productively-are-we-using-our-wealth.

Wohl, A.S. 1983. *Endangered Lives: Public Health in Victorian Britain*. Cambridge, MA: Harvard University Press.

Wright, R., I. Watson, and E. Erdem. 2022. "Uyghur Families Demand Answers Over Fire That Triggered Protests." CNN. Accessed January 11, 2023. https://www.cnn.com/2022/12/01/china/china-protests-urumqi-fire-deaths-covid-dst-intl-hnk/index.html.

Yach, D., and D. Bettcher. 1998. "The Globalization of Public Health." *American Journal of Public Health* 88 (5): 735−744.

Design part I: Artificial intelligence + financing

2.1 Overview of current global public health financing

Before you build a home, you need a design. And that design must be bounded by the budget (along with the people who will help you fund it). What are you trying to get out of what you are putting your money into? The classic management formulation of this basic principle is "no money, no mission." Therefore, to reengineer and regenerate the artificial intelligence (AI)-transformed global public health ecosystem, we will consider in this chapter an overview of the ecosystem's financing, and how AI is improving (and complicating) it—because no funds means no healthcare or public health. Impoverishing or catastrophic health spending plagues nearly 2 billion people globally, with most of the world's healthcare systems and public health agencies struggling to sufficiently and sustainably fund even essential operations (which perpetuates ongoing inequalities, especially for low- and middle-income countries [LMICs] struggling to break out of the cycle of health underfunding and its related worse population health outcomes; WHO 2023a). The World Health Organization (WHO) therefore articulates the broad and influential consensus that the essential health financing objective should be attaining universal health coverage (UHC). This is one of the 17 sustainable development goals (SDGs) targets adopted by the worlds' nations at the United Nations (UN) 2015 General Assembly as a central requirement for sustainable development of the global population's political, economic, and thus social well-being. The WHO notes that nearly 90% of UHC interventions can be achieved through healthcare systems' primary health care, through which 75% of the health-focused SDGs can also be attained (though the COVID-19 pandemic disrupted 92% of countries' essential health services). The WHO thus advocates for healthcare systems worldwide to join the current historic rebuilding period by shifting their primary strategy in health financing to a primary healthcare focus, providing greater population health benefits at lower cost and greater equity. Accordingly, the operational equation (of local healthcare + public health at scale = global public health) is achieved financially through primary care–driven UHC. In it, global public health is delivered locally through public health's interface with healthcare systems at the point of service for their patient and population service.

Historically though, the fundamental hurdle to successful financing is operationalizing this strategy, as there have been signals of progress but a lack of substantive and sustained improvements at scale (WHO, 2023b; Monlezun 2023). Given its global scope, complexity, and expenses, global public health requires sufficient funding if it is to be equitably effective, and

Responsible Artificial Intelligence Re-engineering the Global Public Health Ecosystem. DOI: https://doi.org/10.1016/B978-0-443-21597-1.00002-0

that requires a critical mass of funders (typically richer nations and institutions) with deep enough pockets to pull together the resources needed to achieve verifiable progress toward a shared vision of international well-being (in collaboration with—rather than imposing on—poorer nations and institutions). Yet outcomes and cooperation do not come cheap. So financing is a helpful place to start the consideration of how AI is revolutionizing the global public health ecosystem given its promise (and early progress) helping unite funders and stakeholders through more efficient means to get to more and faster empirically verifiable improvements. The WHO influentially articulates this pivotal point in global public health as seeking a "measurable impact," which is "at the heart of WHO's plans to transform the future of public health," with the "Triple Billion targets" being "fundamental to how this plan will be achieved" (WHO, 2023b). The digitalization of this ecosystem enables such lofty goals by translating the mission of modern global public health (championed by the WHO's 1948 Constitution as the "highest attainable standard of health for all people") into ultimate outcomes which can be tracked, according to an operational plan of concrete intermediate metrics. For example, to reduce a community's excess deaths from cardiovascular disease, you can improve its nutrition through dietary education and support, but only if you know how many people are actually eating more healthy foods after versus before the abovementioned intervention. And so the WHO published its Triple Billion targets in 2019 as a measurable strategic plan for quantifying improvements in global health according to the health-related SDGs: 1 billion more people with UHC (covering essential health services and avoiding health financial hardship, or spending less than 10% of household income on health), protected from health emergencies (through preparedness, prevention, and timely detection and response), and with improved well-being (through 16 indicators including 14 of the SDGs).

But the 2020 emergence of the COVID pandemic stressed the financing of global public health, and so highlighted the shortcomings of its strategy, structures, and mechanisms. *The Lancet* COVID-19 Commission staffed by representatives from the WHO, World Bank, and the health, business, policy, and government sectors published their September 2022 report dissecting those weaknesses (Sachs et al. 2022). After decades of refining its fundamental mission of epidemic prevention, mitigation, and response, this high-level analysis faulted the WHO as "the central organizing body for global cooperation on health" that nonetheless failed to provide sufficiently early warning, guidance, and coordination of resources and partners among the world's nations and institutions to reduce the 21st century's defining global health crisis thus far. The WHO—World Bank report went so far as to assert strategically "we have largely failed in terms of global coordination during the first 2 years of this pandemic." It concretely cited insufficient financing of research and development (R&D), biomedical production capacity, healthcare systems, and public health agencies especially in LMICs. Then it concluded with the central recommendations of WHO-specific "large-scale emergency financing in the case of a global public health emergency," like a credit line particularly for LMICs, on top of the existing operational and financial infrastructures needed for long-term health challenges like noncommunicable diseases. Three layers of financing for the global public health ecosystem is required according to this consensus: local healthcare systems (through UHC for essential services), public health (particularly for disease and disability prevention), and global public health (especially challenges and emergencies like pandemics, climate events, conflicts, poverty, and ecological damage). The committee emphasized further the need for sufficient political empowerment of the WHO coordinating the global public health ecosystem to ensure the financing can be operationalized sufficiently and equitably. Interestingly, the primary committee recommendation was the "strengthening of multilateralism in all crucial dimensions: political, cultural, institutional, and financial." The committee asserted that COVID spotlighted the fundamental political economic structural weaknesses in our global human ecosystem: underfunding of and underutilizing multilateral cooperation on "global public goods," particularly "among the major powers" who are divided by "excessive nationalism." Chapter 1 detailed the WHO's 1990s–2000s liberal capitalist-rooted defense of its policies according to common peace and prosperity. Similarly, two decades later, the commission expanded the defense of this integral approach to enhanced political cooperation on global public health financing by their ultimate recommendation citing the *Universal Declaration of Human Rights (UDHR)* as "the UN's moral charter" in which their ethical and pragmatic considerations were ultimately grounded. So better global health financing is the smart *and* right thing to do according to this consensus position. When the moral, political, and economic convergence translates effective health financing into effective global public health, it becomes effective health governance.

Before we get to how AI is addressing such problems, let us finish up with a more concrete overview of the governance problems facing (and solutions emerging for) global public health financing according to the commission broken down by (1) equity, (2) integration, and (3) resilience (Bartels 2022; Sachs et al. 2022).

2.1.1 Equity

Finance disparities worsen (and are worsened by) health disparities. Further, sicker and poorer populations on one side of the world can undermine the stability and prosperity of healthier and wealthier populations on the other side as our digitalized world is linked through global value supply chains and geopolitical chronic challenges and acute shocks. The global public health ecosystem must spend more to fix deficits in one sector (particularly acute treatment) and region (particularly the Global South), which reduces what they can spend elsewhere (especially more efficient prevention). Emblematically, the commission's Chair, Jeffrey Sachs (Professor at the Harvard and Columbia Universities and the President of the UN Sustainable Development Solutions Network), noted how Japan and sub-Sahara African nations are separated not only by a 30-year life expectancy gap but also by a similar divide in health expenditures. Many LMICs struggle not only to cover the chronic healthcare system costs for essential services (particularly the workforce), but also the acute threats to global public health (like pandemics often requiring adaptive financing) to reduce inequities. To address such operational challenges from inequities, the commission recommended strategically and structurally strengthening national healthcare systems by the dual capacities of effective public health (with its population health interface with systems) and UHC (to ensure a minimum floor for societal well-being). The parallel finance recommendation is "funding for LICs and LMICs" as the "centerpiece of the global response" through a single "Global Health Fund" for the global public health ecosystem. The commission advised it should be "closely aligned with the WHO" and integrate current government, intergovernment, and private funds (including the COVAX, Pandemic Preparedness Financial Intermediary Fund, TB and Malaria, Global Fund for AIDS, and Gavi). Think of such national health ecosystems (bridging healthcare systems and public health agencies) like a worker and the ecosystem financing like the worker's funds. Like most people, the worker to be financially sound must manage their funds such that they uses the steady paycheck to pay for ongoing bills. But the worker needs to also keep some set aside for investments and savings, including an emergency fund for unexpected bills. Similarly, the commission recommended building sufficient finance capacity for the global public health ecosystem to pay for essential health services (for national health ecosystems to collectively keep the global population healthy, principally through preventing and mitigating diseases and disabilities) and public health services (for prevention and emergency responses like for global health crises including pandemics). Mariana Mazzucato (Professor at the University College of London and the Chair for the WHO Council on the Economics of Health for All) argued for such equity-focused finance recommendations (like climate ones) based on the net cost savings for the world. Such savings economically support the WHO's "Health for All" mission that "should be our public purpose…from which we backtrack to design an economy to deliver that goal." Such economic justification is further supported morally by our pluralistic but still objective individual good, pursuant to the unifying ultimate goal of "the common good" (as echoed in the *UDHR* and WHO Constitution).

2.1.2 Integration

Like inequities, disintegration is a further barrier to effective financing and thus performance of the global public health ecosystem. The commission's Mike Ryan (Executive Director of the WHO Health Emergencies Programme) argued for equitable value-based global public health by a "primary health care-led [health] system that is fully integrated and interoperable," providing interlinked "essential healthcare and essential public health services." Such structural integration is key to strategic integration: "the last mile of health delivery—primary healthcare—is the first mile of health security." A shared vision of global well-being articulated as the common good (that is in the pragmatic self-survival and self-determination interests of every state and community) thus drives the reverse-engineered financial design of a global public health ecosystem to achieve it: integrate strategies, structures, operations, and their financing to synergistically leverage the comparative advantages and convergent interests of the ecosystems' partners, countries, and communities.

2.1.3 Resiliency

The basic principles of resilient (equitable, integrated, and so effective) financing for the global public health ecosystem is a bigger version of the responsible money management for the average working adult. Generate enough funds to allow you to save for future emergencies and spend on current needs, allowing you to get the most out of your money while achieving your essential long-term goals. People or ecosystems with sufficient cash flow, assets, emergency funding (and partners), and responsible spending generally, are sufficiently resilient to long-term challenges and sudden shocks. What are the essential and defining operations, programs, traits, and so related challenges to such resilient financing for the global public health ecosystem? (WHO, 2023c).

2.1.3.1 Main levels

Ecosystem financing historically has occurred at the international and national level. The former occurs mostly through the WHO and parallel organizations like the World Bank, dominated by donor-directed funds from richer nations driving the agenda on how they are spent. The latter occurs generally through domestic revenue mostly in richer nations generating foreign aid to poorer countries for their healthcare systems, and to a lesser extent their public health agencies. Historically, there has been limited investment linking the two to reduce program redundancy and excess administrative costs.

2.1.3.2 Core functions

The WHO, as the most prevalent and active global public health agency, influentially has advanced an integrated health delivery and financing infrastructure to deliver public health programs through and in conjunction with local healthcare systems, leaving the strategic objective of local UHC linked with global public health programs. The "core functions" of such integrated financing through healthcare systems therefore include revenue raising (out of pocket, insurance, aid, and government funding), fund pooling (of prepaid monies for part or all of a population), and service purchasing (compensating health providers and managers, preferably by value not volume). There remains high variability within and across countries in these functions, challenging the identification and translation of best practices.

2.1.3.3 Main state funder

The United States by far is the largest donor of global public health through foreign aid as "development assistance for health" (DAH; KFF 2023; GBDH Health Financing Collaborator Network 2019). 70% of the public sector investment, 45% of the total investment, and 55% of the products in global health R&D are contributed by the US government, which represents less than 0.01% of US gross domestic product that is spent on global health R&D (NIH 2023). Although representing a significant absolute amount of funding, the relative concentration of funding to one of just 193 countries does challenge its sustainability.

2.1.3.4 Main overall funders

Among 195 countries from 1995 to 2016, the states' domestic health investments and capacities delivering integrated healthcare and public health increased as their reliance on DAH fell (GBDH Health Financing Collaborator Network 2019). By 2016, only 0.4% of health spending worldwide was spent in low-income countries (LICs), despite them constituting 10% of the global population. The majority of DAH funding was for HIV/AIDS. The top DAH funder aside from the United States noted earlier was private philanthropy separate from corporate charity. The 2016 difference in per capita health spending for high-income countries (HICs) versus LICs ($115 spent by HICs for their citizens for every $1 LICs spend on their citizens) is projected to remain constant through 2050, though LICs are increasing their share of the global population by 5.7%. Domestically, governments tend to spend more on health as their economies grow, allowing them to prioritize interrelated economic and health development (as they additionally respond to greater popular pressure to do so). A substantial percentage of LICs are expected to remain dependent on foreign nations' DAH for domestic health financing for the foreseeable future. Concurrently, higher income nations typically in the Global North are expected to face increasing headwinds sustaining their internal health financing, caught between the competing demands of declining domestic populations and growing global pressure to reduce North–South financing disparities.

2.1.3.5 Main trends

The COVID-19 pandemic highlighted how the decades-long panic–neglect cycle continues to plague global public health financing (GBDH 2023a, 2023b, 2023c). Underinvestments during periods of relative global stability are associated with worse outcomes in the face of acute crises like pandemics and conflicts, as the ecosystem has limited capacities to quickly surge the needed funds to address them (without addressing the serious need for capacity-building to appropriately predict, prepare, and respond to future crises). Similarly, the latest pandemic pressured shifting financing from capacity building in global public health such as with UHC and DAH to "pandemic preparedness and response" (Brown et al. 2022).

2.2 Overview of health artificial intelligence + financing

2.2.1 Artificial intelligence essentials

Now that we have covered an overview of global public health financing, let us pivot to how AI is transforming it (beginning with a more detailed overview of what AI is and its derivative health AI). The 20th-century British mathematician, Alan Turing, is credited with inventing not only computer science but also the modern computer (Van Duin and Bakhshi 2017; IBM 2023a; Monlezun 2023; Watson 2012). This includes the first programmable digital computer, the Bombe, which broke the Nazi's Enigma encryption device during World War II. It in turn set the stage for his creation of "artificial intelligence" (as intelligent computers) when he proposed and attempted to answer the landmark question "can machine think?" detailed in his seminal 1950 paper on the "Turing test" or "imitation game" published in *Computing Machinery and Intelligence*. He articulated the now-canonical definition of AI as "the science and engineering of making intelligent machines, especially intelligent computer programs." AI since has largely been algorithms or step-by-step instructions that human data scientists and engineers create. They allow computers to subsequently automate decision-making to perform tasks that approximate, match, and in some cases, even exceed human intelligence. "Intelligence" typically denotes in subsequent similar definitions the tasks of sensing (using typically large datasets or Big Data), reasoning (based on the data to identify patterns, associations, causes, and effects), engaging (solving problems by determining how to achieve a certain effect with a particular action), and learning (doing the abovementioned cyclical processes progressively better based on iterative improvements more likely to generate the desired outcomes).

In its current form, AI can be understood from the different classes of its different types, to expand on the introduction of them in Chapter 1 (IBM 2023a; Van Duin and Bakhshi 2017; Monlezun 2023).

2.2.1.1 Spectrum types

AI exists on a spectrum between weak and narrow AI (artificial *narrow* intelligence [ANI]) and strong or broad AI (artificial *general* intelligence [AGI]). The former is the most popular version now as it is designed and deployed to do specific tasks like autonomous vehicle driving, IBM Watson, Amazon's Alexa, and Apple's Siri. The latter is the ultimate goal of AI—a self-aware machine that can think and learn tasks on its own, on par with humans (and even exceed us when it reaches the theoretical highest level of AGI, namely artificial super intelligence or simply "superintelligence"). The first AI that potentially broke out of narrow AI into its "twilight zone" to become "transitional AI"—but not yet achieve the level of AGI—was OpenAI's 2020 GPT-3 language model (Grossman 2020). This natural language processing (NLP) performed numerous tasks without explicit training, from creating its own computer code to math calculations, to language translations, and to convincing narratives, using its 175 billion parameters (or model variables). The progress toward AGI is hypothesized to be realized once the AI parameters reach 1 trillion, closer to the number of our human brain's synapses (or number of connections between nerve cells or neurons). Although there is still a sizeable gap, GPT-3 surged at a greater-than 10-fold parameter increase from its predecessor a year prior. It serves as likely the largest artificial neural network (ANN; and AI algorithm more broadly) and the underlying AI program for its widely popular generative AI web app of ChatGPT (which triggered a multibillion dollar bonanza R&D race among the US technology companies and the Chinese military playing catchup in 2023 to the Microsoft bankrolled OpenAI firm that produced it).

2.2.1.2 Learning types

Within ANI, the primary types are defined by their computational scope or how they adapt to data including machine learning (ML), NLP, ANN, and deep learning (DL; IBM 2023b). Picture ML as a big bucket in which the smaller bucket of ANN exists and DL is an even smaller bucket within it (leaving NLP as a parallel brand of similar buckets but focused on language rather than other data types). NLP is ML and/or DL applied to computer understanding and/or generation of written and spoken language, like asking your smartphone to give you directions to work (IBM 2023c). ML uses more structured and labeled data along with more detailed instructions for identifying, learning, and predicting based on the data patterns. Conversely, DL uses less structured and labeled data with less detailed instructions for doing the abovesaid tasks. ANNs are modeled off the human brain (with its nerve cells or neurons connected by synapses) and is a precursor to DL (differentiated by DL having more than three layers). ANNs characterize a series of relationships among data points segmented by an input layer of nodes (or points or neurons) and an output layer which together form the "bread" that sandwich the "meat" of one or more hidden layers. Each node is like a discrete linear regression model, a traditional statistical formula or model. It predicts a dependent variable or outcome based on (an) independent variable(s) by fitting a straight line from one to the other, while minimizing the difference between the predicted and actual values of each variable.

2.2.1.3 Process types

Within supervised ML as the major workhorse of modern AI, the four types of AI understood as a process include the sequential stages of producing model results. Raw data is first cleaned (i.e., making numbers meaningful by linking numbers with names and grouping such variables as continuous data [like blood pressure] or categorical data [like the presence or absence of hypertension], while also excluding erroneous values as applicable). The processed data is then typically split into a larger training and smaller test subdata sets (with the AI model trained on the former and tested on the latter for accuracy through multiple iterations to refine its performance accurately predicting outputs based on inputs). Model predictions are produced and then the AI model optimized through multiple iterations for retraining until it reliably produces the desired results.

2.2.1.4 Algorithm types

Within ML, there are supervised, unsupervised, semisupervised, and reinforcement algorithms distinguished by their type of data processing and training. Supervised learning uses labeled datasets with manual human interventions to adjust its weights (like the beta coefficients in traditional statistics' regression) representing the strength of input and their output variables' associations (or how well input variables predict output or outcome variables). This process is meant to avoid overfitting (producing a model that is overly complex and includes irrelevant or "noisy" information, therefore predicting the trained data perfectly but unable to generalize to new data) and underfitting (producing a model that is overly simple and includes very little relevant information and so unable to predict trained data sufficiently). Overfitting is signaled by low error rates (percentage of inaccurate prediction) and high variance (variability of models' predictions particularly on new data). Underfitting is signaled by a high bias (difference between the correct predicted value and the model's average prediction) and low variance. Linear regression (predicting continuous numerical variables), logistic regression (predicting categorical variables), decision trees (predicting either type of outcome by predictors represented as linked sequences of binary decisions or options shaped like a tree), and random forests (predicting either type but using multiple decision trees) are examples of supervised learning. Unsupervised learning uses unlabeled datasets without human intervention like ANNs to find patterns or associations among data points. Examples include ANNs (noted earlier) and clustering (grouping variables by patterns of association). Semisupervised learning falls in between the abovementioned two types generally using smaller labeled datasets from larger unlabeled datasets, often when labeling more of the original data is too expensive or not feasible otherwise. Reinforcement learning is in a sense parallel to unsupervised learning, but it is trained using a stream of data rather than a sample dataset to learn through trial and error.

2.2.1.5 Adoption types

AI can finally be classified according to its degree of organizational adoption as either discrete or mature. The former is where most organizations are as they use AI for specific tasks they typically want to automate to solve specific problems, often to make human operators more efficient. The latter is where the most efficient organizations are as they embed an organization or enterprise-wide AI strategy, data infrastructure, and workflow to sync human and AI tasks for synergistic boosts in faster results with less resources.

2.2.1.6 Health artificial intelligence

This term refers broadly to AI applied to health, particularly its applications separately in healthcare systems (more developed) and public health agencies (less developed) and the growing integration of both in the global health ecosystem (even less developed, but with the greatest potential for efficiency and equity advancing global well-being as the prerequisite for the world's political stability and economic prosperity irrespective of countries' ideological blocs; Monlezun 2023). The abovementioned work provided the first known comprehensive ecosystem book on healthcare AI; this one now provides the first known one for global public health AI.

2.2.1.6.1 Health finance artificial intelligence state of the art: research overview
The WHO's 2023 rapid literature review provides a concise summary of the last 20 years of AI research for health financing defining its current state of the art (with particular focus on global public health's UHC objective; WHO, 2023d). Of the over 2 million AI studies in that timeframe, there were only 38 such studies for health AI financing. This significantly hampers identifying best practices and standards for this topic, despite the fundamental need outlined earlier for enhanced equitable efficiency to improve ecosystem performance. Among the 38 studies, the predominant AI technique use domains were ML for claims and fraud management (34%), health expenditure prediction (24%), targeted household policies (16%), risks adjustment and selection scoring (13%), personalized benefit packages (8%), and health coverage impact on service utilization (5%). These domains, mapped to the abovementioned core functions for health finance, serve the UHC's intermediate objectives (efficiency, equity, and transparency) for its final objectives: proportionality (utilization according to need), quality, and protection (financially). In these empirical analyses, AI generally improved the intermediate objectives compared to traditional statistical techniques, including by identifying higher than expected service utilizers and fraudulent claims and generating cost savings through early appropriate action (i.e., respectively tailoring more effective preventive services for higher utilizers and blocking fraudulent claims). Yet there were several challenges and disadvantages noted from AI in health financing, particularly in its data and

application. Nearly 70% of the studies were from Asian and US data sources, and only 3% were from LICs, thus limiting the generalizability of the results to populations outside these regions. In addition, the data was largely restricted to private or commercial healthcare insurance, reflecting significant underinvestment in AI for the vast majority of financing schemes for populations globally (publicly or noncommercially insured) and for global public health. Finally, the ML technique limits its broader application (as the models have less utility the more other datasets vary from the ones they were trained on, especially given the income and geographic limitations noted earlier), as does the likelihood that its primary advantage of more efficient analyses lends itself to funders restricting payment for services rather than finding better ways to fund more care for more of the population.

2.2.1.6.2 Emerging trends in health finance artificial intelligence

The landmark 2019 USAID report on global health AI introduced in the Chapter 1 outlined the key emerging trends in health finance AI in terms of use cases informing strategic best practices (USAID 2019). It built on the WHO strategy for primary care–focused UHC by advancing its actionability through integrating best practices from private industry. These include standardizing value assessment frameworks (to identify the most promising AI programs by their health benefit of quality [including service experience] and access [according to each unit of cost], in addition to financial return on investment [ROI]), agile financing of AI R&D (identifying, optimizing, and rapid scaling of effective programs using the abovementioned framework across diverse partners), competitive investment process (using the above to fund pilot cases for scale-up nationwide or worldwide), blended public–private funding sources (underwriting the above to keep costs contained and value maximized), strategic purchasing (particularly for LMICs governments consistent with their long-term priorities, constraints, and procurement processes), and particularly relevant for this book, "ecosystem capacity for ongoing AI use at scale" (leveraging the comparative advantages of the diverse public and private partners from government to industry, to intergovernment, and to nonprofit organizations). The report highlights the use cases informing these strategic recommendations by emphasizing the developments that appears to have the highest value-add (best health improvements for lowest affordable cost): AI-enabled population health, virtual health assistance (for providers and patients), and physician clinical decision support tools, which appear to have the biggest bang for the global public health buck thus far. Yet the key barriers to effective health financing and its related scale-up of success cases in AI-enabled global public health, particularly for LMICs, appear to remain now and for the foreseeable future to be data and algorithm challenges. These are especially focused on interoperability (and the derivative issues of ethics, ownership, quality, availability, privacy, trust, regulation, and standards), business model sustainability, and integration with health systems and local public health agencies.

A year after this report, the COVID-19 pandemic's emergence provided a potent example of the emerging trends in health finance AI highlighted by the WHO and USAID. The US government's Operation Warp Speed was a bright bipartisan spot amid the otherwise widely recognized hyperpolarizing politicization of the COVID-19 pandemic. This program was heralded by the *New England Journal of Medicine* (NEJM) as a "miraculous" "new breed of public−private partnerships" that produced two of the fastest, safest, and most effective commercially made vaccines (including using mRNA and for COVID-19 specifically) in the record time of 8 months—compared to the typical process of up 10 to 15 years (Shulkin 2021). The government provided the concrete measurable strategic outcome (a safe, effective, and mass produced and distributed COVID-19 vaccine), sizeable $18 billion investment (set as an appropriate tax payer ROI given the projected $8 trillion pandemic cost to the US economy), "integrated command structure" (streamlining rapid decision-making and collective accountability), agile parallel development process (i.e., allowing concurrent rather than slower sequential safety then efficacy testing), and cooperative competition (in which multiple private biotechnology companies deployed their scientific and technological expertise using vaccine candidates with diverse mechanisms of action to increase the likelihood of success). One of the two successful candidates was from the AI-driven Moderna company based outside of Harvard University which produced the first vaccine design, just 48 hours from its genetic sequence being published online by the Chinese virologist, Zhang Yongzhen (who did so reportedly in violation of the Chinese government's publication ban; Cyranoski 2020; Ransbotham and Khodabandeh 2021; Neilson et al. 2020). Significant justified critique was levied against its limited initial global public health impact. By design it was narrowly focused on the US public health, despite the pragmatic reality (that an unmitigated global pandemic will inevitably plague even boosted national viral defenses) and the ethical reality (of unaddressed global inequities in access to safe and effective vaccines particularly for LMICs). Yet Operation Warp Speed does provide a significant success case in how efficient funding for R&D with scale-up, particularly of AI-accelerated health products for modern crises, can be translated for global public health by applying this national paradigm for an international collaboration.Global public health public−private partnerships have been proliferating to advance successful and scalable AI-enabled and ecosystem-based use cases including with the WHO, Gates Foundation, and the private industry. The WHO and the global private venture firm, OurCrowd, launched the $200 million Global Health Equity Fund in 2021 as a "financial-first impact venture capital investment fund, focusing on breakthrough technology solutions that can impact healthcare globally," with particular focus on reducing LMIC disparities (Press 2022). The WHO leveraged its global public health experience and collaboration capacity while OurCrowd provided its data platform and finance experience to identify and fund the most promising health products for global health benefit (channeling $1.9 billion commitments across its 215,000 members, 195 countries, and 347 portfolio companies). Its ecosystem understanding (targeting traditional disease-specific and more recent broader social determinants of health including energy and food) and structure (uniting government, industry, health, and community partners) provide a promising way to bridge the current gap between countries' health needs and their domestic revenue generation paired with foreign aid. The US-based Gates Foundation first-in-class ecosystem partnership with the Chinese government, universities, and companies provides another key example of more innovative and agile health financing, particularly on AI-enabled drug discovery, testing, and deployment (Gates 2023; Tsinghua 2023). Only 10% of international spending on drug R&D focuses on the primary infectious diseases facing LMICs, though they shoulder 90% of the disease burden. Beijing and Tsinghua University's Global Health Drug Discovery Institute previously provided its open-access AI drug discovery and Big Data platform to allow researchers internationally to accelerate COVID-19 therapeutics. Its Gates partnership expanded the financing and operational infrastructure to focus on TB and malarial interventions for LMICs. Finally, the Merck Global Health Innovation Fund demonstrates a private industry–driven global public health finance model as an "evolving corporate healthcare venture capital" guided by its "healthcare ecosystem strategy" (Merck 2023). It deploys its internal agile R&D, strategic empathy-based design thinking (understanding the needs and aversions of the consumer and thus the desired results for them from the products reverse engineered to produce them), outcomes-driven investment selection, and global value supply chains and ecosystem partners. Doing so, it amassed over $500 million across 60 investments in innovative products for underserved regions globally to fill local healthcare systems and public health agencies' otherwise overstretched financing and capacity gaps. The abovementioned emerging trends therefore demonstrate how the WHO may articulate the grand financing strategy for the global public health ecosystem of primary care–focused UHC, and the abovementioned private–public partnerships (government driven as with the United States and Chinese governments, or intergovernment and nonprofit institutions as with the WHO and Gates Foundation, or private industry–driven as with Merck) may show the operationalizable strategy for how to realize that vision on the ground.

2.3   Emblematic artificial intelligence use cases in the global public health ecosystem

Within the context of the abovementioned emerging trends in the global public health ecosystem, we can now analyze AI use cases that exemplify key elements in how stakeholders are advancing equity, integration, and resilience in effective and efficient financing.

2.3.1 Translational artificial intelligence public–private partnerships

Annual health funding for AI-enabled digital health startups in the United States alone exploded by over 7600% to $10 billion annually by 2021 from a decade prior, with 70% of the AI-enabled devices approved by the US Food and Drug Administration being in radiology followed by 12% in cardiology (Leonard and Reader 2022). The significant private-sector competition for the state-of-the-art AI and its workforce is beginning to translate as noted earlier into the diffusion of this technological innovation for global health benefit, but without the higher R&D costs. The abovementioned emblematic examples of public–private partnerships are opening more of the AI final products for deployment and optimization in national healthcare systems with their interlinked public health agencies worldwide, particularly with dozens of private firms and academic institutions extending their AI products (especially in population health management and virtual health assistance to extend limited health workforces; USAID 2019).

2.3.2 Artificial intelligence—enabled finance tracking

The surge in private investments in health AI and its organic spillover and strategic expansion into global public health requires better coordination within its ecosystem. To avoid a chaotic traffic jam of global public health funding (oscillating between redundancy and irrelevance, including even imperial), Duke University partnered with Berlin's Open Consultants to generate random forest supervised AI/ML and NLP models to accurately, rapidly, and automatically categorize 10,534 DAH financing projects according to the established global common goods for health framework (Dixit et al. 2022). This appears to serve as the first instance of automatic AI tracking of global public health funding. Thus it enables international coordination across diverse stakeholders to identify financing gaps and redundancy, in turn informing more efficient resource allocation that better responds to the self-identified essential health services and public health needs of local communities.

2.3.3 "Research economies of scale"—artificial intelligence—augmented embedded adaptive clinical and public health trials

Getting to proven health products faster can make them significantly cheaper and fairer and so their populations healthier. This larger health trend additionally has been playing out in the global public health ecosystem which witnessed a historic explosion in translation research innovation during the first 2 years of the COVID-19 pandemic. The REMAP-CAP multicenter clinical trial demonstrated improved survival among critically sick patients with the virus using a new Bayesian inference model (rather than the traditional frequentist statistical approach) with reinforcement learning to achieve more rapid, accurate, and personalized results through preferential, perpetual, response-adaptive randomization of multiple patient subgroups to multiple intervention arms (Yoon et al. 2022; ATTACC Investigators et al. 2021). A typical randomized clinical trial features one group randomized to receive an intervention whose outcomes are then compared to another group randomized as the control to the standard treatment. The upshot is this gold standard of health research generally allows robust conclusions about any difference in outcomes to be attributed to the intervention as the cause. The (significant) downsides are that such trials are historically and often prohibitively slow, expensive, and uninformative (with results generalizable to a small group of patients with limited variability of the treatment, i.e., only to that dosage tested in the trial). Many fail to show what is the best treatment for patients at the most precise subgroup possible enabling appropriate treatment at the individual level. Instead, REMAP-CAP represents a new AI-enabled generation of translational health research. Its innovative design enabled the trial to inform unprecedented response to a multifaceted health crisis, including a pandemic gripping the world's national healthcare systems and public health agencies, bound by the urgent need to identify and deploy affordable evidence-based treatments with limited resources. This new platform trial design allowed much more flexible and wide-ranging patient enrollment across more clinical sites (including in traditionally underrepresented communities) embedded in existing clinical care. Patients were matched faster and more precisely to the adaptive treatment that was most likely to benefit them. These results then fed back into the adaptive randomization scheme to guide each sequential enrolled patient so the best data can be used closer to real time (rather than patients and populations having to wait the historic multi-year mandatory period between a fixed traditional clinical trial's commencement and its conclusion). Far from being a fringe research theory, the world's most prestigious and cited medical journal, NEJM, published its findings similar to the related platform trial, the UK-based RECOVERY, which showed a largely affordable treatment for COVID-19 (namely the oral steroid, dexamethasone) was able to reduce its mortality (RECOVERY Collaborative Group et al. 2021). Rather than newer intravenous drugs costing thousands of dollars per patient or protracted population-wide lockdowns seemingly costing LMICs more lives and billions than they saved (according to World Bank and OECD analyses), such AI-informed innovative translational research may provide a powerful new evidence-based paradigm for the global public health ecosystem (Ma et al. 2021; Eyawo et al. 2021). Accordingly, distributing the otherwise often prohibitive research costs across multiple sites in this trial design increased the translational research capacity for including lower income and traditionally underrepresented communities. It also facilitated more rapid dissemination of results for communities in which the trials were not conducted but the populations are similar, achieving "research economies of scale."

2.3.4 Cost savings

The US National Bureau of Economic Research released their 2023 report demonstrating that nationwide application of existing AI health technologies is projected to reduce US healthcare spending (as the highest globally) by up to 10%, or $360 billion annually (Sahni et al. 2023). These domains (and use cases) include AI-enabled care continuity (with patient transfers and referral), value-based care (matching resources with risk and need stratification), network insights (boosting provider quality), clinical operations (optimizing practice flow and supply chains), clinical analytics (designing care pathways and seamless clinical decision supports), safety and quality (reducing readmissions, errors, and regulatory non-compliance), compensation (streamlining coding, claim, and denial management), and organizational management (of talent, governance, and profit optimization). This notable finding on collective AI use cases suggests how national health ecosystems—networking healthcare systems and public health agencies—can deploy current health AI, but without the high R&D costs for new cutting-edge technologies, to improve global health financing through greater organizational efficiencies. This echoes the larger sector consensus that AI's primary economic benefit is lowering accurate prediction costs (Agrawal et al. 2018). Our societal, economic, and global public health ecosystems have to make decisions with limited information that can undermine effective long-term strategy and short-term operations. AI enables more rapid, accurate, and (often self-) improving predictions to allow smarter decisions that over time generally allow better performance, iteratively driving smarter strategy, operations, and predictions.

2.3.5 Embedded value-based funding models

The UK NHS (National Health Service) Wales embedded a value-orientated capitation-based financing infrastructure integrated with its data infrastructure to enable real-time population health management for value-based care that allocates resources based on population need formulas (WEC, 2023a). Sicker communities get more cost-efficient resources to narrow the gap with their healthier peers. Both at the patient-provider and community-healthcare system levels, performance is rewarded financially based on who provides greater value (highest quality for lowest cost). Across multiple communities, payment is linked to outcomes to incentivize improved quality, affordability, and appropriateness (by resource utilization based on need) of essential health services.

2.3.6 Standardized analytics for global public health investments

DAH funds for global public health tripled from 2000 to 2020 up to $54.8 billion (increased by 36% from just the previous year), with nearly all coming from Western governments and majority-controlled institutions (WEC, 2023b). Yet there is no international consensus on transparent analytic frameworks to inform which investments are made. This critical problem is worsened by the rapid development of rising geopolitical blocs threatening the AI-enabled global public health products and services shared among them (whose technical complexity even further complicates nontechnical audiences deciding on what to fund). The "Impact Investment Matrix" translates best practices in private industry's R&D process (maximizing cost-efficient value creation and market share or how a stakeholder "owns" a unique niche) into global public health, especially in their public—private partnerships in which major technological players lend their products for health partners to adapt and deploy them. The matrix is additionally designed as a decolonizing product to facilitate more transparent codesign of health products including their AI-enabled ones through "design hygiene." Systematic evaluation seeks to fit these global products to the local needs of communities using them, while scrubbing away historical structural power imbalances. Impact potential (*y*-axis) and needed investment (*x*-axis) are therefore mapped in this matrix to triage, identify, and select the most promising investments.

2.3.7 Artificial intelligence—automated integration of cost, equity, and causal inference

The first nationally representative AI (DL and ML-based) model integrating clinical, equity, and cost analyses—the AI-driven Computational Ethics and policy analysis—demonstrated that in the United States alone $2.2 billion could be annually saved reducing racial inequities while saving hundreds of more lives through more targeted utilization of cardiac catheterization following cardiac arrest among patients with cancer (Monlezun et al. 2022). This provides a novel use case for the global public health ecosystem, particularly given how cardiac arrest is one of the most fatal and expensive medical complications often of undermanaged chronic comorbidities (which cost-efficient public health interventions including healthy diet, exercise, and risk factor avoidance can otherwise significantly prevent, reduce, and mitigate). By building the AI model using a nationally representative dataset using ICD (International Classification of Diseases)-10 codes, it demonstrates how it can be embedded in electronic health records (EHRs) to help rapidly and accurately risk stratify patient subgroups (who likely will have the greatest clinical benefit individually) and the local healthcare system (saving resource intensive interventions for them). AI links population health and public health through an automated causal clinical, ethical, and cost analyses in a seamless framework. It runs optimally through real-time clinical care with EHR-enabled health communities, but still effectively in lower income communities without EHRs by leveraging the model predictors refined through local use worldwide.

2.3.8 Resilient revenue cycles

AI is further assisting local healthcare systems to more efficiently, affordably, and accurately capture appropriate charges for health services (allowing more resilient local revenue cycles for self-funding of their essential health and public health services, thus making UHC more attainable, substantive, and sustainable; Montroy and Rakes 2022). Even in the US national health ecosystem, which has among the world's most complex and changing legal, regulatory, and financial infrastructures, AI has numerous use cases optimizing eligibility and benefit verification (with 72% of AI-enabled healthcare systems confirming payor coverage for health services), complete provider records, appropriate charge capture for compensation (through NLP grabbing ICD-10 and current procedural terminology codes from provider documentation with less and even no human intervention), preventing denials (through confirming accurate claims prior to systems submitting them to payors), and extending care to the uninsured (through better matching of financial aid to need).

These emblematic use cases therefore flesh out the emerging finance trends in the AI transformation of the global public health ecosystem. Within it, there is a growing critical mass consensus on a unifying actionable strategy of primary care–based UHC. This is operationalized through more efficient data, finance, and practical integration particularly through public–private partnerships. They leverage the latest AI, profitability, and organizational innovations for local healthcare systems and public health agencies backed by their supportive national governments and global institutions. We discussed earlier how the COVID-19 pandemic highlighted the gaps in the ecosystem's financing, echoing the overarching strategic gaps in how the ecosystem planned to realize its noble and ambitious goal of equitably optimizing global well-being. To get more value out of each dollar in the global public health ecosystem, there are concrete signals that the major influential power players (particularly the US and Western governments, nonprofit organizations, and intergovernment organizations) are increasingly becoming more collaborative and creative with other value blocs and ecosystem partners to advance greater integration of stakeholders (particularly private–public partnerships) and infrastructure (through more interoperable data and interrelated financing), thus optimizing the impact of efficient and equitable resource allocation throughout the ecosystem. Such efforts are meant to ultimately boost the resilience of the global public health ecosystem's financing currently. This is especially true for essential health services and public health needs, both through population health and projected future crises spanning pandemics, famines, and conflicts (potentially complicated and in some ways even worsened by AI and related disruptive technologies impacting global supply chains).

This chapter's overview of these trends, use cases, and basics in health AI sets the stage for us to explore in Chapter 3 the AI-enabled integral sustainable development in the global public health ecosystem, including how political economic forces are placing additional structural pressures on financing advancements to move toward more proactive improvements in the adaptive ecosystem design. We will thus explore the recurrent theme of how the future's emergent vision of the AI-empowered global public health ecosystem entails a clearer focus on its ultimate goal—global well-being, based on the common good of the global human family, bounded by scientific, ethical, pragmatic, and technical demands to protect both human dignity and security, within the societal constraints of navigating the cooperative but also competing interests of the main international power brokers. And through this sharper focus, we can reverse engineer the ecosystem's design that begins with the most efficient, equitable, and so transparent and effective financing mechanisms to achieve those outcomes. As we get through more of the basic theory and frameworks, we will be able to focus on the more concrete details of the different perspectives of the ecosystem with each of the upcoming chapters. But to achieve those outcomes, we need to move to Chapter 3 to understand who is the subject and object of the outcomes we are seeking to optimize with AI-enabled global public health, namely the human person. Chapter 1 introduced how the 2023 book, *Thinking Healthcare System*, provided to be the first comprehensive book on AI-enabled healthcare (Monlezun 2023). We will continue with Chapter 3 to build up to the case how this is the first comprehensive book on the parallel AI-enabled global public health ecosystem by integrating this novel three-dimensional vision of the scientific, ethical, and societal perspectives that explains how global public health actually works today and how to make it work better together in our AI tomorrow.

References

Agrawal, A., Gans, J., and A. Goldfarb. 2018. *Prediction Machines: The Simple Economics of Artificial Intelligence.* Boston, MA: Harvard Business Review Press.

ATTACC InvestigatorsACTIV-4a InvestigatorsREMAP-CAP InvestigatorsLawler, P.R., and E.C. Goligher, et al., 2021. "Therapeutic Anticoagulation With Heparin in Noncritically Ill Patients With COVID-19." *The New England Journal of Medicine* 385 (9): 790–802.

Bartels, J. 2022. "Health Leaders Discuss Mechanisms and Coordination Of Global Health Governance and Finance." Sustainable Development Solutions Network.

Brown, G.W., B. Tacheva, M. Shahid, N. Rhodes, and M. Schäferhoff. 2022. "Global Health Financing After COVID-19 and the New Pandemic Fund."

Cyranoski, D. 2020. "Nature's Ten People Who Helped Shape Science in 2020: Zhang Yongzhen."

Dixit, S., Mao, W., McDade, K.K., Schäferhoff, M., Ogbuoji, O., and G. Yamey. 2022. "Tracking Financing for Global Common Goods for Health: A Machine Learning Approach Using Natural Language Processing

Techniques." *Frontiers in Public Health* 10, http://journal.frontiersin.org/journal/public-health/section/public-health-education-and-promotion#archive. https://doi.org/10.3389/fpubh.2022.1031147.

Eyawo, O., Viens, A.M., and U.C. Ugoji. 2021. "Lockdowns and Low- and Middle-Income Countries: Building a Feasible, Effective, and Ethical COVID-19 Response Strategy." *Globalization and Health* 17 (1)13.

Gates. 2023. "Creating an Innovative Collaborative Model for Global Health Drug Discovery." Bill & Melinda Gates Foundation. Accessed March 25, 2023. https://www.gatesfoundation.org/our-work/places/china/creating-an-innovative-collaboration-model-for-global-health-drug-discovery.

GBDH Health Financing Collaborator Network. 2019. "Past, Present, and Future of Global Health Financing: A Review of Development Assistance, Government, Out-of-Pocket, and Other Private Spending on Health for 195 Countries, 1995–2050." *Lancet* 393 (10187): 2233–2260.

GBDH. 2023a. "Global Investments in Pandemic Preparedness and COVID-19: Development Assistance and Domestic Spending on Health Between 1990 and 2026." *The Lancet Global Health* 11 (3): e385–e413.

GBDH. 2023b. "AI vs. Machine Learning vs. Deep Learning vs. Neural Networks: What's the Difference?" IBM. Accessed March 17, 2023. https://www.ibm.com/cloud/blog/ai-vs-machine-learning-vs-deep-learning-vs-neural-networks.

GBDH. 2023c. "What is Natural Language Processing?" IBM. Accessed March 17, 2023. https://www.ibm.com/topics/natural-language-processing.

Grossman, G. 2020. "We're Entering the AI Twilight Zone Between Narrow and General AI."

IBM, 2023a. What is artificial intelligence? IBM. https://www.ibm.com/topics/artificial-intelligence (accessed 14 March 2023).

IBM, 2023b. AI vs. machine learning vs. deep learning vs. neural networks: What's the difference? IBM. https://www.ibm.com/cloud/blog/ai-vs-machine-learning-vs-deep-learning-vs-neural-networks (accessed 17 March 2023).

IBM, 2023c. What is natural language processing? IBM. https://www.ibm.com/topics/natural-language-processing (accessed 17 March 2023).

KFF. 2023. "Breaking Down the U.S. Global Health Budget by Program Area." Kaiser Family Foundation. Accessed March 13, 2023. https://www.kff.org/global-health-policy/fact-sheet/breaking-down-the-u-s-global-health-budget-by-program-area/.

Leonard, B., and R. Reader. 2022. "Artificial Intelligence was Supposed to Transform Health Care."

Ma, L., G. Shapira, D. de Walque, Q.T. Do, J. Friedman, and A.A. Levchenko. 2021. "The Intergenerational Mortality Tradeoff of COVID-19 Lockdown Policies." *SSRN*. https://www.ssrn.com/index.cfm/en/.

Merck. 2023. "Leadership in Digital Health Investment."

Monlezun, D.J., Sinyavskiy, O., Peters, N., Steigner, L., Aksamit, T., Girault, M.I., Garcia, A., Gallagher, C., and C. Iliescu. 2022. "Artificial Intelligence-Augmented Propensity Score, Cost Effectiveness and Computational Ethical Analysis of Cardiac Arrest and Active Cancer with Novel Mortality Predictive Score." *Medicina* 58 (8): https://doi.org/10.3390/medicina58081039.

Monlezun, D.J. 2023. *The Thinking Healthcare System: Artificial Intelligence and Human Equity*. United States: Elsevier, pp. 1–309. https://www.sciencedirect.com/book/9780443189067, https://doi.org/10.1016/C2022-0-00639-5.

Montroy, T., and G. Rakes. 2022. "What is AI, and How Can It Benefit the Healthcare Revenue Cycle?" *Journal of the American Health Information Management Association*. Accessed March 26, 2023. https://journal.ahima.org/page/what-is-ai-and-how-can-it-benefit-the-healthcare-revenue-cycle.

Neilson, S., A. Dunn, and A. Bendix. 2020. "Moderna's Groundbreaking Coronavirus Vaccine was Designed in Just 2 Days." Business Insider. Accessed March 25, 2023. https://www.businessinsider.com/moderna-designed-coronavirus-vaccine-in-2-days-2020-11.

NIH. 2023. "Analysis Shows Return on Investment for Global Health R&D." National Institutes of Health Fogarty International Center. Accessed March 14, 2023. https://www.fic.nih.gov/News/GlobalHealthMatters/january-february-2017/Pages/roi-global-health-randd.aspx.

Press, G. 2022. "The WHO Foundation and OurCrowd Launch $200 Million Global Health Equity Fund."

Ransbotham, S., and S. Khodabandeh. 2021. "AI and the COVID-19 Vaccine: Moderna's Dave Johnson." MIT Sloan Management Review.

RECOVERY Collaborative GroupHorby, P., Lim, W.S., Emberson, J.R., Mafham, M., and J.L. Bell, et al., 2021. "Dexamethasone in Hospitalized Patients With COVID-19." *The New England Journal of Medicine* 384 (8): 693−704.

Sachs, J.D., Karim, S.S.A., Aknin, L., Allen, J., Brosbøl, K., Colombo, F., and G.C. Barron, et al., 2022. "The Lancet Commission on Lessons for the Future from the COVID-19 Pandemic." *The Lancet* 400 (10359): 1224−1280. https://doi.org/10.1016/S0140-6736(22)01585-9, http://www.journals.elsevier.com/the-lancet/.

Sahni, N., Stein, G., Zemmel, R., and D.M. Cutler. 2023. "The Potential Impact of Artificial Intelligence on Healthcare Spending." *SSRN Electronic Journal* https//doi.org/10.2139/ssrn.4334926.

Shulkin, D. 2021. "What Health Care Can Learn from Operation Warp Speed." *New England Journal of Medicine Catalyst* https://doi.org/10.1056/CAT.21.0001.

Tsinghua. 2023. "Global Health Drug Discovery Institute and School of Pharmaceutical Sciences, Tsinghua University Join Forces to Provide Drug Discovery Capabilities." Tsinghua University. Accessed March 26, 2023. https://www.tsinghua.edu.cn/en/info/1399/9796.htm.

USAID. 2019. "Artificial Intelligence in Global Health: Defining a Collective Path Forward." United States Agency for International Development. Accessed February 18, 2023. https://www.usaid.gov/cii/ai-in-global-health.

Van Duin, S., and N. Bakhshi. 2017. "Artificial Intelligence Defined."

Watson, I. 2012. "The Universal Machine: From the Dawn of Computing to Digital Consciousness." http://doi.org/10.1007/978-3-642-28102-0.

WEC, 2023a. Global health and healthcare strategic outlook: Shaping the future of health and healthcare. World Economic Forum. https://www3.weforum.org/docs/WEF_Global_Health_and_Healthcare_Strategic_Outlook_2023.pdf (accessed: 14 March 2023).

WEC, 2023b. How to boost inclusive investment decision-making in global health. World Economic Forum. https://www.weforum.org/agenda/2022/03/inclusive-transparent-investment-global-health/ (accessed: 14 March 2023).

WHO. 2023a. "Universal Health Coverage."

WHO, 2023b. The Triple Billion targets. World Health Organization. https://www.who.int/data/stories/the-triple-billion-targets-a-visual-summary-of-methods-to-deliver-impact (accessed: 19 March 2023).

WHO, 2023c. Health financing. World Health Organization. https://www.who.int/health-topics/health-financing#tab=tab_1 (accessed: 19 March 2023).

WHO, 2023d. The implications of artificial intelligence and machine learning in health financing for achieving universal health coverage. World Health Organization. https://www.who.int/publications/i/item/9789240064010 (accessed: 19 March 2023).

Yoon, J.H., Pinsky, M.R., and G. Clermont. 2022. "Artificial Intelligence in Critical Care Medicine." *Critical Care* 26 (1)75.

Design part II: Artificial intelligence i(ntegral +) s(ustainable) development

3.1 Development as global public health's future?

As Chapter 1 broadly sketched, modernity moved from its early era of the Industrial Revolution—supercharged competition of European global empires, followed by the late-modern era of the post—World War II (WWII) US-led postcolonial industrialization, democratization, liberalization, and early capitalist globalization. This brings us to our current post—Global Recession and COVID-19 ideological restructuring (according to the democratic West, authoritarian East, and developing South), underlying the global artificial intelligence (AI)-accelerated ecosystem's digital or late globalization. Accordingly, we moved from the first concerted international collaboration on a peaceful and prosperous world order in the mid-1900s (characterized initially by the unipolar US-led West leveraging it to contain the Soviet's communist rise and thus producing public health as foreign diplomacy) to our current multipolar cooperative competition in the early 21st-century period dominated by a shared focus on well-being (championed by global public health and comprised by the global powers technically and financially fueling it). We analyzed in Chapter 1 how politics then economics and now health became the prioritized grand strategic focus in the evolution of the modern world order following WWII. As the world becomes healthier, it generally becomes wealthier and safer (as conflict undermines all three domains, and so my neighbor's well-being as an intrinsic good is also not just practically good for them but also for me and vice versa).

Human and ecological health, justified morally by the common good and pragmatically by the need for collaborative survival, while rooted in human security (connecting health and national security), may generally serve as our common language and world view that can cross even the increasingly sharp though still shifting borders of our nations and communities' ideological and value blocs. But to maximize well-being (individually and at scale internationally), Chapters 1 and 2 have progressively considered how not just the medical but also the societal determinants of health must be considered, addressed, and done so with an increasingly broad ecosystem of partners and stakeholders. They simultaneously affect and are affected by individual and global well-being (trends that are only intensified with greater complexity by the cross-sector disruption of AI-driven digital technologies). And no health framework is better known, used, or impactful as the United Nations (UN) sustainable development goals (SDGs).

The SDGs are our modern world's integrated health-based, equity-orientated, and UN-driven political economic grand strategy for global peace through just and secure prosperity (Morton et al. 2019). They concretely articulate our integrated health determinants in their economic, social, and environmental dimensions. The SDGs can be understood as an ecosystem approach characterized as a comprehensive whole-of-government (WoG) and whole-of-society (WoS) dual-level strategy to achieve global public health at the local level, through synergistic cross-sector international and local partners (Brolan 2022). The COVID-19 pandemic accelerated greater widespread understanding of the fundamental strategic and structural failings in global public health (principally driven by governments and "experts") to address global crises affecting us all. The deepening and broadening interest and investment in SDGs demonstrate what appears to be a global trend, consisting of a sustained institutional transformation of global public health to a whole-of-world (WoW) approach integrating and scaling internationally WoG and WoS approaches. This trend reflects the shifting design of the global public health ecosystem that complements the financing shifts explored in Chapter 2. It comes down to clarifying what we are trying to achieve and how we are going to achieve it (including paying for it). If the *Universal Declaration of Human Rights* (*UDHR*) is the UN's moral vision for humanity, the SDGs are its practical strategy (as this post-COVID period may be the future of AI-electrified global public health). The SDGs also serve as the highest profile development framework, adopted by the world's nations in 2015 as a "shared blueprint for peace and prosperity for people and the planet," consisting of 17 goals spanning 169 constitutive targets and 232 indicators (UN 2015). The top goal just after the eradication of poverty and hunger is global health (to "ensure healthy lives and promote well-being for all at all ages"), including 13 targets and 28 indicators (i.e., maternal−child health, communicable diseases, noncommunicable diseases [NCDs], substance use, and financing particularly universal health coverage [UHC]), with five adjacent goals (i.e., eliminating poverty and hunger, reducing inequality, and boosting marine wildlife sustainability and clean water and sanitation). As our epoch continues with greater AI digitalization and globalization (notwithstanding the ideological and political economic tensions), and political economics increasingly becomes integrated with health and policy (foreign and domestic), health in general and global public health in specific are framed in terms of development. We typically conceptualize health as static and individual (even with global public health as individuals collectively try to influence other individuals). In contrast, development is dynamic and societal. But there are still normative and collaborative aspects to it. Personal well-being requires proper internal functioning of organs and external functioning with others. Development requires sustainable progress within its frameworks moving toward consensus goods it aims to eventually reach. And as we have increasingly considered, AI is our time's great accelerant from A to B. We will therefore analyze how AI is transforming human development within the global public health ecosystem.

3.2 Integral versus sustainable development

We need to begin by clarifying what human development is before we understand how AI is transforming it in the global public health ecosystem. The two dominant modern conceptual frameworks describing it are (1) "integral development" and (2) "sustainable development," which will set the stage for our more comprehensive approach of "integral sustainable development."

3.2.1 Integral development

This concept was formally introduced in the 1960s during the intensifying decolonization process, as India and other nonaligned developing nations chartered a course between the competing democratic West (particularly the United States and Western Europe) and communist East (particularly the Soviet Union and China) (UN 2023a; Paul 1967). When the UN was founded over 20 years before, one of every three people globally lived in colonized territories dependent on colonial powers. As dozens gained their right to self-determination, they had to decide who that "self" was and what development of its people meant for them, sandwiched between the competing ideological-based political economic systems of the West and East. And 20 years before the UN embraced the integral development concept to support this process, it was defined by the Catholic Church's Pope Paul VI in his 1967 *Populorum Progressio*: "Development cannot be limited to mere economic growth. In order to be authentic, it must be complete: integral, that is, it has to promote the good of every man[/person] and of the whole man[/person]." According to this account for justice or right ordering of any society to be achieved (including good health individually and communally), the integral good of the person had to be understood, protected, and included equally across persons. Paul VI invoked Aristotle's classic philosophical description of the human person for this account to advocate states respect the integral development individually (body, mind, and soul including health, education, and flourishing through relationships with self, others, and the divine [or at least being societally and politically allowed in one's self-determinism to choose such]), and communally (avoiding the potential extremes of capitalism's radical individualism on one side and communism's radical collectivism on the other that both reduce and so lose the uniqueness and dignity of the person to either the autonomous agent or faceless crowd, respectively). Integral development rather requires societal protection of the minimum basic goods required for individual and therefore communal flourishing.

The world's nations invoked and adapted this concept in its 1986 General Assembly Resolution 41/128 on the "Declaration on the Right to Development" (UN 1986). It articulated their consensus on 10 development articles by first grounding its primary mission of world peace via global economic and social progress on the foundational concept of integral development of the person:

Recalling…the United Nations and its specialized agencies concerning the integral development of the human being *[emphasis added], economic and social progress and development of all peoples, including those instruments concerning decolonization, the prevention of discrimination, respect for and observance of human rights and fundamental freedoms, the maintenance of international peace and security and the further promotion of friendly relations and co-operation among States in accordance with the Charter...proclaims the following declaration.*

This integral development relies on the assumed underlying Aristotelian realist metaphysics, or objective truth of the human being as a unique person. Their dignity is realized in contributing to the community's common good, which in turn encapsulates and is meant to safeguard through justice the individual's unique good (as each is given what is due to them as each gives themselves to the community). This classical metaphysics is translated into the modern social contract of the UN's global charter that unites the world's diverse states and belief systems. Accordingly, the UN articulated this concept in a different complementary manner:

An inalienable human right [emphasis added] by virtue of which every human person and all peoples are entitled to participate in, contribute to, and enjoy economic, social, cultural and political development, in which all human rights and fundamental freedoms can be fully realized. The human right to development also implies the full realization of the right of peoples to self-determination [emphasis added], which includes, subject to the relevant provisions of both International Covenants on Human Rights, the exercise of their inalienable right to full sovereignty [emphasis added] over all their natural wealth and resources (Article 1).

Integral development (which occurs in community as an operation of and necessity of the common good) articulates the dignity of the person from which rights are derived individually (to goods required for personal flourishing) and so self-determination and sovereignty societally (in which that individual flourishing occurs at scale). The General Assembly thus asserted that the "human person is *the central subject of development* [emphasis added] and should be the active participant and beneficiary of the right to development" (Article 2). It is therefore unjust and should be collectively prohibited from international colonial or domestically repressive powers using persons (and their resources) solely as a means to their ends. All people by reason and consensus have the right and need to this integral development. Therefore, decolonization is development. Yet the General Assembly noted that integral development does not just mean weaker states self-governing by differentiating themselves from prior colonial overseers, but also those states effectively governing to optimize the societal context needed for development: "States have *the primary responsibility* [emphasis added] for the creation of national and international *conditions favourable* [emphasis added] to the realization of the right to development" (Article 3). Paul VI's Aristotelian framing of integral development further echoes in the UN's advocating of the common good. The state must be empowered and act toward securing the goods necessary for their people's full flourishing or development. The UN invoked an early ecosystem framework to assert "sustained action" is a prerequisite for "effective international cooperation" empowering "developing countries" to "foster their comprehensive development" as part of their duty to their people's development (Article 4). Individuals and states have a duty to each other to make the positive realization of their rights possible—not simply considering them in their negative dimension alone as things to be protected from assault but rather also as capacities to be fulfilled.

3.2.2 Sustainable development

The UN developed this concept further supporting "sustained action" on integral development that is "comprehensive" (both internally for states and internationally across them) in its landmark 1987 Report of the World Commission on Environment, or *Our Common Future* (UNWCE 1987). It was known as the Brundtland Report after its Chair, Gro Harlem Brundtland, whom we will return to shortly. The report defined "sustainable development" as "development that meets the needs of the present without compromising the ability of future generations to meet their own needs." It specifies its two constitutive "key concepts" as "needs" (especially the "essential needs of the world's poor" who are least able in society to develop without assistance) and that of "limitations" (placed by "technology and social organization" on "the environment's ability" to satisfy such needs). The 1986 General Assembly Resolution applied Paul VI's integral development to how it can be *strategically* achieved through global collaboration and why ethically it should be (for global peace through collective prosperity and security, achieved by equitable personal development at scale, which is in everyone's pragmatic interests). And the 1987 report showed how it can be *practically* achieved by prioritizing global resources according to present need and future resource shortages. The evolution of the concept of development is fundamentally influential in our emerging AI-enabled global public health ecosystem, especially when we consider the public health pioneer after whom the 1987 report was named. Chapter 1 introduced Brundtland as the 1998−2003 WHO Director-General whose influence can be seen in the earlier sections detailing the embrace by the UN and WHO of the eventual "Sustainable Development Goals," the practical operationalization of integral development through sustainable development, and the central actionable WoW societal strategy of global public health.

3.3 Integral sustainable development of health

From the 1960s' integral development to the 1980s' sustainable development, we are approaching what may be its latest iteration including for the global public health ecosystem as "integral sustainable development." This is seen as with the 2023 UN working group coordinated by the Vatican's Pontifical Academy of Social Sciences under Paul VI's successor, Francis (PASS 2023). Along with Jeffrey Sachs' UN Sustainable Development Solutions Network, Columbia University's Center for Sustainable Development, and the Enel Foundation (the nonprofit charity of the Italian energy corporation, Enel), they launched in February 2023 the first of the workshops planned for 3 years on the "The Fraternal Economy of Integral and Sustainable Development," the first such cross-sector global collaboration on this emergent ecosystem model of integral sustainable development (kicked off in the same year as the WHO's 75th anniversary). The collaboration is meant to respond to the COVID-19 pandemic critique of the SDGs and global public health's purported widespread failure strategically, structurally, and operationally by proposing "the institutional and ethical basis of a new economic framework fit for the challenges of the 21st century." As decolonization gave way to development's evolution, it opened the global discourse, governance, and power sharing to underrepresented voices and their values and belief systems. This expansive inclusion of different cultures informs this emergent international consensus on new paths forward in the same shared direction of global well-being. Within this trend, the UN is seeking to unite integral and sustainable development, and so diverse peoples, beliefs, and perspectives in the abovementioned workshops, through "an actionable synthesis based on scientific findings, philosophical wisdom, and theological teachings" for religiously affiliated and unaffiliated, South and North, East and West.

The vision for this synthesis as a novel foundation for this "new economic framework" begins with such development that "first…promote[s] the happiness (*beatitudo*) of current and future generations" in a way that still "respect[s] the planetary boundaries of Earth's physical systems." Its accompanying concrete mission is "the fulfillment of the…*UDHR*" through its primary actionable strategy of "the SDGs." But this happiness is a more comprehensive description than the influential modern (particularly in the Western) description simply as a passing subjective feeling or experience. It is rather a more multicultural, comprehensive, and ancient description of fulfillment as an abiding state of well-being. This *beatitudo* is framed according to the UN working group as the ultimate objective of integral development which must be made sustainable to be successful. It invokes Paul VI's 1967 formulation in the philosophical tradition of the concept's principal architect, the 13th-century Catholic Aristotelian philosopher, Thomas Aquinas (Müller 2013). Aquinas himself synthesized Christian, Islam, and Jewish thought along with the secular or pagan thought of the earlier Greek philosophers to argue that all of us seek a common ultimate end in all our choices: happiness. Pleasure, power, and prestige are desirable and helpful, but as means to rather than being our final end (without excessive embrace of them that harms us, others, and our pursuit of this fulfillment). We ultimately desire and act toward them and any perceived or real good ultimately to attain integral happiness, our ultimate good that is desired for itself—namely union with goodness itself—like the lover united through love with the beloved. We desire the good and increasingly are united with it the more we know it. A physician for instance becomes an increasingly good physician the more they understand what being a good physician is (i.e., competently and compassionately facilitating patients' progress toward the healthiest state possible) and increasingly becoming it through actions that conform to that standard and destination. Aquinas (along with the abovementioned Abrahamic monotheistic belief systems) describes goodness itself, or the ultimate end or Supreme Good as God in ways that have substantive convergence with Buddhism' *nirvana* or union with the universe and thus liberation from the cycle of rebirth, and Hinduism' *moksha* or union with *Brahman* or God (generally speaking; Juergensmeyr 2006). Aquinas further describes *beatitudo* as a refinement of Aristotle's *eudaimonia*, echoing modern secular conceptions emphasizing self-actualization through self-authenticity, but expanding it in his secular philosophy to describe integral happiness as personal fulfillment. It is achieved by living a truly human life, excelling in the intellectual and moral virtues, chiefly, human reason's ability to know the good and the will's consistent choice of living justly in society with others according to it (Müller 2013). By anchoring collaboration in our deeper and more foundational belief systems and derivative values (religiously affiliated and unaffiliated), such global cooperation in integral sustainable development may therefore mature into the more substantive, enduring, and shared framework of our common good (animating the derivative societal frameworks to achieve it, including the AI-enabled global public health ecosystem).

Why is this postcolonial, multicultural, cross-sector, foundational collaboration important for global public health and its AI transformation? Because the post-COVID global consensus indicates how it is not enough to have ethical principles described in the *UDHR*, or a strategic plan to realize them through the SDG, or the global public health ecosystem using AI to make them efficiently operationalizable. We had all these things. But still millions died, billions were made poorer, and trillions were lost according to this line of widespread critique explored earlier. So as Jeffrey Sachs, one of the leading global figures in sustainable development, moved from the 2022 *Lancet* Commission on COVID described in Chapter 2 to the 2023 UN working group with the Vatican mentioned earlier, we can see a concerted institutional push in the global public health ecosystem to develop a better formula for a better common future and home (by considering more diverse perspectives in this dialogue). An early formulation of this more substantive integral sustainable development framework, particularly focused on global health, emerged in the same year the SDGs were affirmed with Francis' proposal in *Laudato Si'* ("On Care for our Common Home") outlined by the 2015 World Economic Forum for a pluralistic global audience (WEC 2015). It refined Paul VI's early integral development work and broadened the SDGs to consider how the human toll of the global poverty and climate crises arise from (or at least are worsened by) societal, political, and economic inequities perpetuated by developed and developing countries' elites: corruption, short-sightedness, ineptitude, and selfishness not only morally violate the common good but also jeopardize the practical effectiveness of today's capitalism (including its state centralization and even autocratic formulations) that built and dominates our modern world. According to such a critique, elites to maintain power must cultivate durable population support by short-term gains, often at the expense of much larger long-term losses—including worsening societal inequity, polarization, disintegration, and unsustainable ecological damage. Radical attempts to change this societal structure have often ended radically unsuccessfully, including with genocide and wars. But gradual attempts have also been derided broadly as excessively slow and ineffective. Growth, consumerism, and individualism must again be bounded by the common good according to this line of argument. This proposal concludes we have a common home and thus must safeguard our common good within it, without which individual good is compromised and even cancelled for billions globally today and tomorrow.

Like Chapter 3 on financing described with the AI codesign transformation of the global public health ecosystem, the societal and ecological (not just economic) impact must be considered prior to product deployment and organizational changes, rather than reacting to them after launch. Integral sustainable development at scale and through the global ecosystem requires an ethically weighted ecological vision (bounding the short-term goals for new products and innovations within acceptable impact on humanity and our home and future), rather than a narrow economically focused vision on an organization or group's return on investment solely. Francis therefore advocates for an "integral ecology as an ecologically minded, holistic human-centered theory of development. It unites societal, political, economic, and environmental dimensions to frame and address problems for equitable and comprehensive development, personally and globally (sharing the overarching objective of humanity's well-being with the global public health ecosystem, synced with such ecological considerations even further with the ecosystem approach). Francis grounds his approach in and while citing the UN's SDG 2015 consensus and Paul VI's *Populorum* in his *Laudato* to accelerate their realization (Francis 2019). He does so by making sustainable development more inclusive through multicultural integral ecology spanning diverse states, sectors, and belief systems to describe this new integral sustainable development, the ultimate goal of which is the same as global public health, namely the holistic health of all amid our ongoing threats to human security:

> *The challenges are complex and have multiple causes; the response, therefore, must necessarily be complex and well-structured, respectful of the diverse cultural riches of peoples. If we are truly concerned about developing an ecology capable of repairing the damage we have done, no branch of science or form of wisdom should be overlooked, and this includes religions and the languages particular to them...Religions can help us along the path of authentic integral development, which is the new name of peace.*

Integral sustainable development—echoing the abovementioned global institutional and structural ecosystem pivot demonstrated by the UN and WHO—appears to be gaining traction as the emergent strategic framework not only for the global public health ecosystem but also our global human ecosystem more broadly as public health, domestic policy, foreign policy, and corporate governance converge on the common good (Monlezun 2022, 2023). The SDGs and Francis's related framework advance this multicultural normativity in development to invest in families (as the central building block of society in which we develop as persons) at the microlevel, in addition to social cooperation (through inclusion, environmental sustainability, and economic prosperity anchored in national and interdependent human security, while respecting national security needs) at the meso- and macrolevels (Schmieg et al. 2018). The WHO shares a compatible ecosystem vision of integral sustainable development in its 2020–2025 *Global Strategy on Digital Health* (WHO 2021, pp. 7–8, 10). It unites the WHO's Triple Billion target in general and the UN's SDGs in particular by promoting public–private partnerships. Through them stakeholders' more narrow individual interests are orientated to the common good, bounding them by larger societal and ecological concerns to keep us on a sustainable path to it. Not pitting the public against the private sector, nor individual freedom against collective security, nor growth against the environment, this more comprehensive development approach to health at least implicitly replaces radical individualism with personalist communitarianism, destructive consumerism with responsible stewardship, unbridled capitalism with principled free markets, and utopian progress with sustainable development (Monlezun 2022, 2023). The major social determinants of health and those of development overlap: economic, social, and environmental. Thus integral sustainable development may accelerate the design and so the actionable grand strategy of an affordable and accessible global public health ecosystem by uniting local integral (personal-level) development with global sustainable (population-level) development, like the ecosystem unites healthcare (individually) with public health (collectively). An AI algorithm must be mathematically and practically sound before it can be scaled throughout an organization or sector. Similarly, integral sustainable development may provide a theoretically and experientially sound global anthropological vision that allows us to scale health programs, policies, and innovations through this ecosystem for our benefit today, without sacrificing our children's tomorrow, by having an accurate understanding of the persons and personal communities it serves.

3.4 From 20th-century development to 21st-century artificial intelligence × Sustainable Development Goals

Now we can drill down more concretely in how this ecosystem design particularly applies to and is influenced by AI. We introduced earlier how government and corporate interests particularly in the United States—Chinese arms race have driven the majority of AI developments thus far. Yet there is a growing push within the abovementioned overall global focus on the technical development of "socially good AI" or AI for social good (AI4SG). Within this, larger societal well-being is advanced not simply as an effective means to greater power by the abovementioned stakeholders, but as an end unto itself particularly in human and ecological health (Cowls et al. 2021; Monlezun 2023). This trend is powered by AI's technological and ecosystem effects: it generally allows greater efficiency through more rapid, complex, accurate analytics and predictions driving better decisions and innovations, while facilitating greater synergistic collaboration among ecosystem partners, as seen with modernity's globalization accelerating our multisector interconnectedness even amid competing value blocs. Aside from the positive aspects of these trends, their inverse is true for the negative effects: AI can be equally destructive and divisive as its efficiency can be used for effective power grabs, exponentiated through leveraging synergistic ecosystem partners. To amplify the good and avoid the worrying bad, AI4SG enjoys a rising global societal interest and investment.

Yet until recently, it has lacked a clear definition, normative benchmark, and systematic analysis of current best practices and gaps (Cowls et al. 2021; Monlezun 2023). Oxford University's Saïd Business School therefore launched their Initiative on AI4SG as an academic–private partnership (including with Facebook, Google, and Microsoft) and subsequently produced their 2021 *Nature* study to reverse the abovementioned deficits with the first such high-profile integrated proposal. They began by formally defining AI4SG:

The design, development, and deployment of AI systems in ways that help to (i) prevent, mitigate and/or resolve problems adversely affecting human life and/or the wellbeing of the natural world, and/or (ii) enable socially preferable or environmentally sustainable developments, while (iii) not introducing new forms of harm and/or amplifying existing disparities and inequities.

The Oxford team further argues that the optimal global normative benchmark for AI4SG so conceptualized is the UN SDGs. This is because they represent the highest level, longest running, and broadest consensus on an internationally agreed empirical framework to define and evaluate progress toward equitable, socially beneficial collective action that maximizes the greatest well-being for the greatest number—without sacrificing individual good for collective gain (or devolving into irrelevance, relativism, or reductionism). Finally, the Oxford team produced the first global systematic analysis from 2018 to 2020 of AI4SG codified and measured by the SDGs to identify 108 use cases. The top domains (by the number of AI use cases) included health (44), responsible consumption and production (31), sustainable cities (31), climate change (28), and industry and infrastructure (24) (with some projects addressing more than one SDG). All 17 SDGs already by 2018 had established AI use cases, with gender equality, just institutions, and effective partnerships having the fewest AI projects. The analysis additionally highlighted the ecosystem benefit of translational AI: repurposing of business and academic AI into global public health generally and SDGs specifically that in turn empirically enables the greatest AI4SD growth (through a "funneling in" process of considering multiple AI options for particular SDG targets then "fanning out" of iteratively scaling successful use cases within and across adjacent domains). How concretely is AI × SDGs changing global public health?

3.5 Artificial intelligence × Sustainable Development Goals institutional momentum

As health AI × SDGs lead the way ahead of other domains, there is concerted growth in their greater institutionalization and related use cases through international nongovernmental organizations (NGOs) and academic sectors collaborating with private industries. This momentum is building with the empirical evidence underling high-level consensus about AI's efficacy technologically accelerating the realization of the SDGs according to the current use cases. A 2020 *Nature* study suggested that AI may help achieve 79% of SDG targets, with particular benefit for poverty, education, clean water/sanitation, affordable/clean energy, and sustainable cities. Although it may also inhibit the remainder according to AI's societal, economic, and environmental impacts, especially if there are insufficient institutional and regulatory measures and multisector buy-in to prevent and mitigate these impacts (Vinuesa et al. 2020). A 20% risk for 80% gain seems like a straightforward win for AI × SDGs. But the study emphasized how AI's efficiency underscores its concurrent risks weighted by their severity, especially in healthcare. Bigger data can mean better health AI effectiveness. But it also entails a greater likelihood of more powerful abuses of this technology—especially with governments and corporations undermining data privacy and ownership for their personal gain, generating even such significant adverse outcomes as "technological totalitarianism" as is already present according to its critics in autocratic states like Russia and China (Polyakova and Meserole 2019). Who should regulate what and how it will be enforced are thus key questions we will take up in Chapter 5 on political economics and Chapter 6 on ethics. But for development in this chapter, let us focus on how institutional domains are nonetheless moving forward to optimize the benefits and minimize the risks for AI × SDGs, keeping its efficacy bounded by the dual duties to our common humanity and home.

3.5.1 International NGOs

The UN may be coordinating the highest profile, best funded, and most influential global public−private partnerships focused on AI × SDGs thus far. The collaboration among the UN Human Rights, Danish Institute of Human Rights, and private Danish corporation, Specialisterne, produced the Universal Human Rights Index (UHRI), the largest AI-enabled comprehensive database on human rights for implementing the SDGs (UNHR 2022). It features over 180,000 individual observations, mechanisms, and recommendations while saving thousands of manpower hours annually on manual entry and analysis. UHRI accomplishes this through its "TextClassify" algorithm, built for rapid multidimensional sorting. The AI model arranges millions of phrases across thousands of categories within seconds on a standard personal computer or PC, accelerating the translation of high-level global strategy into more agile local policy. A more immediate actionable approach to international AI × SDGs is the Istanbul-based SDG AI Lab (UNDP 2023a). It serves as the UN's technical and advisory accelerant applying AI digital technologies along with geographic information systems (GIS, or computer-based technologies to visualize and analyze geographic data) to SDG programs and policies. This public−private partnership by the UNDP (which Chapter one introduced as the generator of the "human security" concept) and the Turkish government's Istanbul International Center for Private Sector in Development coordinates private sector stakeholders and societal organizations and government agencies to develop the AI technologies and their organizational deployments for their target audiences, while allowing the identification of best practices that can be applied by the international community through the UNDP. It additionally strengthens capacities within the global SDG community, as seen with its ongoing education through a webinar series with Koç University on real-time AI advances, including ChatGPT's risks, benefits, and SDG impact shortly after the technology was released (UNDP 2023b).

3.5.2 Academics

Universities are increasingly partnering with such international organizations to help define and develop the standards for AI × SDG concepts, products, and deployment processes, especially given the wide-ranging societal impact of such innovations. As noted in the previous section, Oxford's AI × SDGs codified the seminal AI4SDG definition, benchmark, and analysis with its 2019 *Nature* study. Their focus is on AI's technical advancement of SDGs along with enhanced ecosystem collaboration on AI-enabled SDGs (Oxford 2023). Similarly, University College London (UCL) offers a graduate degree in "Artificial Intelligence for

Sustainable Development," taught by the UNESCO-affiliated Computer Science department and marketed for private technology companies (UCL 2023). What is notable with both of these high-profile initiatives is that they are orientated toward enhancing AI × SDGs within private industry. Oxford's program is housed in their business school and UCL's program is marketed as a means of boosting graduates' desirable skill sets for corporations (given tech companies generally struggle to find workers not only trained in societally responsible AI but also in the foundational technical skills to create them). Within this cross-sector intersection, the political scientist, Henrik Skaug Sætra at Norway's Østfold University College, advanced this growing corpus with his 2022 textbook *AI for the Sustainable Development Goals*, which appears to be the first such academic standard (Sætra 2022).

3.6 Artificial intelligence × Sustainable Development Goals local use cases

The global public health ecosystem is riding the growing health-focused institutional wave of AI × SDGs. It spans a range of local use cases manifesting what appears to be the contours of that ecosystem's emergent future, intersecting with the health aspects of (1) food/poverty, (2) climate/maritime, (3) energy, (4) financing, (5) and equities according to their SDG (and number; WEC 2022).

3.6.1 Poverty—Hunger (SDG2—3)

AI-driven remote sensors, drones, cameras, and autonomous robots (linked through deep learning (DL) algorithms processing real-time data from these cheaper Internet-of-Things hardware) are informing variable-rate technologies (VRTs). These optimize cost, time, and resource efficient crop yields through customized land management decisions down to the foot (already in use in up to 40% of US farms by 2016), all within the "next agricultural revolution" of "precision agriculture" (BIS 2022; Itzhaky 2021). Less seed, water, fertilizer, pesticides, land, and human workers can make more affordable food. This is especially true and needed as Russia's 2022 large-scale invasion of Ukraine and systematic bombing of its agriculture infrastructure (as Ukraine before 2022 was among the world's largest grain suppliers including donors to developing African countries) threatens what the UN describes as a worsening global food shortage crisis (UN 2023b). This antihunger approach is additionally relevant for the SDG poverty target as lower income communities' greatest immediate health threat is healthy food shortages (directly increasing morbidity and mortality, while increasing malnutrition and undermining gainful employment that otherwise could ameliorate poverty). Public health's vaccines and hospitals' antibiotics are not much use if poor patients and populations lack even sufficient healthy food to sustain life. One such global public—private—academic partnership for VRT to build global agriculture resilience includes a UK-government grant funder, US-based biotech company, and Imperial College London (ICL) to produce point-of-use remote sensors with short-term memory recurrent artificial neural networks (ANNs; Grell et al. 2021). These AI digital technologies accurately predict crop conditions up to 12 days out from just one remote measurement, without the need for expensive dedicated instruments in the field, and so reduce guess work, waste, and yield inefficiencies.

3.6.2 Climate/maritime (SDG13/14)

The probabilistic DL model, IceNet, generated the longest accurate predictions to date at up to 6 months out of monthly average sea ice concentration maps (Andersson et al. 2021). These are concurrently thousands of times faster than the traditional statistical models, enabling more actionable early-warning systems to protect at-risk coastal communities and wildlife. Increased global temperatures and extreme weather are associated with increasingly destructive and fatal climate conditions and acute weather events, especially for populations on the coast (the majority of our planet). As more coastal human communities are threatened by climate change geographically and financially, such precise modeling can inform better medium- and long-term policies. A related AI climate use case is explained in the energy domain.

3.6.3 Energy/industry (SDG7/9)

The Global South bears a disproportionate burden from climate change than the North, as the former are typically less industrialized, consume less, and have less resources to transition to carbon neutral and renewable energy sources longitudinally, while also addressing the impact of climate changes on their people currently (Ülgen 2021). A 2022 Oxford study supports consensus estimates of how the global transition to cleaner renewable energy away from fossil fuels such as coal and oil can produce net savings of $12 trillion by 2050; meanwhile, a 2022 Stanford study similarly demonstrates $11 trillion in annual global savings for such a global transition, along with a net creation of 28.4 million long-term full-time jobs (Way et al. 2022; Jacobson et al. 2022). This means that within just 6 years we would break even on this investment with the total $62 trillion transition cost, before saving over $60 trillion within another six. The cost of inaction according to a 2021 Boston Consulting Group analysis is $5 trillion annually by human-influenced climate change and ecological decay, undermining earth's $150 trillion estimated value (twice our global GDP) from biodiversity and healthy ecological function from stable food systems to freshwater filtration, leading to the popular critique that "the biodiversity crisis is a business crisis," and thus looming health crisis (Kurth et al. 2021). Yet these costs are notoriously difficult to estimate accurately and can be politically polarizing, while the price of failed estimates can be grossly unaffordable for high-income countries (HICs) and even crushing for low- and middle-income countries (LMICs). There are prominent critics who point out that there is so much data from so many sources required to develop even a rudimentary picture of what climate change is occurring, let alone to what degree we are affecting it and how if at all we can meaningfully reverse or mitigate that damage. There is therefore a growing worldwide push across the UN-coordinated international institutions, governments, and academics to deploy AI (including across 37 use cases by 2023) to answer such questions according to the same Oxford team that produced the abovementioned seminal AI $\times$ SDGs study. AI is uniquely situated (and showing early substantive breakthroughs already) among all our technological tools to integrate diverse data sources in real time, provide a more comprehensive picture of reality, inform actionable predictions, and guide rapid feedback to optimize agile policies and programs (Cowls et al. 2023).

3.6.4 Financing/equity (SDG3/10)

For the global public health ecosystem to effectively advance its provision of needed services, it must find sustainable financing to extend UHC for complementary essential health services (usually for acute treatment) and public health services (usually for chronic prevention). A global public–private–academic partnership among Google's DeepMind, Northwestern University, ICL, and the NHS demonstrated how a DL ANN algorithm based on 29,000 women's mammograms successfully detected breast cancer more effectively than radiologists, while reducing physician workload by 88%—while still preserving performance even with successfully scaling of the model to different countries' populations (McKinney et al. 2020). Replacing physicians with such an algorithm to read the 39.7 million mammograms annually performed in the United States alone could produce upward of $1.71 billion in annual savings (O'Donoghue et al. 2014; FDA 2023). Given the worsening physician shortages in HICs and already pervasive understaffing from insufficient medical training in and brain drain migration out of LMICs, safe and reliable AI may potentially help fill the global gaps in the healthcare workforce to extend lower cost but effective preventive measures in population health.

3.6.5 Equities/partnerships (SDG10/17)

This chapter detailed the growing AI $\times$ SDGs ecosystem of academic–private–public partnerships to lower costs and improve equitable value that boosts global public health. Emblematic high-profile examples of this include mRNA vaccines and digital diagnostics to plug the gap in healthcare systems and public health agencies lacking affordable alternatives for the provision of essential health services. Chapter 2 on finance highlighted how Moderna's infusion of United States government funding enabled the AI-driven creation in record time of its safe and effective mRNA vaccine for COVID-19 (Ransbotham and Khodabandeh 2021). This was accomplished through its unique design process (rapidly arranging mRNA sequences based on prior and current viral DNA) and robotic automation (accelerating monthly creation of mRNAs as the vaccine's molecular building block to number in the 1000s, up from only 30 created manually before). These operations accelerated the company's strategic value differentiation by enhanced product availability and affordability through faster vaccines generated at scale with lower research and development costs. The Digital Diagnostics for Africa Network (a private–academic partnership between Ghana's MinoHealth AI Labs and the United Kingdom's ICL Global Development Hub) produced a handheld lab-on-a-chip test that allows unprecedented inexpensive, accessible, and agile testing for a range of diseases, especially for remote and underserved communities who lack such local resources (DDAN 2022). MinoHealth's brand of "democratizing quality healthcare" through "artificial intelligence powered solutions" addresses severe physician shortages felt particularly severely in the Global South, undermining UHC and the capacities of local public health agencies and healthcare system to deliver their essential health services (MinoHealth 2023). This partnership pioneers early use cases including in scaling up better AI radiology diagnostics. The impact is significantly more affordable and immediate than waiting 20 years to train more radiologists, as the current rate is one radiologist for every 800,000 Ghana residents (compared to the over 20-year process for educating and training to create new radiologists). AI × SDGs thus augments rather than replacing humans by plugging holes, building capacities, and bridging divides (technical and political economic).

3.7 Polycrises versus AI4SDGs: the Great Divergence, Global South, and Ukraine

Despite such promise with health AI, its evolution and scale up is framed—and potentially even bounded—by the emerging negative synergy of modern crises. The UN Secretary-General at the 77th General Assembly in January 2023 declared urgently that "the Sustainable Development Goals are issuing an SOS," noting that Russia's February 2022 full-scale invasion of Ukraine following the COVID-19 pandemic's emergence have created a perilous one-two punch, not only to global public health, but also to the stability and sustainability of the post-WWII modern international order, built on collective defense of rights, sovereignty, self-determination, and collective action for global well-being (UN 2023b). As such, the very crises threaten to disrupt and even endanger the previous decades-long progress in the collaborative relationship of humanity's development, technology, and global public health. Further, they demonstrate how fragile and intensive long-term development and investment in global public health investment can be. Hard-won health gains can and have been wiped out and even reversed with unpredictable geopolitical shocks, particularly when they are seemingly driven by a smaller number of actors with limited domestic and international accountability. How does any country in the Global South (or North) develop their peoples' well-being within their borders if pandemics and wars can rip through them with limited warning? For example, Putin's ordering of the full-scale invasion by Russia (as one of the handful of permanent members of the UN Security Council) forced in just 12 months nearly 20 million (or half) of Ukraine's population into depending on humanitarian assistance for survival, displaced one in three (creating one of modernity's largest refugee crises), killed up to 300,000 people, and destroyed or damaged over 1200 health facilities, including through deliberate and sustained Russian bombing attacks on Ukrainian infrastructure, hospitals, and homes (UN 2023b; HPW 2023). But world leaders also highlighted at the abovesaid 77th General Assembly how this geopolitical shock is triggering a growing global health crisis. From raising the risk of World War III and even nuclear war to its highest point in decades, to unleashing what appears by early 2023 to be looming global food, fuel, and finance crises, the 2020s appear to mark a new postpandemic era of conflict and uncertainty, especially in the Global South. Vaccines, diets, and mammograms may be the last on the docket for national priorities in such a world.

With hunger, poverty, and disease (the primary immediate products of the war), all other SDGs are compromised, propagating from Ukraine outward with political economic ripples throughout the entire global community. Initially begun by Russia after it and China declared their "unlimited friendship," the invasion is described in the West as Russia and China seeking to replace including by force the modern democratic Western-led world order with an autocratic order in their image (Fidler and Gordon 2023; Bo 2023; Russell 2023). Russian commentators rather argue it is Russia's existential defense against the encroaching West. Chinese voices (including that of a prominent former senior colonel in the country's People's Liberation Army) assert the war has "nothing to do with China" or "the global south"—though their own food and fuel security, on which their health and economy depend, are progressively undermined by this increasingly global conflict (with a historic degree of destruction from its advanced AI and digitally enabled weapons). This is all occurring while the UN through its General Assemblies in the first year consistently reflected the global consensus of its condemnation of Russian aggression and destruction (yet without any clear ability to deter further devastation or facilitate a prompt, durable, and just peace). The massive surge of advanced Western weapons coupled with the wide-scale social media for Ukraine's defense, at the historical intersection of an emergent multipolar world, makes this conflict the first large-scale AI digital war—and the one that may make or break post-COVID international development, so dependent on global security, stability, and prosperity.

The global pandemic and conflict are forging Ukraine into what increasingly appears to be modernity's most intense and impactful case study, historical precedent, and real-time laboratory of a WoW approach to AI-accelerated development in global public health (WHO 2022; Monlezun 2023). It is seeking to rebuild back better a national health ecosystem in real time within an SDG framework, supported by the WHO coordinating in conjuncture with Ukraine's government over 190 global and local partners. This ecosystem is regenerating the strategic, organizational, operational, and data infrastructures to deliver essential health services through a development assistance for health—supplemented UHC, alongside critical public health services including vaccines, all the while resisting regular Russian bombardments. The WHO affiliates were often the first humanitarian convoys, including the first civilians, in just hours after Ukrainian military forces liberated previously Russian-occupied territories of Ukrainian sovereign territory. They coordinated public—private partners to link global supply chains with air—rail—car bridges and logistic hubs back into war-torn Ukraine areas to surge resources and personnel according to the SDG pillars—food, basic living needs, health kits, and so on, as progressively higher order needs were met. Within the first year, this ecosystem approach reached 8.4 million people across 1175 health facilities, providing 41,000 vaccines and 6 million civilians with NCD care, 38,000 with trauma and emergency care, and 23,000 with mental health services while the longitudinal health infrastructures were rebuilt.

What does the Ukrainian example mean for our shared future and that of development in the global public health ecosystem? It may represent a historic moment not only for Russia and Ukraine, but also for the Global North and South, West and East, and even the United States and China to consider what a mutually beneficial postcolonial world order looks like.

Can a new one be generated, one that is orientated toward global peace through integral sustainable development, ordered by a robust network of interest-focused institutions (explored in Chapter 4), addressing the deficiencies in the existing international order (of the West-dominated UN and related structures), and grounded in the sovereign self-determination of nations, accountable to their self-determining citizens as unique persons, bound in a common global human family by the common good in a common home? (Feltman 2023; Monlezun 2023; UN 2023b). Simply put, it is an international order built on the founding principle of personal dignity (with its derivative societal implication of national sovereignty), that therefore deploys development as the means to reach its destination of global well-being (manifested as peace, prosperity, and equality at international scale, managing the competing interests of diverse value blocs). It is a development that is not the exclusive property of democracies or autocracies, the North or the South, the rich or the poor. About 96.6% of the world's nations appear to support (or at least not oppose) such an order, and its development design for our global human ecosystem (along with its embedded global public health ecosystem), as reflected in the consensus of nearly every country in the UN 2023 General Assembly vote declining to side with Russia's seizure by military force of Ukrainian territory. Nonetheless, the West faces justifiable criticism from the South when it attempts to rally support for the defense of Ukraine under the banner of democracy over autocracy and dignified sovereignty over imperial conquest, especially at a time when the West failed to adequately support the rest during COVID-19 (especially in the early pandemic phase with its mRNA vaccines at scale), 60% of workers globally have lower real incomes than prepandemic, and 60% of low-income countries are near or at debt distress by early 2023 (before the likely full force of the abovementioned global food, fuel, and health crises strike). Yet from India to China, to Africa, and to South America, there appears to be a bare minimum design vision for an international order of development over destruction. No shared rules mean only divisive conflict at best and collective abandonment at worst. Losing the global institutional and sustained push for deciding border disputes diplomatically means they must be done so militarily. If COVID-19 and the Russian invasion are enough to threaten the stability and even survivability of the health ecosystem and nations globally, it may practically be that we must strengthen our international political economic order for peace—constituted by equitable integral sustainable development at scale, as necessary for the derivative global public health ecosystem. Or we must prepare for the "geopolitical jungle" where survival of the fittest is the dominant or even sole organizing principle (in which health is a luxury for the elites alone and global development was a passing phase of history). In a world of diminished resources and greater needs, AI may be the critical force-multiplier and enabler for a sufficient sustained response for solving (or worsening) local and global health crises and challenges. Leveraging AI-enabled global public health assets for such development rather than domination may thus boost not simply local health on moral grounds, but also its global prosperity and synergistic stability (through more efficient global value supply chains) on pragmatic political economic grounds.

A WoW approach to health's AI × SDGs for development may therefore be good for global public health and necessary for humanity. The International Monetary Fund estimated that COVID-19 will cost the global economy $12.5 trillion by 2025, with Russia's invasion pushing these global crises' price tag to $18 trillion (OECD 2022). The extreme pandemic rescue funding from governments globally created an explosion of global debt to an unprecedented $281 trillion, nearly three times our global GDP (Pesek 2021). The OECD joined growing multisector global warnings about such modern "polycrises" where successive global challenges create compounding negative effects, worsened by our increasing international structural interconnectedness (and related tensions limiting global cooperation addressing them). Such shocks can lock in longitudinally the Great Divergence between typically the poor South and rich North. Beginning in the 1500s, the European then American nations emerged from the 1500s with liberal democratic capitalist reforms in their political economics (informed by the Protestant Reformation then Enlightenment emphasis on the individual) and technical industrialization (powered by the related Scientific Revolution then Industrial Revolutions empowering them). We previously considered how such historic forces accelerated the early modern age of empires before the post-WWII decolonization period witnessed "the American empire," reportedly by invitation rather than invasion, as a first of its kind alliance-based world order facilitating the shared political economic and technical innovations globally. And now with the AI digital revolution from the early 21st century onward, we are entering new waters where power is diffused to a degree no prior period has seen. And yet without greater collaboration on equitable development (ensuring this late-modern world order delivers on its ambitious vision of integral human development), the Great Divergence can persist, worsen political instability, and precipitate "the Great Dissolution" of this order (to regress to our characteristic pre-WWII international [dis-]order driven by regional imperial conflicts—but now supercharged by exponentially more powerful weaponization of AI digital technologies with worldwide reach and impact). The OECD particularly cautions that multidimensional polycrises can be a potent existential threat or unifying challenge to our world, as understood through the SDGs: climate change (environmentally threatens SDG13 especially if global warning exceeds 2°C this century), Ukraine war (politically threatens SDG16 and growing cataclysmic conflict with Russia and China versus the United States and Europe, with over 50 million expected victims of acute hunger), poverty (socially threatens SDG1 as insufficient North support of the South can result in over 100 million facing extreme poverty and inequality from these polycrises), crises transmission (economically threatens SDG17 as insufficient public—private and North—South partnership can translate polycrises' impact long-term to the global economy, indefinitely blunting or preventing LMICs growing to become HICs), and COVID-19 (as this and future pandemics healthwise threaten SDG3 and millions of deaths acutely and even more chronically by blunting the necessary structural reforms to the global health ecosystem to make it sufficiently resilient, effective, and efficient for the global population). If the war drags on in short, so will the risk of the permanent Great Divergence—but not the realization of the SDGs or the global public health ecosystem's mission.

Conversely, the Great Convergence may thus begin with Ukraine, ripple through the Global South, and out through the rest of the world, accelerated by the global public health ecosystem's investment in a WoW approach to AI × SDGs. As a template technically and institutionally, Ukraine appears (at least at the time of writing this chapter in early 2023) to paradoxically be at the epicenter of this emergent future order. After China brokered a landmark "peace" agreement between the traditionally warring Saudi Arabia and Iran in March 2023, it offered the early steps to similarly mediate an end to the active conflict between Russia and Ukraine (compatible with the expressed wishes of India, Brazil, and influential figures in the Global South for prompt peace). It did so in a strategically competitive way that nonetheless complements the West-led diplomatic, defense, and development investments in these regions (Aboudouh 2023). By largely avoiding the rights-focused strategy of the West (with military and development aid often tied to mandated liberal political economic reforms), China offers a potentially effective synergy in its foreign policy of more interest or economic-focused strategy (leaving domestic political systems largely untouched). Consider how WoW AI $\times$ SDGs can be framed by and influence this emergent synergistic world order starting from Ukraine (as the most intense flashpoint and investment epicenter for our current great power conflict within this order). Its President Zelenskyy adopted the SDGs as government policy in 2019 (UNDP 2022). Subsequently, 6.7 million were lifted out of poverty to less than 45% of population in just 3 years prior to Russia's 2022 invasion, followed by a projected doubling to 90% of the population if the war continues for at least 2 years. The WoG approach (marshalling Ukrainian political, economic, societal, and military leaders in the unified strategy of national survival) complements the WoS approach (as decentralized efforts across diverse regions, sectors, and belief systems similarly unified around this mission through the means of their diverse skills and capacities). So integral human development via the SDGs integrates these dual dimensions to allow the first "rapid recovery phase of critical social and economic infrastructure" to enable resettlement, setting the stage for the second phase of "mid-term and long-term recovery and development" (projected to be the largest foreign aid development in modern times post-WWII, and the most sophisticated SDG-based actionable development strategy for how to generate a sustainable modern state in our globalized world; UN 2023c; HPW 2023; WHO 2022).

Emblematically, the most critical AI $\times$ SDG in this early recovery phase thus far has been mine clearing, to literally and analogically clear the ground for the construction of this state of the future (which previously counted China, Russia, India, and Turkey as among its biggest trading partners, while modelling its societal and political system on the United States and Western Europe). The UNDP by early 2023 is leading the way in this SDG to enable the subsequent SDGs (through funding primarily by Europe and Japan; UNDP 2023c). The World Bank estimates that just the first year of mine clearing would cost $37 billion, as Ukraine remains among the most heavily mine-contaminated countries with the highest related casualty rate in the world, particularly among civilians. Russia mined largely civilian areas that indefinitely prevents resettlement. The UN and its public—private partners including in parallel with American universities and nonprofits increasingly utilize efficient AI-linked drones to map and clear such hidden mines more safely than done by humans alone using less time and resources (Robinson and Smith 2022). Concurrently, Ukraine has already been the world's test lab for war AI, as it is the first large-scale use of combat AI from drones to facial recognition, to precision targeting, to cyberwar and counterdisinformation, and to decentralized internet connectivity and rapid health system triage of civilians—all implications for AI $\times$ SDG when such technologies can be shifted from destruction to development especially following the conflict (given the preexisting skilled labor and infrastructure both digitally, technically, and organizationally; Allen 2022). If the SDGs are already WoG policy, the critical lifeline for WoS recovery and rebuilding efforts, and AI for the technology-driving concrete deliverables, Ukraine may thus become the successful health AI $\times$ SDG model in the global public health ecosystems for the Global South as a way out the Great Divergence as their bridge with the North, enabling (or at least no longer hindering) the Great Convergence.

3.8 From financed development design to data architecture framework

Chapter 2 on and the current development chapter by now provide us a more complete overview for the future's emerging design of the global public health ecosystem, respectively understood through its economic pressures and historic trajectory, allowing us to progressively move into the daily on-the-ground concrete reality of AI facilitating health progress at the personal and population levels. Key to rounding off this design vision has been the historical arch informing its strategic future articulated as a development framework. We therefore considered how the 1990s US-led unipolar liberal world order of democratic globalization closed the chapter on public health's WHO monopolization (and subsequent rebranding and restructuring as a collaborative enabler in public health's 2000s pivot to global public health; Brolan 2022; Monlezun 2023). Then the Great Recession capped off by COVID in the 2010s into the 2020s closed the global chapter of Western government and expert-driven dominated global governance. And now, we may be witnessing the beginning of the WoW approach to governance with global public health now as a more inclusive decolonizing ecosystem designed for development. Such an ecosystem is increasingly united strategically through the SDGs toward this goal of the common good or global well-being, technically through AI as its capacity enabler, and structurally through the necessary common data architecture which Chapter 4 will explore. Financially, this may be the global strategy we can afford (and cannot afford politically and economically to avoid given the failure to find alternatives after the last decades of searching).

This trajectory is supported by the WHO's 2020−2025 strategic plan for AI-accelerated digital health. It asserts there is a "growing consensus in the global health community" that this AI $\times$ SDG approach is rapidly becoming "an essential enabling factor" to ultimately achieve the primary objective of this ecosystem, articulated by what the report explicitly cites generally as the WHO's Triple Billion target and specifically as the SDGs (WHO 2021, pp. 7−8, 10). This strategic convergence linking the government, intergovernment, academic, private, and community sectors, foreign and health policy, and the UN and the global public health ecosystem is manifested in the evolution from the UN General Assembly's 1986 adaptation of Paul VI's 1967 integral development formulation, to its translation into sustainable development by the 1987 Brundtland Report, to the post-Brundtland WHO's embrace of the

2015 SDGs, and to the post-COVID 2023 UN/Vatican working group on integral sustainable development. But as the WHO's 2020−2025 strategic plan on digital health emphasizes, this grand strategy requires fundamental ecosystem interoperability so partners can effectively collaborate with and benefit from each other to justify and sustain their partnership longitudinally. We will therefore continue this book's own evolution to propose how this interoperability can be achieved strategically through the design of the global public health ecosystem's twin finance and development in Chapters 2 and 3, structurally through the ensuring Chapters 4 and 5 on data architecture (internally) and political economic (externally), functionally in Chapter 6 through the cultural values and demographics populating this structure as well as foundationally through the security and ethics in which the above are grounded. As the WHO celebrates its 75th year the same year this book is published, let us continue its movement away from the 20th-century destruction into this direction of 21st-century development it pioneered, facilitating public health's adaptation to changing social situations— but with the constant mission fixed on global well-being. There is no sustainable development without equity (via efficiency) or integral development (via comprehensive cross-sector multicultural collaboration). And neither may there be a sustainable global public health ecosystem without the AI that organizationally and technically facilitates this efficient collaboration of public−private−academic partnerships, central to the development that increasingly frames this ecosystem that flourishes by it. This financed development design of the ecosystem in summary therefore may provide a promising strategic design for global public health with the SDGs (informed by wider multicultural and cross-sector cooperation) as a health-based WoW approach. It is framed by the economic and social determinants of health, formed by these dimensions of our global societies, and united by the UN's political economic grand strategy through stability and prosperity for shared peace. Within this model, our future's emergent AI (as we will increasingly fill out its structure and functions) "IS" development that is as integral (whole person and whole society) as it is sustainable (measurable and mutually beneficial). A WoW approach may thus be required to break the global political economic impasse across financing constraints and competing great powers (and their proxies and partners). The SDGs may be needed as an effective actionable strategy to optimize global public health. And AI may be the prerequisite to efficiently operationalize the above.

References

Aboudouh, A. 2023. "China's Mediation Between Saudi and Iran is No Cause For Panic in Washington." Atlantic Council. Accessed April 20, 2023. https://www.atlanticcouncil.org/blogs/menasource/chinas-mediation-between-saudi-and-iran-is-no-cause-for-panic-in-washington/.

Allen, G.C. 2022. "Across Drones, AI, and Space, Commercial Tech is Flexing Military Muscle in Ukraine." Center for Strategic and International Studies. Accessed April 6, 2023. https://www.csis.org/analysis/across-drones-ai-and-space-commercial-tech-flexing-military-muscle-ukraine.

Andersson, T.R., Hosking, J.S., Pérez-Ortiz, M., Paige, B., Elliott, A., and C. Russell. 2021. "Seasonal Arctic Sea Ice Forecasting With Probabilistic Deep Learning." *Nature Communications* 12 (1): 5124.

BIS. 2022. "Applications of Variable Rate Technology In Precision Agriculture at Different Stages of Farming." BIS Research. Accessed April 16, 2023. https://bisresearch.com/news/applications-of-variable-rate-technology-in-precision-agriculture-at-different-stages-of-farming.

Bo, Z. 2023. "Caught Between Russia and the West, China is Treading a tightrope on Ukraine. *Financial Times*. Accessed April 8, 2023. https://www.ft.com/content/c012270e-f89c-4ca8-8533-357204dc432f.

Brolan, C.E. 2022. "Public Health and the UN Sustainable Development Goals." Oxford University Research Encyclopedias. Accessed April 6, 2023. https://oxfordre.com/publichealth/display/10.1093/acrefore/9780190632366.001.0001/acrefore-9780190632366-e-327;jsessionid = 81116DE2AD757929 E4610ADAD05B3254.

Cowls, J., Tsamados, A., Taddeo, M., and L. Floridi. 2021. "A Definition, Benchmark and Database of AI for Social Good Initiatives." *Nature Machine Intelligence* 3 (2021): 111−115.

Cowls, J., Tsamados, A., Taddeo, M., and L. Floridi. 2023. "The AI Gambit: Leveraging Artificial Intelligence to Combat Climate Change—Opportunities, Challenges, And Recommendations." *AI & Society* 38 (1): 283−307.

DDAN. 2022. "The Potential of Digital Molecular Diagnostics for Infectious Diseases in Sub-Saharan Africa." *PLOS Digital Health* 1 (6): e0000064.

FDA. 2023. "MQSA National Statistics." United States Food and Drug Administration. Accessed April 17, 2023. https://www.fda.gov/radiation-emitting-products/mqsa-insights/mqsa-national-statistics.

Feltman, J. 2023. "War, Peace, and the International System After Ukraine." Brookings Institute. Accessed April 19, 2023. https://www.brookings.edu/articles/war-peace-and-the-international-system-after-ukraine/.

Fidler, S., and M.R. Gordon. 2023. "Russia, China Challenge U.S.-Led World Order." *The Wall Street Journal*. Accessed April 8, 2023. https://www.wsj.com/articles/russia-china-challenge-u-s-led-world-order-3563f41d.

Francis. 2019. "Listening to the Cry of the Earth and of the Poor. Vatican. Accessed April 6, 2023. https://www.vatican.va/content/francesco/en/speeches/2019/march/documents/papa-francesco_20190308_religioni-svilupposostenibile.html.

Grell, M., Barandun, G., Asfour, T., Kasimatis, M., Collins, A.S.P., Wang, J., and F. Güder. 2021. "Point-of-Use Sensors and Machine Learning Enable Low-Cost Determination of Soil Nitrogen." *Nature Food* 2 (2021): 981−989.

HPW. 2023. "Ukraine War Sparks Global Health Crisis." Health Policy Watch. Accessed April 8, 2023. https://healthpolicy-watch.news/ukraine-war-sparks-global-health-crisis/.

Itzhaky, R., 2021. "Artificial Intelligence and Precision Farming: The Dawn of the Next Agricultural Revolution." Forbes. Accessed April 16, 2023. https://www.forbes.com/sites/forbestechcouncil/2021/01/07/artificial-intelligence-and-precision-farming-the-dawn-of-the-next-agricultural-revolution/?sh = 2eb92a9f1dbe.

Jacobson, M.Z., von Krauland, A.K., Coughlin, S.J., Dukas, E., Nelson, A.J.H., Palmer, F.C., and K.R. Rasmussen. 2022. "Low-Cost Solutions to Global Warming, Air Pollution, and Energy Insecurity for 145 Countries." *Energy & Environment Science* 2022 (15): 3343−3359.

Juergensmeyr, M., ed. 2006. *The Oxford Handbook of Global Religions*. Oxford: Oxford University Press.

Kurth, T., G. Wübbels, A. Portafaix, A.M. zum Felde, and S. Zielcke. 2021. "The Biodiversity Crisis is a Business Crisis." BCG Group.

McKinney, S.M., Sieniek, M., Godbole, V., Godwin, J., Antropova, N., Ashrafian, H., and T. Back, et al., 2020. "International Evaluation of an AI System for Breast Cancer Screening." *Nature* 577 (7788): 89−94.

MinoHealth. 2023. "About." MinoHealth AI Labs. Accessed April 5, 2023. https://www.minohealth.ai/#about.

Monlezun, D.J. 2022. *Personalist Social Contract: Saving Multiculturalism, Artificial Intelligence, and Civilization*. Newcastle upon Tyne: Cambridge Scholars Press.

Monlezun, D.J. 2023. *The Thinking Healthcare System: Artificial Intelligence and Human Equity*. New York: Elsevier.

Morton, S., Pencheon, D., and G. Bickler. 2019. "The Sustainable Development Goals Provide an Important Framework for Addressing Dangerous Climate Change and achieving Wider Public Health Benefits." *Public Health* 174, 65–68.

Müller, J., 2013. "Aristotle's Legacy and Aquinas's Conception of Human Happiness. In *Aquinas the Nicomachean Ethics*, edited by T. Hoffmann, J. Müller, and M. Perkams. Cambridge: Cambridge University Press.

O'Donoghue, C., Eklund, M., Ozanne, E.M., and L.J. Esserman. 2014. "Aggregate Cost of Mammography Screening in the United States: Comparison of Current Practice and Advocated Guidelines." *Annals of Internal Medicine* 160 (3): 145.

OECD. 2022. "From the Great Lockdown to the Great Divergence." Organisation for Economic Co-operation and Development. Accessed April 19, 2023. https://www.oecd-ilibrary.org/sites/e445a79d-en/index.html?itemId = /content/component/e445a79d-en.

Oxford. 2023. "Oxford Initiative on AI × SDGs." Oxford University. Accessed April 4, 2023. https://www.sbs.ox.ac.uk/research/centres-and-initiatives/oxford-initiative-aisdgs.

PASS. 2023. "The Fraternal Economy of Integral and Sustainable Development." Vatican City's Pontifical Academy of Social Sciences. Accessed April 5, 2023. https://www.pass.va/en/events/2023/fraternal_economy.html.

Paul V.I. 1967. "Populorum Progression: On the Development of Peoples." Vatican. Accessed April 5, 2023. https://www.vatican.va/content/paul-vi/en/encyclicals/documents/hf_p-vi_enc_26031967_populorum.html.

Pesek, W. 2021. "Covid-19's $24 Trillion Cost (So Far) Means Economics Will Never be the Same." Forbes. Accessed April 19, 2023. https://www.forbes.com/sites/williampesek/2021/02/26/covid-19s-24-trillion-cost-so-far-means-economics-will-never-be-the-same/?sh = 600746024844.

Polyakova, A., and Meserole, C. 2019. "Exporting Digital Authoritarianism." Brookings Institute. Accessed April 15, 2023. https://www.brookings.edu/research/exporting-digital-authoritarianism/.

Ransbotham, S., and Khodabandeh, S. 2021. "AI and the COVID-19 Vaccine: Moderna's Dave Johnson." MIT Sloan Management Review. Accessed March 25, 2023. https://sloanreview.mit.edu/audio/ai-and-the-covid-19-vaccine-modernas-dave-johnson/.

Robinson, A., and Smith, D. 2022. "To Clear Deadly Land Mines, Science Turns to Drones and Machine Learning." *Scientific American*. Accessed April 6, 2023. https://www.scientificamerican.com/article/to-clear-deadly-land-mines-science-turns-to-drones-and-machine-learning/.

Russell. 2023. "AI Weapons: Russia's War in Ukraine Shows Why the World Must Enact a Ban." *Nature* 614 (2023): 620–623.

Sætra, H.S. 2022. *AI for the Sustainable Development Goals (AI for Everything)*. Boca Raton, FL: Taylor & Francis CRC Press.

Schmieg, G., Meyer, E., Schrickel, I., Herberg, J., Caniglia, G., Vilsmaier, U., Laubichler, M., Hörl, E., and D. Lang. 2018. "Modeling Normativity in Sustainability: A Comparison of the Sustainable Development Goals, the Paris Agreement, and the Papal Encyclical." *Sustainability Science* 13 (3): 785–796.

UCL. 2023. "Artificial Intelligence for Sustainable Development MSc." University College London. Accessed April 4, 2023. ucl.ac.uk/prospective-students/graduate/taught-degrees/artificial-intelligence-sustainable-development-msc.

Ülgen, S. 2021. "How Deep is the North–South Divide on Climate Negotiations?" Carnegie Europe. Accessed April 16, 2023. https://carnegieeurope.eu/2021/10/06/how-deep-is-north-south-divide-on-climate-negotiations-pub-85493.

UN. 1986. "General Assembly Resolution 41/128: Declaration on the Right to Development." United Nations. Accessed April 6, 2023. https://www.ohchr.org/en/instruments-mechanisms/instruments/declaration-right-development.

UN. 2015. "Transforming Our World: The 2030 Agenda for Sustainable Development." United Nations. Accessed April 5, 2023. https://sdgs.un.org/2030agenda.

UN. 2023a. "United Nations and Decolonization." United Nations. Accessed April 8, 2023. https://www.un.org/dppa/decolonization/en/about.

UN. 2023b. "Global Impact of War in Ukraine on Food, Energy and Finance Systems. United Nations. Accessed April 8, 2023. https://unsdg.un.org/resources/global-impact-war-ukraine-food-energy-and-finance-systems-brief-no2.

UN. 2023c. "Warning 'World is in Peril,' Secretary-General Stresses Countries Must 'Work As One' to Achieve Global Goals, at Opening of Seventy-Seventh General Assembly Session." United Nations. Accessed April 8, 2023. https://press.un.org/en/2023/ga12487.doc.htm.

UNDP. 2022. "Sustainable Development Goals an Integral Part of Ukraine's Recovery Plan." United Nations Development Programme. Accessed April 4, 2023. https://www.undp.org/ukraine/press-releases/sustainable-development-goals-integral-part-ukraines-recovery-plan.

UNDP. 2023a. "SDG AI Lab." United Nations Development Programme. Accessed April 4, 2023. https://www.undp.org/policy-centre/istanbul/sdg-ai-lab-0.

UNDP. 2023b. "SDG AI Lab Dives Into the Latest Technologies Behind ChatGPT." United Nations Development Programme. Accessed April 16, 2023. https://www.undp.org/policy-centre/istanbul/press-releases/iicpsds-sdg-ai-lab-dives-latest-technologies-behind-chatgpt.

UNDP. 2023c. "Making Ukraine Safe Again." United Nations Development Programme. Accessed April 4, 2023. https://stories.undp.org/making-ukraine-safe-again.

UNHR. 2022. "Artificial Intelligence and the Sustainable Development Goals." Office of the United Nations High Commissioner for Human Rights. Accessed April 4, 2023. https://www.ohchr.org/en/stories/2022/05/artificial-intelligence-and-sustainable-development-goals.

UNWCE. 1987. "Report of the World Commission on Environment and Development: Our Common Future." United Nations World Commission on Environment and Development. Accessed April 5, 2023. https://sustainabledevelopment.un.org/content/documents/5987our-common-future.pdf.

Vinuesa, R., Azizpour, H., Leite, I., Balaam, M., Dignum, V., and S. Domisch. 2020. "The Role of Artificial Intelligence in Achieving the Sustainable Development Goals." *Nature Communications* 11 (1): 233.

Way, R., Ives, M.C., Mealy, P., and J.D. Farmer. 2022. "Empirically Grounded Technology Forecasts and the Energy Transition." *Joule* 6 (9): P2067–P2082.

WEC. 2015. "What's the Pope's View on Sustainable Development?" World Economic Forum. Accessed April 6, 2023. https://www.weforum.org/agenda/2015/06/whats-the-popes-view-on-sustainable-development/.

WEC. 2022. "Why Artificial Intelligence is Vital in the Race to Meet the SDGs?" World Economic Forum. Accessed April 5, 2023. https://www.weforum.org/agenda/2022/05/artificial-intelligence-sustainable-development-goals/.

WHO. 2021. "Global Strategy on Digital Health 2020–2025." World Health Organization. Accessed June 11, 2022. https://www.who.int/docs/default-source/documents/gs4dhdaa2a9f352b0445bafbc79ca799dce4d.pdf.

WHO. 2022. "WHO's Response to the Ukraine Crisis." World Health Organization. Accessed April 8, 2023. https://www.who.int/europe/publications/i/item/WHO-EURO-2023-5897-45662-68308.

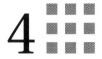

4

Framework part I: Artificial intelligence + data architecture

4.1 Basic concepts and terms

The global public health ecosystem lives and dies by its data, as the better the data, the better typically the algorithms and the decisions they drive (and conversely). The growth in data volume, velocity, and variety progressively distinguished the 19th-century public health, then the early 20th-century international health, and then the 21st-century's global public health —to the point it is now considered the "Big Data" that makes powerful health AI possible (Laborde 2020). And as that ecosystem digitalized with the Fourth Industrial Revolution and the global economy in the 1990s onward, artificial intelligence (AI) became an increasingly integral means of meaningfully understanding and using this otherwise overwhelming Big Data whose unprecedented scale and speed outstrips traditional analog and manual approaches. But the World Health Organization (WHO) or any global public health agency does not simply sit in a dark office and get thousands of boxes of paper files or millions of emails filled with zero's and one's. Even if fragmented and immature (which describes most of ecosystem stakeholders), there is some structure or "data architecture" within and across them organizing how data flows into an organization and the ecosystem and then is stored, analyzed, and reported to drive decisions. Generally, the more streamlined and mature a data architecture is, the more data AI can analyze, the more comprehensive and accurate an organization or collaborative understands the world, and the more accurate their predictions and thus data-informed decisions are Chapters 2 and 3 on finance and development, respectively, described the emerging design of the future's AI-enabled global public health ecosystem. This chapter will now consider its internal digital structure, before moving on to Chapter 5. So let us start with an overview of the basic terms and concepts for its data architecture, and then consider its current challenges, emerging solutions, and leading use cases for this ecosystem (bearing in mind the rich variety of you, the readers, with a wide range of backgrounds, perspectives, and familiarity with this content, thus requiring a broad overview this book will attempt).

4.1.1 Data versus information

Typically, data refers to raw facts without organization, context, or meaning (think of a paper in front of you filled with zero's and one's). Information is data that is attached to a larger organization or context by stringing multiple data points together according to a unifying data "key" or language allowing their meaningful interpretation (like being given the abovesaid

Responsible Artificial Intelligence Re-engineering the Global Public Health Ecosystem. DOI: https://doi.org/10.1016/B978-0-443-21597-1.00004-4

page with a key which says each data point is a "no" or zero and "yes" or one, describing whether each sequential hospitalized patient is alive). There can be a blur between the two because there is often a spectrum of specificity attributing facts with context, such that data is often the predominant entity described when discussing facts before they are processed, analyzed, and reported on. Data also contains several key higher order distinctions.

4.1.2 Data infrastructure versus data architecture

Infrastructure versus architecture are the main organizing data domains within an organization or collaboration (IBM 2023a, 2023b).

1. *IT (information technology) infrastructure* is the overarching technological hierarchy of hardware and software comprising a physical–digital network, which includes data architecture. Hardware includes computers, servers (computers enabling users to share resources), hubs (computer network devices broadcasting a data "packet" or group through electrical signals to all ports or end destinations across network devices), switches (a "smarter" hub that sends the packet to its intended port), routers (the "smartest" hub that dynamically directs packets like an air traffic controller for airplanes to the intended port across local area networks (LANs) and wide area networks (WANs), according to the packet's IP or "internet protocol" address), and facilities (data centers, servers, and hardware). Software can be system software (including operating systems and database management systems which coordinate resources of the overarching computer system) and application software (coordinating a computer's particular functions like Microsoft's Word or Google's Gmail). The two main types of IT infrastructure are traditional (dominated by a greater number and cost of physical assets) and cloud (where end users use the internet to access the infrastructure remotely through virtualization, which is the process of dividing up access to the capacities of physical services from users' multiple physical locations). An effective IT infrastructure ideally has effective virtualization (for server provisioning), zero downtime (minimizing disruptions), dynamic WANs (prioritizing traffic by need), security (against cyberattack breaches), low latency (minimizing delays in data flow), and high performance (reliably performing functions with robust postdisaster recovery).

2. *Data architecture* is the structure for raw facts that organizes how they flow into an organization or interorganizational data space (collection), often from different sources to then be processed (transformed into a standard format then distributed to other digital parts of the architecture and/or stakeholders), stored, analyzed (consumed), and then utilized for decisions. An effective data architecture ideally has effective data collection (particularly through the Internet of Things [IoT]), integration (across different data silos, domains, sectors, and geographic regions), efficiency (minimizing required energy and storage usage through deduplication and cleansing to avoid data redundancy and poor quality), capabilities (particularly through the lower cost, force-multiplying, scalable cloud platforms dynamically fitting cloud resources for users' needs), and management cycle (of creation, storage, sharing, use, archival, and deletion).

4.1.3 Data meshes versus fabrics

These are the main architecture types according to the hierarchical structure of the data (or how data points and partners relate to each other).

1. A *data mesh* is a decentralized architecture organized according to the economic sector or domain of an entity's data.
2. A *data fabric* is a more centralized architecture that automates integration of data from diverse sources according to identifiable patterns or metadata (general data descriptions of specific data's origins, creation, ownership, location, and meaning) into a "data value chain" between data producers (i.e., smartphone users) and consumers (software firms producing apps based on user preferences), ultimately reducing integration, deployment, and maintenance time, respectively, by 30%, 30%, and 70%.

4.1.4 Data lakes, warehouses, and marts

Data lakes, warehouses, and marts are the different data management systems that collectively generate the abovementioned data meshes and fabrics.

1. *Data lakes* store raw-structured and unstructured data and thus are typically cheaper and more useful for more advanced AI and machine learning (ML) than the belowmentioned alternative data repositories. Data lakes are like our earlier pluripotent stages of pregastrulation embryonic development in which our various stem cells have a much wider range of differentiation (in which cells become more specialized in later stages of development according to their ultimate development destination such as a heart vs skin cell). As data is "poured" into lakes from its different data "streams," its largely undifferentiated state is more like a blank canvas for data scientists to do data exploration, back up, recovery, test, and generation of analytic AI and ML models.
2. *Data warehouses* collect data from different streams and sources into a data pipeline, which transforms and sorts it according to predefined relationships, specified by the predefined data model required for specific applications and tasks. A data lake often allows data scientists to build "proof-of-concept" data models once they determine what data they need for specific applications. The data can then be exported from the lake into the more differentiated warehouses in a process that can eventually be automated to scale with related applications more cheaply and efficiently.
3. *Data marts* are the final step in repository differentiation in which the smallest subset of data for the narrowest focus allows the smallest number of human users (often in single teams like a public health agency's immunization staff) to accomplish tasks using the data most relevant to them.

4.1.5 Primary needs: interoperability and onward

The primary functionalities include connectivity (uniting diverse ecosystem stakeholders and data sources), computing capacity (particularly AI driven), and hardware (required for the above; Broadband 2020, p. 78). The primary needs that practically enable the above include the following (IBM 2023a, 2023b):

1. *interoperability* (extensible decoupling between standards and services which allow diverse data to be structured according to organizational needs)
2. *integration* (linking data into these structures often through standard APIs or application programming interfaces which allow multiple software components to communicate through standard data definitions and use protocols)
3. *enablement* (real-time data classification, validation, management, and governance that allows an architecture to meaningfully structure data according to organizational needs and communicate this structure to users who in turn can adapt it for those needs)
4. *portability* (of scalable data pipelines that allow cognitive analytics in intelligent workflows to dynamically integrate and transport data, while also communicating the performance of the abovementioned tasks to users in an iterative process, which in turn generates organizational applications by moving the relevant data as efficiently as possible to where it is needed)
5. *scalability* (of cloud-enabled and cloud-native IT infrastructure to elastically adjust or "right-size" access to the data management and analytic capacities, proportional to shifting applications and organizational needs)
6. *standardization* (in which structural and governance interoperability integrates with technical data standards, including with common data domains [digital spaces defined by a shared range of data values for the attributes or features in data models], events [changes in data states such as patients placing desired appointments in their digital shopping cart in the healthcare system app on their smartphone], and microservices [particular intermediate process applications triggered often by an event such as booking the abovementioned appointment once the request event is placed in the cart] allow diverse data to meaningfully communicate with each other and users in the architecture).

4.1.6 Primary exchange types: centralized, federated, and hybrid architectures

The primary exchange types of health data architecture include the following (HIMSS 2023):

1. *centralized* (in which data is stored in a single repository where the primary exchange organization generally has full control over it)
2. *federated* or decentralized (in which independent but interdependent data repositories from different partners grant access to others on a predefined need-to-use basis such as through APIs)
3. *hybrid* (combining the two above).

4.2 No data architecture, no global public health ecosystem

Chapter 3 summarized the historical development of public health into the global public health ecosystem in the institutional dimension: diverse stakeholders from varied sectors, levels, and regions leverage their synergistic capacities for the shared ultimate objective of global well-being with individual mutual benefit. The technical dimension that enables this complex collaboration structure is its underlying data architecture. The WHO's Global Strategy 2020−2025 on Digital Health highlighted how global public health's primary mission or end is "to achieve the health-related Sustainable Development Goals" (WHO 2021, p. 10). Its primary means of this "global strategy" is "person-centric digital health solutions," as AI efficiency in programs and policies gives way to health effectiveness. Yet such solutions require three principles according to the WHO: political economic (sustained institutionalization and investment), ethical (doing the above mentioned prudently given limited resources and equitably for mutual benefit, especially for the most vulnerable starting at a lower societal point), and technical (an effective data architecture). The WHO thus emphasizes how "the digital health ecosystem" can generate "sustainable health systems and universal health coverage" to accelerate global well-being—but only if effective stakeholder collaboration is "underpinned by standards and an architecture which enables this integration" (p. 15). For multiple people to work together, there must be some degree of common human, institutional, and technical language among them (with standard meanings of words and structures for the related sentences exchanging them) so they can communicate and coordinate their actions. And for different data systems to work together, there similarly must be some degree of a common digital language and means of communicating by it. The WHO emphasizes that such a global data architecture facilitates this needed "syntactic and semantic interoperability" among ecosystem stakeholders or partners as the "cornerstone" empowering the "sharing of information in a connected world" (p. 16). The architecture enables this interoperability through its format or structure (syntactically) of the uniform data exchange for data to flow among stakeholders, while also allowing it to be interpreted (semantically) using standardized meanings or "vocabulary" of the coded data (WHO 2021, p. 16; HIMSS 2023). The WHO endorsed ICD-10, HL7's Version 2.x (the world's top healthcare information exchange among healthcare systems across over 35 countries), and Fast Healthcare Interoperability Resources (FHIR, an internet-based suite of APIs expanding on Version 2.x using more web services and technologies for greater adaptability and faster interconnectivity among different systems), respectively, as influential interoperable standards semantically, syntactically, and foundationally (HL7 2023). The standards and resultant interoperability within the global public health ecosystem's architecture is so critical according to the WHO that it represents the "digital determinants of health" without which the medical and social determinants of health cannot be adequately addressed for global well-being (WHO 2021, p. 16).

The United Nation's (UN's) Broadband Commission elaborated on the WHO's strategic report detailing the importance and role of this global data architecture. The Commission was created by UNESCO and the International Telecommunication Union as a public–private–NGO partnership, cochaired by Microsoft and Novartis corporations, and driven by its Working Group members from the African Union, World Bank, and WHO. To effectively and equitably accelerate the AI-empowered global public health ecosystem, the Commission highlighted the needed development of the data architecture as one of the six critical areas for "AI maturity in health," alongside sufficient workforce, governance, design, partnerships, and business models to operationalize that technical capacity (Broadband 2020, p. 9). But implementing this needed architecture requires more than just the above-mentioned three layers of interoperability according to the Commission, which additionally specified the need for "consent-driven policy frameworks" advancing "a strong data and AI strategy" for mature AI-driven equitable optimization of global health. The influential US-based nonprofit organization, the Healthcare Information and Management Systems Society (HIMSS), defined this as the fourth or organizational level of interoperability in which good governance through social, legal, and policy mechanisms—like the United States' Health Insurance Portability and Accountability Act or the European Union's (EU's) General Data Protection Regulation (GDPR)—facilitate user and societal trust and engagement with the data architecture through adequate safeguards on user privacy and data security. The global health ecosystem's data architecture (when it works the way it should) crystalizes the unique value proposition of health AI. It puts accelerant intelligence to work for the global common good (instead of worsening inequities). It does this by filling human capacity gaps in prediction (through pattern detection, Big Data analysis, statistical reasoning, and iterative improvement) for human-identified concrete health objectives as the means of measurable progress to the ultimate end of our common good, according to our common values (p. 20, 31). Trustworthy AI-driven data architecture for the global public health ecosystem therefore must be the technical enabler of and safeguard for the standardization, interoperability, and strategic alignment that keeps the ecosystem together, growing, and progressing toward equitable global well-being.

4.3 Overview of challenges and solutions

The primary operational challenges slowing the realization of this needed global data architecture include its (1) heterogeneity, (2) silos, and (3) vulnerabilities (Martins 2021). The COVID-19 pandemic acutely demonstrated the chronic absence of an effective unifying data architecture for the global public health ecosystem (or its European subecosystem). Therefore, the EU commissioned a 2021 study on how to remedy this strategic capacity gap. It concluded that the abovementioned challenges were the predominant culprits and had to be addressed through the primary related solutions of (1) interoperability, (2) integration, and (3) security. For COVID and similar global health challenges, there is generally widespread heterogeneity in data sources, streams, pipelines, lake, indicators, semantics, regulations, risk management systems, governance mechanisms, strategies, and categories (including communicable diseases and noncommunicable diseases [NCDs]). If data remains stuck as unitless digits rather than meaningful information, then it remains useless. The data must be integrated to allow coordinated exchange, communication, and decisions. But all the abovesaid functions must be secured from internal threats (including inaccuracies from "dirty" data) and external threats (from cyberattacks, hacking, weaponization, and data theft).

The EU study therefore proposed an AI-driven "health data centre" driven by the unifying "common strategy" of achieving global well-being, empowered to sufficiently "influence Member State[s] public-health-relevant data ecosystems," and technically equipped with an effective data architecture that spans a "central coordination and support structure with advanced digital public health functions" (Martins 2021, p. iii). The political economic strategy of integration institutionally (that is consent based and mutually beneficial) would form the concrete structure for the data architecture to digitally complement, accelerate, and be governed by the consensus of all partners. Data sources (from the health and nonhealth sectors), data elements (matched to care processes), data sharing (both interorganizational and interlevel), technical and semantic requirements (enabling the above), data quality and interoperability (generated by the above), accountability (safeguarding cybersecurity and privacy), and strategic investment (achieving the above according to measurable development milestones) are the hallmarks of this strategy, translated and operationalized by the resultant data architecture. At the center of this data architecture, the data center would therefore define, reinforce, and optimize the networked digital structures, indicators, semantics, and governance. The report emphasized how this secure hybrid architecture can balance the need for a centralized subarchitecture (in which the data center acts as the "brain" that standardizes, integrates, coordinates, and directs data) and a decentralized federated subarchitecture (in which local healthcare systems and nations acting like the "nerves" traveling through the ecosystem's "body" have defined, secure, and consent-based exchange of their individual data repositories on a need-to-use/know basis), all safeguarded through centrally coordinated "minimum privacy and cyber-security preserving processes" that ensure "minimum standards for interoperability and health data quality control" (p. IV).

The Broadband Commission additionally highlighted how these solutions require (1) consensus-based architectural standards, with related legal and institution-facilitated compliance for adequate interoperability, (2) streamlined data sharing for real-time actionable intelligence for integration, and (3) minimized threats to data security with maximized AI explainability and interpretability (Broadband 2020, p. 77). The Commission underscored how the Global South and low- and middle-income countries (LMICs) have the most to gain —and lose—from AI. Falling short of such solutions accelerates the worsening of the global public health ecosystem's larger challenges or "key global and national health issues," including workforce shortage, emerging threats (pandemics, antimicrobial resistance, climate change, finance shortages, etc.), chronic disease burden, inequities (by poverty worsening affordable access to essential health services), urbanization (rapidly shifting populations from rural areas which thus worsens the abovesaid inequities), and misinformation (with AI-accelerated propagation of divisive disinformation; p. 7). Recent academic research in security has additionally emphasized the need for "a decolonized global health data architecture" that is "led by the very people who 'populate the dataset'" (Qato, 2022; Monlezun 2023). This approach proposes a "Community-based Participatory Research" model (with interventions developed *with* rather than imposed *on* the community), codesign and cogovernance (of programs conceived and run with the local community), architecture and AI transparency and accountability, and concrete mutually desired objectives. All of this requires a consent-based "quality narrative control system" in which local community members—not simply foreigners, executives, and data scientists—are the "humans-in-the-loop" generating and optimizing the AI and its data architecture. A decolonized data architecture therefore is central to the ethical and pragmatic necessity of decolonization (and successful operationalization) of the global public health ecosystem. According to the abovementioned commissions and empirical research, this transformation is required to address the structural health determinants in the ecosystem, namely, the very societal processes and relationships framing what and how data is collected, stored, analyzed, used, and owned. Political stability and ethical justification of such related concepts of locality, diversity, transparency, consent, sovereignty, subsidiary, and solidarity will be later explored throughout the rest of the book (especially in the Chapter 6 on ethics). But let it suffice for now how such high-level consensus as noted earlier in the ecosystem codesign explored in Chapters 2 and 3 requires coownership of the data.

The EU and Broadband reports highlight how failing to unite these interoperability, integration, and security solutions in an effective data architecture for the health ecosystem may continue to fatally undermine accurate, precise, and timely data insights, and so jeopardize or even block effective coordinated action. This in turn perpetuates "smouldering public health crises," like the chronic rise of NCD and inequities in addition to "emergencies" like pandemics (Martins 2021, p. VII). This was particularly problematic and evident for effective and prompt health policy and governance locally, nationally, and globally with COVID as potentially the single defining crisis for our late-modern global public health. If we do not know how many health indicators, disease cases, hospital beds, providers, and resources there are, how can we fit local supply for demand—especially if local health responses depend on global supply chains? This challenge of supply chain vulnerability was elevated as noted in Chapter 1 to an identified national security threat by the US White House and governments globally (Sullivan and Deese 2021, p. 6). And yet public health agencies and governments all over the world have slowly if at all come to address its preceding structural challenge of insufficient data architectures (including for supply chains) that fail to predict, detect, and mitigate shortages before they impact health programs and products.

4.4   Data architecture advances: Artificial intelligence-enabled health use cases

Now that we have considered an overview of the need, terminology, challenges, and solutions to an effective data architecture for the global public health ecosystem, let us finish this chapter by considering the concrete use cases advancing those solutions. The WHO and UN for instance articulate the abovesaid centralized consensus (of thought leaders and leading influential stakeholders internationally driving the standards and strategies for such an architecture). Yet there are a growing number of best-in-class use cases among public–private partnerships showing the impact and practicality of such an architecture (and the organic nature of its decentralized development). They additionally demonstrate ways to operationalize and scale effective and trustworthy data architectures successfully, while also collectively manifesting a budding patchwork of data architectures that increasingly constitute the global public health ecosystem's overarching data architecture (both in their unique value-add to the ecosystem and their relationships to related initiatives). Finally, it should be noted that such architecture advances are often indirect by-products of AI-enabled global public health program and products meant to address a defined health need. By April 2023, for instance, there were only four PubMed-indexed academic publications on "data architecture" for "global health" (even considering variations of such search terms, with none providing empiric assessment of interventions compared to controls; Nadhamuni et al. 2021; Metz et al. 2021; Mackey et al. 2019; Al-Shamsi Govender King 2020). These studies detailed below manifest the larger trend of real-world public–private–academic partnerships seemingly driving the majority of global health innovations and initiatives, which a priori require underlying data architecture improvements to realize their objectives. AI advances in isolation may advance important technical breakthroughs, but to scale and sustain them globally requires linking and leveraging them in an ecosystem approach which this book attempts to detail. So let us explore these architecture advances in breadth, setting the stage for analysis in depth in the subsequent chapters as they enable the other dimensions of the health ecosystem.

4.4.1 Interoperability: the United Kingdom's international hybrid + federated data architecture for COVID-19

Federated data governance particularly in data meshes are accelerating enterprise data architectures that stretch and connect an entire organization or multiinstitutional collaborative, bringing to bear their diverse data, capacities, and perspectives (Jefferson et al. 2022; Monlezun 2023). The data's federated structure and related learning does this by balancing innovation at scale (through decentralized data according to domains and partners) and effective collaboration with it (through centralized data standards enabling secure interoperability and integration across diverse data and its source partners). In the decentralized dimension, each partner and domain own their data and can thus creatively solve problems impacting the entire ecosystem. But they do so internally while sharing the solutions according to the shared standards to communicate that data and solutions in the centralized dimension. The transportation analogy may be that each person can drive their own vehicle (they choose, maintain, modify, replace, and use according to their internal objectives and external traffic patterns), but with such behaviors also bound externally by shared traffic rules and roads (that states define, generate, maintain, and enforce). Local autonomy generates innovation, while shared communication generates collaboration.

The United Kingdom's CO-CONNECT hybrid data architecture demonstrates this in action for COVID-19 (Jefferson et al. 2022). The architecture facilitated the collective transition from fragmentation to federation to fair and effective collaboration "at scale and at pace," uniting 56 datasets from 19 organizations and three countries (including hospitals, schools, care homes, and general populations). It spanned nationwide longitudinal demographics and electronic health record data on healthcare provision and outcomes to generate streamlined real-time insights, without the data leaving the secure environments of the individual partners. Accessing secure data from any organization traditionally can take months of bureaucratic steps across multiple organizations and security regulations. Yet their insights are needed in hours to days to treat patients and modify policies. In contrast, CO-CONNECT deployed a GDPR-compliant hybrid architecture as a "one-for-all and all-for-one" approach that placed the entire international data federation at the service of each partner organization, enabling them to serve their communities while their data was kept secure (and securely accessible for all other partners to leverage for their communities). This was accomplished by identifiable data extracted and pseudonymized from each partner within their "identifiable data zone" that was simultaneously sent to each partner's "federated node" or "secure virtual machine" (separate from where identifiable data is stored) in addition to the CO-CONNECT infrastructure as metadata. The centralized infrastructure team applied its self-defined rules to map the data into a shared data standard format or script, and then pushed that mapped data back to each partner's federated node into the pseudonymized data linked to their earlier version of the identifiable data. Each partner who was an approved user could then query the Health Data Research Innovation Gateway or data pipeline to pull aggregated fully anonymous data from across all partners for data discovery (or feasibility analyses) and metaanalyses to inform how they responded to their local community's dynamic needs.

4.4.2 Interoperability: India's enterprise federated architecture for universal health coverage and primary care

One of the four PubMed publications on global health data architectures focused on the design of an LMIC-wide enterprise architecture as India's National Digital Health Mission, a national digital health ecosystem enabling the organizational equivalent of the country's national health ecosystem (Nadhamuni et al. 2021). The Mission is working to digitally and institutionally connect the existing data platforms into a single national or enterprise-wide federated architecture to advance the sustainable development goals (SDGs). It seeks to balance decentralized needs (for local adaptation of national standards and resources) with centralized needs (for interoperability-by-design that integrates diverse IT systems). In doing so, it seeks to ultimately preserve the digital continuum of care, undergirding and more accurately mirroring the clinical continuum and its overarching organizational continuum (financed by universal health coverage). It is meant to do this according to regulation-by-design ensuring data quality, accessibility, and compliance. These are manifested as robust role-based access, user authentication, data consent and management ultimately for an "efficient national digital health ecosystem." The architects of these existing platforms go so far as to assert that the "fundamental building block" of this ecosystem is this "enterprise architecture" that "will determine the...trajectory of the nation."

4.4.3 Interoperability: swarm learning architecture—the "preferred choice" for Big Data?

Swarm learning may be the next generation improvement on even the competitive advantages of federating learning (i.e., keeping partners' data private but still learning from partners' data securely) by instead utilizing a decentralized ML generating more sophisticated data models and analyses with greater security and privacy protections (Näher et al. 2023). Consider the two dominant federated learning approaches of horizontal and vertical architectures. The horizontal approach enables local ML models to be created from data partners' unique datasets such as through aggregation and averaging. The vertical approach allows models to be united from the same datasets but with diverse features. Yet the partners' different models and data features must combine linearly (limiting their higher level modeling) and are vulnerable to back calculation to approximate identifiable data (such as with outliers in federated linear regression). Swarm learning instead eliminates the need for a centralized architecture coordinator and server through blockchain (securing data instead through pseudonymization) and edge computing (locally driven calculations). These architecture features facilitate secure peer-to-peer data communication and thus iterative improvements in local models within partners' own IT infrastructures (the following sections will further detail both blockchain and edge shortly). A 2021 *Nature* empirical study in precision medicine demonstrated that such swarm learning utilized local ML to unite such diverse diseases and quality of studies (as 16,400 blood transcriptomes and 95,000 chest x-rays from 127 studies including in COVID-19, leukemia, and tuberculosis) to outperform individual sites' disease classification, while still complying with data privacy by design (Warnat-Herresthal et al. 2021). The study postulated that since swarm learning's dynamic optimization of data traffic, security, and privacy reduces "data sharing" and increases "knowledge sharing," it "will become the preferred choice" for the global health ecosystem's dominant data architecture model.

4.4.4 Integration: public–private application programing interface platforms as "augmented public health intelligence"

API-enabled platforms are facilitating a growing number of public–private partnerships improving data architectures in service of global public health. The 2018 health interoperability report by the US-based National Academy of Medicine, the country's top independent medical advisory body, highlighted how "data interoperability is absolutely critical to this transformation" digitally of "health...organizations" to ensure their "future sustainability and competitive advantage," by delivering "safe, efficient, and economical care" (NAM et al. 2018, p. xix). The report singled out the US military's Department of Veterans Affairs (VA) as the nation's largest healthcare system, connecting hundreds of academic medical centers. It is therefore an influential driver of "national interoperability" through their use of AI and an open API platform to facilitate private−public partnerships uniting stakeholders and their data-driven insights including through swarm computing, blockchain, and federation learning use ML-based pseudonymization (with metadata and aggregation). And such partnerships use APIs as their web-based analogous tool to securely integrate their IT systems through these secure analytic techniques. Similarly, the WHO Hub for Pandemic and Epidemic Intelligence (or the "WHO Pandemic Hub") features the WHO as a central facilitator of a multisector global partnership from over 150 countries, streamlining a translational global data architecture into faster and more effective decisions to preempt, detect, manage, and mitigate emergent global public health crises (WHO 2023).

The related initiative of the WHO's Epidemic Intelligence from Open Sources or EOIS is "powered by artificial and augmented intelligence" that "lead[s] and coordinate[s] the evolution of a global eco-system of connected information, systems, and people" to "provide timely actionable intelligence for health emergency prevention, preparedness, response, and recovery activities" through "a complex information network" (EOIS 2023). EOIS focuses on a global data architecture integrating the patchworks of partners' local architectures through an iterative cycle of global infrastructure generation for intelligence sharing. It in turn facilitates enhanced real-time data capture, syncing, and analytics, which then informs data-driven policy and management decisions (that finally feed back into improved infrastructure design to restart the cycle). The data architecture thus strategically and technically is the backbone for this model and an emblematic demonstration of the global public health "ecosystem." The WHO emphasizes it as the ecosystem's defining structural framework and AI as its predominant enabling technology. This model of AI-accelerated public health creates what the WHO terms "augmented public health intelligence." It is constituted by a public health intelligence or "PHI Knowledge Network" of data-driven insights facilitating "collaborative learning." It utilizes a federated learning platform of "Big Data Analytics" deploying AI to generate insights from partners' health data, media, and social networks.

This model of augmented public health intelligence is additionally represented by UNICEF's Magic Box which began as an Ebola-focused data architecture. It fed real-time health Big Data into its architecture before expanding its technical capacities (through its private partnerships with Google, IBM, Telefónica, Amadeus, and Vodafone) and thus its health applications (to COVID-19, Zika, dengue, and yellow fever, the latest for which it achieved 95% precision identifying cases and thus effectively predicting future new cases proximate to current ones; Broadband 2020, p. 42). Its real-time modeling allowed it to empirically assess the possible role of COVID-19 physical distancing policies and net benefit for global public health particularly for LMICs. In parallel like the abovementioned Indian platform, the US-based Mayo Clinic Platform is seeking to establish the modern health standard for an integrated data platform as a "data behind glass" model through a federated architecture that makes integration profitable and scalable for augmented public health intelligence globally (Joseph 2023). Mayo's three-dimensional platform organizationally unites data network partners (including healthcare systems providing their data and learning from collaborative collective architectures), solutions developers (private companies using secure deidentified data to create AI analytic approaches using that data), and healthcare providers (licensing or sharing those data-driven solutions), all supported by the "construction partners" who generate the overarching IT infrastructure and derivative data architecture for the platform. Within the Platform, "Mayo Clinic Platform_Accelerate" spurs private early-stage health tech AI start-ups to efficiently scale up solutions. This ecosystem approach to interoperable integrated data architectures therefore accelerates the economies of scale and financial sustainability for such initiatives within the larger global health ecosystem, which is especially critical given the need to diffuse such innovations through LMICs facing less resources to codevelop and apply them locally.

Growing proof-of-concept cases for integrated data architectures are similarly demonstrating enhanced dynamic advantages through multisector collaboration. Syncing relatively new partners in multiomics, environmental, and community data partners with the global public health ecosystem concurrently demonstrates the novel synergistic effects of this approach (Rowe 2019). It also shows the greater organizational urgency for an enterprise-wide data architecture like the Indian and Mayo examples, complete with data hubs or command centers to coordinate the complex data that is generally new to the public health community. Failure to adopt an effective federated or at least federated-like data hub (coordinating decentralized partners, which may apply even to swarm learning) often can produce "shadow IT" in which pockets of smaller IT teams create IT infrastructure and constitutive architectures. These in turn not only fail to advance the organization or collaborative's unifying strategy, but they also divert needed digital resources to such limited impact initiatives to the point that the net outcome is ineffective enterprise architecture and unnecessary privacy and security failings. In contrast, another one of the limited PubMed studies on global health data architecture leveraged an enterprise-wide integrated federated platform approach in the India-based international HIV data architecture (Metz et al. 2021). It united tablet-based electronic survey data, point-of-care and laboratory testing, an inventory management system, and automated data processing across its architecture partners to generate daily and weekly data uploaded to its central data warehouse via open, custom, and vendor software. From the warehouse, the architecture populated survey-monitoring dashboards and timely test reporting across 450,000 subjects, spanning 30,000 files, 6000 aliquots (or portion of a biological sample weekly per country), 13 nations, and 25,600 viral loads total. This secure, scaled, and streamlined platform integrates 14 data architectures constructed and maintained by 17 full-time equivalent staff.

4.4.5 Integration: deep versus shallow learning and architectures

The bigger the data, the more advanced the architecture, the greater the computation needs for more advanced modeling. Accordingly, there are increasingly rapid developments in shallowing learning as a novel AI modeling approach alongside stream, batch, and quantum computing. A 2023 *Nature* study from an Israeli team demonstrated that "shallowing learning" may be superior in certain key regards to the current state-of-the-art AI algorithms, namely those using "deep learning" or DL (Meir et al. 2023). As introduced earlier, DL algorithms generally are "artificial neural networks" or ANNs modeled after our own brain's neural networks in which the strength of the connection or synapse between two neurons or nerve cells are modified based on their related activities. In a simplistic example, a group of neurons in a physician biologically power the electrical transmission or thought that a patient clutching her/his chest and crying in pain may be having a heart attack which requires urgent medical intervention. The more times a physician sees and treats this correctly, the stronger the connection among those related neurons (with the input of seeing the patient's behavior travels through the physician's "layers" of neurons to the output of identifying the appropriate treatment). But to improve ANN performance, algorithms have become increasingly complex, often spanning up to hundreds of convolutional hidden layers between inputs and outputs (in which such layers attempt to identify localized patterns in the input and large-scale partners in its subsequent layers to ultimately produce an output that reliably characterizes different inputs). The greater the model complexity (and related data architecture), the greater the time, computational power, cost, and expertise required, thus limiting the scale up and adaptation of such models for wider use. The Israeli team instead considered how biologically our brains have only a few yet effective neuron layers for particular functions. So instead of "deep learning," they demonstrated successfully how "shallow learning" can use a fixed depth ratio between the first and second convolutional layers that thus ultimately required only five layers, while also demonstrating the error rates "decay as a power law" relative to the first layers' filters. The seeming universal behavior of this power law additionally appeared to crack the code on explaining how complex DL data architectures work by showing the "quantitative hierarchical time-space complexity." Essentially, this power law determines how shallow learning architectures can more accurately resemble our simpler but more efficient neural networks to perform just as well (with comparable error rates), but with significantly less time, energy, data, software, hardware, and thus cost (suggesting a way forward to better democratize powerful AI computing for more users in more regions and sectors).

4.4.6 Integration: stream, batch, and quantum computing

Such advances highlight the importance of right-fitting the data architecture for the AI required for an organization or collaboration's needs. In addition to the predominant algorithm types, we must also consider the way architectures integrate data to be eventually used for such modeling. A key hurdle in the ultimate value, relevance, and reliability of a data architecture is how well it performs such computations by first processing, integrating, and analyzing data. A Morocco-based team in 2018 showed how the combination of batch and stream computing can power a health data architecture to effectively manage a healthcare system's Big Data (El Aboudi and Benhlima 2018). Batch computing consumes, processes, and analyzes data in "chunks" over a defined time period when there are less time constraints for doing so. Stream computing instead does the abovementioned functions in real-time as data "flows" from when and where it is created to where its data-driven insights are required for decisions in a continuously updated manner. The first method often gives more complex insights, but the latter gives more timely ones. By uniting them, a health ecosystem can have a more complete and actionable picture of reality. This in turn informs what they must do to achieve their objectives within it, similar to how the Morocco team demonstrated how this integrated computing detected alarm cases (when measurements such as blood pressures exceeded accepted averages or thresholds) and produced real-time updates (warning clinicians of potential patient worsening) as clinical decision support tools (to more efficiently and safely triage and manage a patient population by focusing the right resources at the right time on the right people according to need).

Balancing stream and batch computing though can be technically difficult for a data architecture and its users. A preferred scenario would be complex data processing, integration, and analysis in real time, which is a tantalizing combination of advantages that "quantum computing" may be poised to progressively deliver in the near future (Davids Lidströmer Ashrafian 2022). In March 2023, Cleveland Clinic and IBM launched the first AI-driven health quantum computer for on-site integrated commercial use—"IBM Quantum System One"—to leverage clinical, drug, and multiomics databases to solve health problems like new drug discovery. Unlike stream and batch computing that focuses on Big Data processing and analysis, quantum computing refers to the more general methodology that uses the quantum states of subatomic particles to solve more complex problems more rapidly than classical computers. Quantum computers use the "qubit" as the basic information unit (and so performs "superposition" in which they can concurrently code the same data point as zero and one, while qubits are additionally entangled or linked to each other), rather than traditional computers' "bit" (coding data points as zero's and one's which are discrete, sequential, and binary). Classical computers run on electronics in classical physics (in which a circuit is in a single on or off state), while quantum computers run on quantum mechanics (of superposition and entanglement allowing multiple concurrent states). Unlike classical computers, quantum computers can therefore generate more rapid, complex, and multidimensional computations. Through massive parallel processing on massive data, quantum computing is increasingly demonstrating how it can generate nondeterministic results by simultaneously exploring an enormous number of solutions (in a way that in a sense combines batch computing's complexity and stream computing's real-time aspects) into the supercomputer or even ultimate computer of the future, facilitating next-generation data architectures and AI.

4.4.7 Integration: liquid neural networks

"Liquid neural networks" suggest a potent breakthrough in the underlying mathematics making AI more effective by more efficiently integrating diverse data sources, times, and types to better adapt to real-world dynamics in real time (Chahine et al. 2023). In contrast to older neural networks, liquid models modify their fundamental differential equations to continuously learn and adapt to new data even outside of training data, which is particularly key for time series data including natuural language processing, video, and robotics technically and telehealth diagnostics and autonomous robotic agents practically. In April 2023, a US Air

Force—funded MIT team demonstrated that autonomous flight navigation agents adapted from a real-time stream of visual inputs from different environments to eliminate irrelevant features and fine-tune their decision-making for flying to targets, even surpassing previous best-in-class DL models.

4.4.8 Security (and privacy by design): zero-trust prevention and dual-defense containment

Three key security advances for health data architectures include a zero-trust strategy, block-chain technology, and a data solidarity framework. Interoperability and integration in data architectures can enable scale and speed, but they need security and privacy to be trusted. "Zero-trust architecture" is an emerging model for the healthcare cloud as more health agencies and collaborations move to cloud computing on safe IT infrastructures (with a projected $33.59 billion increase in cloud migration revenues in the US market alone up to 2025; Siwicki 2021). Yet the transition exposes their data to greater external cybersecurity and internal data integrity threats as they migrate to a cloud-based model from their local sites where data is generated. Even before widespread cloud adoption, at least a third of healthcare organizations are annually targeted by ransomware attacks (with 40 million patients' data breached), amid their rich sensitive data and often subaverage security safeguards compared to other societal and economic sectors. The more clinics, hospitals, public health agencies, and other data partners joining a regional, national, or global health ecosystem's overarching data architectures (often provided by multiple vendors) mean there is more diversity in the degree of overall data security and security interoperability within and among them. Less secure partners make it easier for cyberattacks to infiltrate them and then spread through the larger collaborative's data architecture often undetected. "Zero-trust" is an emergent "assume breach" paradigm shift in contrast to the traditional "just-keep-them-out" approach that focuses on dual-defense of prevention and containment. It protects against intruders' digital entrance into an IT infrastructure and related data architecture. But it also kicks them out as soon as possible if they get in, while mitigating the spread of their damage and data access. Zero-trust practically focuses on two key elements. These include "least-privilege access controls" (allowing users only the necessary information they need while limiting the ability of digital intruders to move much beyond the initial breach or entry point). It additionally emphasizes infrastructure and architecture-wide visibility (monitoring the security weak spots between the overarching hybrid cloud and its constitutive diverse cloud vendors and data centers).

4.4.9 Security (and privacy by design): blockchain

Blockchain is arising as one of the most disruptive technological advances in secure data architectures, driven by consensus, decentralization, and cryptography (advanced encryption; Mackey et al. 2019). This shared distributed digital ledger was popularized in digital finance (with Bitcoin and other cryptocurrencies) and increasingly is growing in the health ecosystem as "fit-for-purpose" optimization of secure streamlining for health outcomes, costs, operations, and compliance. Traditional centralized databases house data in a single site that others cannot view. Blockchain (permissioned to data partners with predefined data participation and access) spreads out the encrypted data (verified, authenticated, and agreed on by all data partners) across multiple databases (nodes) in which all chain partners have copies (ledgers) of transmitted data (transactions) that partners cannot modify. Data chunks (blocks) are "chained" together by a digital signature of random numbers and letters (hashing), providing a full tamper-resistant transaction history or map of how the data flows and from where. It still has vulnerabilities in code exploitation (generating the blockchain), stolen keys (personal digital signatures), and partner computer hacking. But the abovesaid advantages compared to traditional security technologies mean there is no centralized data "authority" that can be a single point of security failure, nor clear domain limitation or technical barriers to a single security interoperability even across data partners' diverse data architectures. Although blockchain is a relatively immature technology with limited adoption, there is still a sharp uptick in blockchain applications in the global health and public health ecosystems including in data architecture interoperability, clinical trial management, IoT, health financing, precision medicine's multiomics, and supply chain management. Meanwhile, multisector consensus including from Big Tech reflect World Economic Forum estimates that blockchain will store 10% of the global GDP by 2025. Specifically in the health sector, the abovesaid 2021 Warnat-Herresthal et al. study on swarm learning emphasized how its secure data architecture runs on blockchain, allowing it "robust measures against dishonest participants or adversaries" through "confidentiality-preserving machine learning by design" that can adapt to "differential privacy algorithms, functional encryption, or encrypted transfer learning approaches." The authors propose that this integration of data partners through interoperable AI-driven swarm learning—safeguarded by blockchain—may be a "a very promising approach to democratize the use of AI among the many stakeholders in the domain of medicine" and health more broadly, while simultaneously "resulting in improved data confidentiality, privacy, and data protection, and a decrease in data traffic."

4.4.10 Security (and privacy by design): decolonization and data solidarity

Finally, data solidarity represents an influential framework for the decolonization of the international data architecture for the global public health ecosystem (Prainsack et al., 2022). The *Lancet* and *Financial Times* Commission in 2022 noted how the "defining features of the current phase of digital transformations" internationally, particularly in the health ecosystem, are "business models based on data extraction, concentrations of power, and viral spread of misinformation and disinformation." Such critique argues that data is often "extracted" from local populations for the disproportionate benefit of the more powerful foreign parties doing the extraction—not wholly dissimilar to the European age of empires drawing raw materials and commodities from the Global South to feed the Global North's manufacturing and consumer markets, with minimal at best political and economic benefit for those "colonies" of the empires (or the current Russia–directed and funded Wagner mercenary group, increasingly labeled as a terrorist organization by a number of countries including the United Kingdom, who have an extensively documented track record of extracting African mineral resources and systematic rape, torture, and murder of civilians globally to prop up autocratic leaders despite widespread popular resistance to them, ultimately to expand Russian foreign influence and profit; Rynn and Cockayne 2023). And consent for modern data extraction is generally insufficient to address such vulnerabilities. In contrast, "data solidarity" is an emerging regulatory and data governance framework for "strengthening collective control and ownership of data" by managing the tension between "public value" and data risks. Accordingly, data use should be supported (when it is low risk with high public value), delayed (when it has high public value and high risk which should be reduced sufficiently prior to use), compensated (through commercial profits when it is low risk and has low public value), and prohibited (when it has low public value and high risk). This data governance should be accomplished through "harm mitigation instruments" and "remedies" operating in all four of those abovesaid matrix domains. The Commission concluded that the definition of secure data architecture thus should be expanded to moral minimums such that technical criteria for effective data architectures (including interoperability and integration) are ultimately conditioned on moral criteria (for the ultimate end or criteria being "global justice," considering the global ethical principle that all of us have equal dignity and thus rights to the goods needed for our full flourishing in and through our global human community). This high-level emphasis on "data solidarity" follows the influential consensus critique noted in Chapter 1 by the African CDC Director's comments in 2021 that the Global North's vaccine nationalism for COVID-19 manifested the "collapse of global cooperation and solidarity" (Myers 2022). Ethical solidarity requires data solidarity and vice versa. The Commission further developed and operationalized the Broadband Commission's 2020 report noted earlier which emphasized data solidarity as a key "enabler" for effective data architectures as part of the six required areas for reaching AI maturity in global health (p. 77). A practical example of this is a 2020 United Arab Emirates (UAE) study seeking to develop effective LMIC health data architectures (Al-Shamsi Govender King 2020). It calculated a Framingham Risk Score (the US-generated cardiovascular risk scale that is among the most widely used and dominant such statistical scores) for every UAE citizen. The team used them to personalize population health measures, only to find that the scores failed to accurately predict cardiovascular risk for its people (because the American data did not generalize to the UAE). Such emblematic findings support the potential benefit of a data solidarity-informed approach for a more AI-accelerated, real-time, localized global data architecture and analytics.

4.4.11 Hybrid cloud–fog–edge blockchain computing: smart environment architectures

Now we can put it all together to envision what an integrated, interoperable, secure model for an ideal data architecture may (already) look like for the global public health ecosystem, based on the advances in "smart cities" especially (Simonet-Boulogne et al 2022). This municipality is like a microcosm of what the global ecosystem intends to do but at worldwide scale: using AI-accelerated digital technologies to more efficiently improve government and community resources for people's well-being. This 2022 French, Norwegian, Spanish, and Greek team outlined a blockchain secured cloud−fog−edge data architecture with hybrid and federated learning to enhance citizen well-being through digital health technologies and policies. Generally, this three-layer architecture featured the cloud layer on top (for Big Data processing, warehousing, and intelligent analytics), the fog layer under it (for nodes and servers facilitating data standardization, visualization, control, pruning, and analysis), and the edge layer at the local end-user level (for real-time embedded Big Data processing of users applications at the point of use, i.e., from IoT sensors, controllers, and devices ranging from smartphones and personal computers to digital service providers, interacting with users through micro or local data storage, visualization, and analysis). A 2022 Palestinian−French team refined this hierarchy to show how a narrow-band IoT allows a larger number of devices (particularly remote home monitoring for health vitals) at the edge, while minimizing computational power, latency, and data processing by higher value data prioritization for transmission to the fog and cloud layers (Daraghmi et al. 2022). In addition, the Microsoft−Ukraine public−private partnership following Russia's 2022 full-scale invasion demonstrates how this three-layer data architecture can safeguard the critical sectors required for public well-being, resilient to full-spectrum multidomain threats including regular Russian cyberattacks and missile barrages against civilian targets and built infrastructure (Microsoft, 2023). Leading up to the invasion and shortly afterward, Ukraine's government migrated its local server-stored data to Microsoft's Azure cloud (physically distributed throughout European data centers), along with its major companies including in agriculture, energy, and banking. Microsoft as a private company leveraged its IT infrastructure, data architecture platform, edge communication (through Microsoft Teams), software as a service, and security functionalities empowered the government to uphold its public goods duty of sustaining these critical sectors and institutions required for its citizens' population health. A final improvement to such a full-spectrum data architecture is the Taiwanese−Pakistani−Indian−Iraqi−Swedish collaborative in the March 2023 *Nature* study showcasing the novel "deep reinforcement learning-aware blockchain-based task scheduling" (DRLBTS) (Lakhan et al. 2023). DRLBTS as a global "distributed mobile fog cloud" data architecture proposes a robust solution to the persistent prioritization problem with the cloud−fog−edge data architecture. It suggested proof-of-concept for managing diverse IoT applications on the edge with differing delay, energy, latency, and cost constraints to ultimately ensure the right data gets to the right data partners in the right layers at the right time (so users can receive their needed timely services within a seamless health workflow).

4.4.12 From data architectures to societal architectures

These use cases demonstrate the general trend of innovative public−private−academic partnerships generating AI advances in global public health, especially through their underlying innovations in the data architectures enabling those advances. And the growth of this organic decentralized patchwork of overlapping data architectures and health programs manifest how they are often pruned and integrated (as more influential architectures and programs become synced or replace lower order ones). We are not at the point of having a centralized data architecture for the global public health ecosystem. But it does look possible if not probable for the deepening federated coordination of subdata architectures in the near term allowing greater data interoperability, integration, and security to drive more efficient, effective, and equitable outcomes for the overarching ecosystem. Technology is rapidly advancing to facilitate this. The major hurdle to it therefore increasingly appears to be the political economic hurdles (as questions of data governance, ownership, accountability, and use or misuse gain prominence in an increasingly divided world). The world's leading influential figures in the ecosystem make explicit their attempts at advancing this centralization of data coordination among decentralized actors and architectures, especially with the WHO at the helm of such efforts including through its 2020−2025 global strategy. The WHO report cites the consensus of the world's nations on the 2010s' SDGs and digital health related General Assembly resolutions that reportedly "encourages [the] WHO, within its respective mandate and strategic plan, to contribute to the outcomes" of related high-level meetings to accelerate the health-related SDGs through AI-accelerated digital technologies (WHO 2021, p. 7). It therefore proposed its "global strategy" in digital health to advance the political economic, institutional, and technical necessities of the needed data architecture that "promotes...interoperability," but specifically "with WHO norms and standards as a cornerstone of health information" (p. 16). In data architecture, standards are power, both in their definitions and enforcement. And there are no clear competitors to its WHO architects. Therefore, Chapter 5 will assess the political economics of the global public health ecosystem to explore the external factors shaping the internal data architecture for this ecosystem, while exploring how it shapes the ecosystem's future and its mission for equitable global well-being.

References

Al-Shamsi, S., Govender, R.D., and J. King. 2020. "External Validation and Clinical Usefulness of Three Commonly Used Cardiovascular Risk Prediction Scores in an Emirati Population: A Retrospective Longitudinal Cohort Study." *BMJ Open* 10 (10): e040680.

Broadband. 2020. "Reimaging Global Health Through Artificial Intelligence: The Roadmap to AI Maturity." Broadband Commission for Sustainable Development. Accessed April 21, 2023. https://www.broadband-commission.org/wp-content/uploads/2021/02/WGAIinHealth_Report2020.pdf.

Chahine, M., Hasani, R., Kao, P., Ray, A., Shubert, R., Lechner, M., Amini, A., and D. Rus. 2023. "Robust Flight Navigation Out of Distribution With Liquid Neural Networks." *Science Robotics* 8 (7). https://doi.org/10.1126/scirobotics.adc889.

Daraghmi, Y.A., Daraghmi, E.Y., Daraghma, R., Fouchal, H., and M. Ayaida. 2022. "Edge−Fog−Cloud Computing Hierarchy for Improving Performance and Security of NB−IoT−Based Health Monitoring Systems." *Sensors* 22 (22): 8646.

Davids, J., Lidströmer, N., and H. Ashrafian. 2022. "Artificial Intelligence in Medicine Using Quantum Computing in the Future of Healthcare." *Artificial Intelligence in Medicine* 308 (1): 423−446.

El Aboudi, N., and L. Benhlima. 2018. "Big Data Management for Healthcare Systems: Architecture, Requirements, and Implementation." *Advances in Bioinformatics* 2018 (4059018): 1−10.

EOIS. 2023. "Epidemic Intelligence From Open Sources Collaboration." World Health Organization. Accessed April 21, 2023. https://www.who.int/initiatives/eios/eios-collaboration.

HIMSS. 2023. "Interoperability in Healthcare." Healthcare Information and Management Systems Society. Accessed April 28, 2023. https://www.himss.org/resources/interoperability-healthcare.

HL7. 2023. "HL7 Version 2 Product Suite." Accessed April 28, 2023. https://www.hl7.org/implement/standards/product_brief.cfm?product_id = 185.

IBM. 2023a. "IT Infrastructure." IBM. Accessed April 21, 2023. https://www.ibm.com/topics/infrastructure.

IBM. 2023b. "Data Architecture." IBM. Accessed April 21, 2023. https://www.ibm.com/topics/data-architecture.

Jefferson, E., Cole, C., Mumtaz, S., Cox, S., Giles, T.C., Adejumo, S., and E. Urwin, et al., 2022. "A Hybrid Architecture (CO-CONNECT) to Facilitate Rapid Discovery and Access to Data Across the United Kingdom in Response to the COVID-19 Pandemic." *Journal of Medical Internet Research* 24 (12): e40035.

Joseph, S. 2023. "Building Bridges Between Data Silos: Mayo Clinic Platform's Ambitious Endeavor to Enable a Learning Healthcare System." Forbes. Accessed April 28, 2023. https://www.forbes.com/sites/sethjoseph/2023/02/01/building-bridges-between-data-silos-mayo-clinic-platforms-ambitious-initiative-to-enable-a-learning-healthcare-system/?sh = 62acfa283511.

Laborde, R. 2020. "The Three V's of Big Data: Volume, Velocity, and Variety." Oracle. Accessed April 24, 2023. https://blogs.oracle.com/health-sciences/post/the-three-vx27s-of-big-data-volume-velocity-and-variety.

Lakhan, A., Mohammed, M.A., Nedoma, J., Martinek, R., Tiwari, P., and N. Kumar. 2023. "DRLBTS: Deep Reinforcement Learning-Aware Blockchain-Based Healthcare System." *Nature Scientific Reports* 13 (1): 4124.

Mackey, T.K., Kuo, T.T., Gummadi, B., Clauson, K.A., Church, G., Grishin, D., Obbad, K., Barkovich, R., and M. Palombini. 2019. "'Fit-for-Purpose?'—Challenges and Opportunities for Applications of Blockchain Technology in the Future of Healthcare." *BMC Medicine* 17 (1): 68.

Martins, H. 2021. "EU Health Data Centre and a Common Data Strategy for Public Health." European Union Parliament. Accessed April 22, 2023. https://www.europarl.europa.eu/RegData/etudes/STUD/2021/690009/EPRS_STU(2021)690009_EN.pdf.

Meir, Y., Tevet, O., Tzach, Y., Hodassman, S., Gross, R.D., and I. Kanter. 2023. "Efficient Shallow Learning as an Alternative to Deep Learning." *Nature Scientific Reports* 13 (1): 5423.

Metz, M., Smith, R., Mitchell, R., Duong, Y.T., Brown, K., Kinchen, S., and K. Lee, et al., 2021. "Data Architecture to Support Real-Time Data Analytics for the Population-Based HIV Impact Assessments." *Journal of Acquired Immune Deficiency Syndromes 1999* 87, S28–S35.

Microsoft, 2023. How technology helped Ukraine resist during wartime. Microsoft. Accessed April 22, 2023. https://news.microsoft.com/en-cee/2023/01/20/how-technology-helped-ukraine-resist-during-wartime/.

Monlezun, D.J. 2023. *The Thinking Healthcare System: Artificial Intelligence and Human Equity*. New York: Elsevier.

Myers, J. 2022. "From Pandemic to Endemic." World Economic Forum. Accessed February 4, 2023. https://www.weforum.org/agenda/2022/01/covid-19-pandemic-2022-what-next-expert-voices-from-davos.

Nadhamuni, S., John, O., Kulkarni, M., Nanda, E., Venkatraman, S., and D. Varma. 2021. "Driving Digital Transformation of Comprehensive Primary Health Services at Scale in India: An Enterprise Architecture Framework." *BMJ Global Health* 6 (Suppl 5): e005242.

Näher, A.F., Vorisek, C.N., Klopfenstein, S.A.I., Lehne, M., Thun, S., Alsalamah, S., and S. Pujari, et al., 2023. "Secondary Data for Global Health Digitalisation." *The Lancet Digital Health* 5 (2): e93–e101.

NAM. 2018. "Procuring Interoperability: Achieving High-Quality, Connected, and Person-Centered Care." In *National Academy of Medicine*, edited by P. Pronovost, M.E.J. Johns, S. Palmer, R.C. Bono, D.B. Fridsma, A. Gettinger, J. Goldman, et al.,.

Prainsack, B., El-Sayed, S., Forgó, N., Szoszkiewicz, è., and P. Baumer. 2022. "Data Solidarity: A Blueprint for Governing Health Futures." *The Lancet Digital Health* 4 (11): e773–e774.

Qato, D.M. 2022. "Reflections on 'Decolonizing' Big Data in Global Health." *Annals of Global Health* 88 (1): 56.

Rowe, J. 2019. "Comprehensive Data Architecture Critical to AI Success." Healthcare IT News. Accessed April 21, 2023. https://www.healthcareitnews.com/ai-powered-healthcare/comprehensive-data-architecture-critical-ai-success.

Rynn, S., and K. Cockayne, 2023 "Where Next for Wagner Group in Africa?" Royal United Services Institute. Accessed September 24, 2023. https://rusi.org/explore-our-research/publications/commentary/where-next-wagner-group-africa.

Simonet-Boulogne, A., Solberg, A., Sinaeepourfard, A., Roman, D., Perales, F., Ledakis, G., Plakas, I., and S. Sengupta. 2022. "Toward Blockchain-Based Fog and Edge Computing for Privacy-Preserving Smart Cities." *Frontiers in Sustainable Cities* 4, 846987.

Siwicki, B. 2021. "Why the Healthcare Cloud May Demand Zero-Trust Architecture." Healthcare IT News. Accessed April 30, 2023. https://www.healthcareitnews.com/news/why-healthcare-cloud-may-demand-zero-trust-architecture.

Sullivan, J., and B. Deese. 2021. "Building Resilient Supply Chains, Revitalizing American Manufacturing, and Fostering Broad-Based Growth." The United States White House. Accessed February 10, 2023. https://www.whitehouse.gov/wp-content/uploads/2021/06/100-day-supply-chain-review-report.pdf.

Warnat-Herresthal, S., Schultze, H., Shastry, K.L., Manamohan, S., Mukherjee, S., Garg, V., and R. Sarveswara, et al., 2021. "Swarm Learning for Decentralized and Confidential Clinical Machine Learning." *Nature* 594 (7862): 265–270.

WHO. 2021. "Global Strategy on Digital Health 2020–2025." World Health Organization. Accessed June 11, 2022. https://www.who.int/docs/default-source/documents/gs4dhdaa2a9f352b0445bafbc79-ca799dce4d.pdf.

WHO. 2023. "The WHO Hub for Pandemic and Epidemic Intelligence." Accessed April 30, 2023. https://pandemichub.who.int/.

Further reading

WHO. 2022. "Strengthening the Global Architecture for Health Emergency Preparedness, Response and Resilience." World Health Organization. Accessed April 22, 2023. https://cdn.who.int/media/docs/default-source/emergency-preparedness/20220324_wha-hepr-concept-note_final-for-publishing.pdf?sfvrsn = cffd8e98_11&download = true.

5

Framework part II: artificial intelligence + political economics

5.1 Part I: Theory

5.1.1 Political economics: metadeterminant of health determinants (and the global public health ecosystem?)

We explored up to this point how the AI-enabled global public health ecosystem, if it to be a common home for humanity, is informed by its design (finance and development) and determined by its framework (technically by its data architecture and societally by its political economics). Having dealt with the other ecosystem dimensions earlier, this chapter will now seek to better understand political economics in more of its present depth and future trajectory concretely. Why does it matter? Politics drives how the ecosystem is formed, governed, and adapts with AI technically in response to societal supplies and demands, while economics defines its funding priorities and constraints (with the abovesaid societal structure manifesting, influencing, and influenced by the underlying substructure of our common values and beliefs). A natural ecosystem like the ocean spans the algae, seagrass, corals, fish, and so on, which collectively give life to the ecosystem that runs on energy (of their individual components) and "rules" (of how they interact and benefit from each other). The health ecosystem similarly runs on financing and agreements. These *consensus* and *constraints* thus frame how the ecosystem lives, adapts, and dies. Although scientifically more complex, artificial intelligence (AI) health digital technologies are in a process sense much more straightforward and predictable: they define material problems and then develop material solutions to them. Its political economics though are significantly more societally complex, as the *how* it creates and uses the *what* of health AI is influenced by significantly greater number of factors, capable of producing significantly greater unpredictable effects and directions. Few at the dawn of 2020 predicted a pandemic and war would fundamentally, rapidly, and maybe even permanently upend our interconnected international society and global public health ecosystem. And yet here we are. From a practical standpoint, the central challenge of this ecosystem may be the *how* we should coexist in it together rather than *what* should be in it. And this challenge has both present and future aspects. Now, ideologically worsened political economic divisions may improve or doom health determinants by undermining needed collective action (particularly through either excessive globalization driving nationalism backlashes or insufficient globalization limiting efficient economies of scale). Tomorrow, the "winner" of the current global political economic competition (and in some domains even

Responsible Artificial Intelligence Re-engineering the Global Public Health Ecosystem. DOI: https://doi.org/10.1016/B978-0-443-21597-1.00005-6

conflict) will decide what kind of AI-driven global public health ecosystem we will have. The rules-based, institutional-driven liberal democratic capitalist West and the power-based, strong man-driven autocratic capitalist East are both fighting to win the support of the sovereignty-based South by arguing which is better able to provide global public goods. The 2022 United Nations Development Programme report highlighted the stakes for both these present and future domains: worsening acute 2020s polycrises from COVID to Russia's invasion of Ukraine (that exacerbate the chronic polycrises from debt distress to climate change to societal polarization) were followed by 9 out of 10 countries backsliding in human development, with 5 years lost in sustainable development goal (SDG) progress in just the first 2 years of the decade alone, with continued development reversals expected (Lusigi 2022). Political economics is so fundamental to health according to global empirical consensus that it may be *the* "meta-determinant" of the determinants of health (Labonté and Ruckert 2019). Therefore, the AI-enabled global public health ecosystem may need to understand and foster the requisite political will and economic financing for its survival, as a prerequisite for the future of our common humanity, home, and future.

5.1.2 Health politics, economics, and values: a societal ecosystem

The health ecosystem's political economics framework is the intersection of the political, economic, and value domains which we will analyze separately to see how they interact and inform the ecosystem's future evolution (Monlezun 2023). The highest profile recent health example of these relationships is the COVID-19 pandemic, as a 2023 nationwide longitudinal *Lancet* study demonstrated that higher rates of poverty and minorities (African American and Hispanics) along with less education, interpersonal trust, and healthcare access were significant and independent predictors of mortality (without any clear association with greater public health spending; Bollyky et al. 2023). Such emblematic research supports how the AI-powered ecosystem requires shared governance structures to politically define and enforce consensus-based authority and spending priorities—and the absence of such undermines effective collective action, while worsening significant global health, political, economic, and equity costs. If we cannot agree what our house should look like, we cannot agree on how to spend our money to design, make, fix, and use it together. Accordingly, the health ecosystem requires a requisite degree of shared beliefs (about who the person is, what the good is, and thus what good health is for the person and their society that in turn generate our cultural values for seeking that vision together). These values then inform how politically and economically we cooperate and compete (and to what degree conflict can occur and how it ends) within that shared societal structure or ecosystem (which generates the subecosystem of global public health). The defining challenges which AI can improve and worsen for the health ecosystem therefore break down into these domains:

1. *Politics*: "Building healthy societies" requires a political economics lens to global public health to foster cooperation, manage competition, and mitigate conflict according to Oxford University's canonical global health textbook (Birn et al. 2017, pp. 565–602).

The positive political challenges to health center on how to best facilitate not just greater global institutional governance top-down (that decentralizes power consensually and transparently in a rules-based system such as the World Health Organization [WHO]), but also healthy contributions from political, economic, academic, social media, and community sectors from the bottom-up. The negative political challenges are how best to reduce the likelihood of competition exploding into conflict, especially accelerated by global stressors such as the US—China great power competition, pandemics, climate change, and Russia's war against Ukraine (especially with its risks spilling into other European nations and to the level of nuclear weapons). Reportedly regarded by Beijing as a "wise man" respected for attempting to reduce unintended conflict escalation, the retired US Marine General and former Secretary of Defense, James Mattis, warned that militaries will spend more on bullets if they do not spend enough on bandages (Stewart and Ali 2018; Mattis 2018). Underinvesting in diplomacy (particularly in global health collaborations, aid, and economic integration) requires making up the difference in deterrence and defense in the "3-D" model of political economics. In this epoch or pivot moment of the 2020s, we are facing our history's first showdown between two global full spectrum multidomain global superpowers, at the same time we are the closest to a truly AI-enabled global public health ecosystem (CFR 2023; Monlezun 2023). And these political economic superpowers are either the biggest drivers or threats to both. Growing international cross-sector consensus warns that the mutually described strategic competition by the United States (as the main global health funder and promoter) and China (as the main engine of global economic growth) would wreck the world if it spills into open armed conflict or economic fragmentation—as appears may be increasingly likely over the semiconductor-rich Taiwan off China's coast (Miller 2022). As Chapter 1 introduced, if China follows through with its repeated threat to change the international status quo through force to "re-unify" Taiwan, as Russia attempted in 2022 to do with Ukraine, then there are broad fears that the plug would be pulled from the global digital economy. The knock-on effects even in conservative estimates would include shuttering global industrialization, trade, basic infrastructure, and even daily life for much of the global population for the foreseeable future. This would call into question even the survivability of such broad societal structures as the global public health ecosystem which runs on global cooperation (the US—Chinese conflict would jeopardize) and AI digital technologies (which depend on Taiwan's semiconductors). Extensive analyses from multiple nations and institutions suggests the United States may subsequently limp along (being the sole largely self-sufficient energy superpower and net food exporter without local security challenges), but China may not just fail but fall (with postinvasion radical decoupling by the United States and China), triggering unprecedented global shocks that may make the Great Divergence permanent and Global South's development indefinitely arrested.

   We will shortly analyze advances to manage this strategic competition, particularly with implications for the health ecosystem. But let us first analyze state cooperation and social media aspects of this ecosystem's political domain. The COVID-19 pandemic again poignantly portrays the headwinds to the effective political cooperation on which the ecosystem depends. A 2023 *Nature* investigation of the United States, Chinese, WHO, and independent academic representatives concluded that the WHO "quietly shelved" the critical second phase of its scientific analysis of the pandemic's origins due to the Chinese Communist Party blocking needed access to the WHO's independent investigators (Mallapaty 2023). A WHO epidemiologist confessed that "the politics across the world of this really hampered progress on understanding the origins." Proponents of the investigation argue that without understanding how one of the most destructive pandemics in modern history began prevents us from halting its inevitable successor. Such investigations within the global public health ecosystem sought to bypass politics so science could unify and solve shared problems. But such efforts failed to disentangle allegations from multiple nations that China blocked WHO investigation efforts, delayed reporting of COVID-19 (losing critical early time to contain or mitigate it), and contributed potentially to its origin (with the WHO unable to finish assessing the lab leak hypothesis from China's Wuhan Institute of Virology, which conducted research on novel coronaviruses and is located minutes away from the first known COVID cases). This follows the WHO Director-General along with 14 countries expressing concerns about China reportedly limiting COVID data access, including the WHO chief emphasizing that the lab leak theory should be sufficiently explored (Gan 2021).

In addition to these fundamental top-down political challenges in global governance, we explored the bottom-up challenges in the prior chapters how locally focused and globally empowered public—private—academic partnerships with greater community engagement are seeking to advance the AI-enabled global public health ecosystem. In addition, social media is increasingly emerging as a key opportunity for and challenge to the ecosystem politically. It is also doing so societally as an accelerator for not only societal progress, but also polarization amplifying individual psychopathology (with more extreme and divisive views being prioritized through AI algorithms to stimulate greater user engagement via fear and anger) and societal disintegration (through such psychopathology and misinformation entrenching greater tribalism within social networks; Anderson et al. 2021; Bremmer and Kupchan 2023). Chapter 6 will further analyze the role of AI-driven social media advancing and dividing cultures with particular implications for health (and its weaponization by strategic state and corporate competitors). We will focus here on a high-level summary of the political challenge it poses to the health ecosystem.

A 2021 Pew study of cross-sector global experts noted their consensus of the mostly negative projected impact of a "tele-everything" world, constituted by increasingly dense digital platforms integrating, engaging, and engrossing people's daily lives (Anderson et al. 2021). These trends are concurrent with the correlate rise in societal misinformation, inequities, and power differentials (with American and Chinese technology companies increasingly influencing and even to some degree "steering" users). After World War II (WWII), the United States became the largest exporter of democracy. But today, it risks becoming the largest exporter of (digital) autocracy as its technology companies are progressively producing powerful centralized AI tools that enable greater autocrat control and influence of societies domestically and globally. Such proponents of this empirical argument note how Putin's Russian government manufactured high national support in a country of nearly 150 million for its full-scale genocidal invasion of Ukraine. It did so principally through traditional and social media pushing effective propaganda (which the United Nations [UN] and hundreds of institutions and governments have since debunked), scaring Russians into believing it was actually Ukraine that was on a genocidal war path to erase the Russians and Russian culture, emboldened by the existential threat supposedly posed by the West against Russia.

Although not with the same unethical severity but at a greater geographic scale, global expert consensus noted earlier additionally highlights how AI-driven technology companies boast expanding international sway with minimal public accountability, regulation, and incentives to deviate from their key profitable objective of user engagement, even if doing so stimulates societal fragmentation of local, national, and global communities. But still amid the general freedom of information flows and their predominant Anglo-American corporate drivers in liberal democracies, a median of 57% of "ordinary citizens" worldwide believe social media for instance is a "good thing for democracy" despite its "expert" and media critics according to a 2022 Pew study (Wike et al. 2022). Although people generally acknowledge its divisive and misinformation risks accelerated by AI engagement algorithms, they mostly view social media positively to inform and unite.

2. *Economics*: The economic challenges to advancing the AI-enabled global public health ecosystem center on integral sustainable development, health delivery, and health financing through AI-accelerated public—private—academic partnerships in the value agenda (Birn et al. 2017; Anderson et al. 2021; Bremmer and Kupchan 2023; Monlezun 2023). And these challenges are more and more intertwined and interlinking all of us. Regardless of political regime, the AI-based Internet of Things on the digital edge— including ubiquitous smartphones spanning the majority of the Global North and South —are driving greater economic and digital connectivity (with digital social networks as noted earlier may then tribalize culturally to varying but still impactful degrees). The already described "Great Retirement" and concurrent "Great Baby Bust" of the richer Global North means that the historic flight of workers and capital in the world economy leaves less government and charity capital for funding global public health (and the AI digital innovations accelerating it). We therefore began exploring in Chapter 2 on finance how public—private—academic partnerships (mostly driven by US aid agencies, health organizations, and technology companies) are restructuring global public health into an AI-enabled ecosystem that reportedly is seeking to leverage synergistic skills, capacities, and funding for global well-being, driven by local representation and buy-in. Concurrently, the WHO and private sector are pushing for global universal health coverage (UHC) to get more health bang for each buck. The political optimism and health advances (particularly with the SDGs noted in Chapter 3 on development) are

articulated by such high-profile experts and consensus as Harvard University's *Business Review*, advocating for this "value-agenda" as "*the* [emphasis added] strategy that will fix health care" (Porter and Lee 2013). This approach is imported from the private sector where it is central to corporate growth. In health, it maximizes return or healthcare quality while minimizing its cost for equitable local and national benefit (through healthcare systems and public health agencies) and global benefit (through the overarching global public health ecosystem). By emphasizing a value-focused future rather than the volume-driven past, this patient- and population-focused strategy prioritizes the sustainable delivery on health needs (i.e., essential health services not simply wants, such as excessive medical imaging or nontherapeutic cosmetics) through common and comprehensive data interoperability (linking health ecosystem partners with standardized data definitions, architectures, and ecosystems). It strategically restructures how health as well-being is defined, measured, organized, and financed. No longer supply and provider driven, this approach is driven by demand and patients, with health products and services enabled digitally and coordinated globally through a force-multiplying ecosystem. America's Mayo Clinic and Cleveland Clinic, Germany's Schön Klinik, and Chinese, Indian, and African digital extensions of their national health ecosystems demonstrate concrete advances in scaling the value-agenda for local needs (Porter and Lee 2013; Monlezun 2023).

Yet significant implementation hurdles remain to a global value-agenda through such partnerships for the global public health ecosystem, including financial constraints in scaling it and political divisions funding it. Three key related economic hurdles include research and development (R&D), regulation, and public funding. The Commissioner for the US Food and Drug Administration (FDA), tasked with protecting public health by regulating the food, drugs, and medical devices for the world's largest health market, reported in 2023 that health AI digital technologies are developing faster than the FDA can regulate them (Lawrence 2023). This additionally extends to the challenge above of social media–spread misinformation (which gained prominence during the COVID-19 pandemic and which the FDA considers an "urgent threat" that has become a primary focus in its regulatory agenda; Kadakia et al. 2023). A Duke University analysis draws attention to the FDA's resultant "regulatory paradigm shift" of "[a]utomating FDA regulation" toward "postmarket surveillance and review" and away from "premarket clearance," allowing greater efficiency and adaptiveness but also risking insufficient scrutiny and public trust (Sharkey and Fodouop 2022, p. 87). The FDA is touted as being "at the forefront of" of the AI health revolution through this strategic external pivot to new AI products, sped up by its internal technologic pivot in which it enhances its regulatory work through AI (including natural language processing [NLP] and "fit-for-purpose" safety data from external device firms standardizing their data for better monitoring; p. 88). This regulatory redesign appears to already be allowing faster and cheaper development, approval, and distribution of AI digital health technologies by viewing them as pipelines of dynamic capacities rather than discrete products. How does a regulator approve an AI product for public use that can then change itself? Often deep learning (DL)-enabled AI tools, for instance, make self-corrections through more data and time, with the FDA increasingly attempting to allow it to do so, but within a trajectory bound by technological parameters that limit the degree of adaptiveness to known variations. Generally, better health AI faster means cheaper health eventually. But funding healthcare systems and public health agencies seeking to deliver it is an additional economic challenge. The failure to fix excessive health costs not only is an inherent health economic constraint, but a larger one on national and global Gross Domestic Product (GDP; with sicker and fewer workers and innovation).

There are complementary (and to some degree conflicting) calls for improving this. Harvard University's David Cutler, for instance, places greater blame on the private sector for excessive administration, prices, and technologies separated from value that drive up health costs which we have already explored in the prior chapters (Cutler 2020). Stanford University's John Cochrane places the blame on governments particularly with cross subsidies (Cochrane 2023). Generally, the US government instead of raising taxes has Medicare, for instance, pay less than what healthcare costs are for their insurees, economically driving healthcare systems to charge more than what care truly costs for privately insured patients (to cross-subsidize government paid patients). Healthier and wealthier workers using less healthcare pay more for their own insurance to cover the generally sicker, poorer, older, higher utilizer Medicare patients. By removing the price check (especially in a free market system), value is increasingly separated from costs. This generates an economic "death spiral" by reducing economic competition among new healthcare systems and companies (who otherwise generally boost efficiency and innovation while reducing costs to compete successfully against each other). This in turn increases healthcare costs, the gap between Medicare payments and those costs, the private insurance costs for the decreasing number of workers able to afford them, and thus the greater government expenditures. Cochrane points to the older cross subsidies in the US airline and telephone industries that have since been slashed (and thus unleashing private competition, lower costs, and better access to affordable services for more people) as a historical template for health economic reform. The solution globally may be some combined version of Cutler and Cochrane's approach, allowing more efficient public–private partnerships competition for higher value in the global health ecosystem as less public health (including financing) means worse healthcare (and costs), and vice versa.

3. *Values*: Ultimately, the global public health ecosystem is determined by its political economics framework, which is determined by its values foundation. Questions of how to organize and fund governance structures and institutions, whether they are more democratic or more autocratic, come down to maximizing utility from limited resources. Does the global public health ecosystem spend the bulk of its budget on lower cost prevention with greater population benefit, or higher cost acute care for lower population benefit? Our values break ties amid competing interests by articulating what we prioritize more as a people and how we balance those interests. They also highlight the fundamental divides between "value blocs" that deter faster development of the global public health

ecosystem. This includes the United States and China championing competing political economic approaches with foundationally different underlying value systems (particularly their post-Christian liberal democratic and post-Confucian/Buddhist ideologies, which nonetheless share significant common ground, moral language, and thus a pragmatic hope for a common future; Labonté and Ruckert 2019). Our values manifest a metaphysical vision, source, and guardrails for the generation, direction, and modification of our political economic structures and how competition and conflict with competitors can be resolved locally, nationally, and globally. Chapter 1 introduced how the political economic model of hyper-globalization was followed by the 2010s nationalist backlashes (including with the Trump's US election, the United Kingdom's Brexit, and China's domestic crackdown on dissent and more aggressive foreign including armed expansionist policy), in addition to the resultant reprioritization of national security, sovereignty, and ultimately self-determination as expression of collective values free of perceived excessive external interference (Lahart 2022). Such latent values help explain the widespread decried sacrifice of community's local needs and identity for global profit and power (centralized to a smaller number of states and corporations). But these values are also weaponizable for political gain. China's Chinese Communist Party (CCP) in 2021 alleged that the Five Eyes alliance of the United States, Canada, Australia, New Zealand, and the United Kingdom are "becoming a racist, and mafia-styled community" with "neo-Nazi" leaders threatening the "diversity of the modern world" (WSJ Editorial Board 2021). Such critique purportedly invoked the West's own "woke" critics espousing "progressive" values that Putin explicitly referenced, including in his May 2023 speech on Russia's Victory Day alleging woke "western globalist elites" are using Ukraine as a proxy to wage "a real war...against us" and Russia's "traditional values" (Sauer 2023). Such polarizing comments come after the International Criminal Court's (ICC's) conviction of Putin in 2023 as a war criminal for his unprovoked genocidal invasion of Ukraine, cited in Chapter 1, in addition to a UN report citing the Chinese government may be committing "crimes against humanity" (Maizland 2022). The report was corroborated by multiple nations' governments and independent journalists (using satellite imaging, testimonies, and leaked Chinese records) documenting China's genocidal campaign against its over 1 million Muslim Uyghur minorities through forcible mass relocation, sterilization, and separation of children from their parents (what Putin was charged by the ICC as doing).

The ambiguity and superficiality of "values" therefore are persistent challenges in the political economics of the global public health ecosystem. They "work" generally well to vaguely defend high-level political economic consensus on health AI (as with the abovesaid chapters' discussions of private, public, and global principles for responsible AI) when there is general alignment of like-minded ecosystem partners. But they also "work" it seems nearly equally well as political economic weapons of rhetoric among global strategic competitors that can precipitate, facilitate, or even "justify" conflicts. Therefore, there is a sustained and systematic need to clarify substantive definitions and convergence of values across the global public health ecosystem and our larger global human community. If globalized political economics are our day's *meta*determinant of health determinants, then our values are the *meaning* behind them. Clarifying what we mean when we use terms and why we are using them become indispensable to break logjams in political economic debates about what the practical framework of the ecosystem's political economics should be today and tomorrow. The prior chapters have progressively described the growing global divides between a global political economic structure that is primarily *rules*-based (democratic generated consensus-based rules governing institutions that decentralize power among the population) and *ruler*-based (autocratic generated control-driven rulers overseeing hierarchies that centralize power among individuals; Monlezun 2023). Both ends of the political economic capitalist spectrum propose they better protect people's values and more fairly distribute greater benefits of globalism (i.e., superior health and wealth) balanced with nationalism (i.e., superior security and self-determination).

There is increased international debate, academic scholarship, and cross-sector policies aimed at what may be termed "local globalism" to determine the optimal balance in governance (within and among competing political economic structures) for what the WHO termed "global public goods" for health (WHO 2002). As Chapter 1 described the public health transition from the second to third millennia, the WHO pivoted from an early post-WWII commander to more coordinator role. This was further evidenced by its then Director General, Brundtland, who oversaw the 1987 report formalizing the SDGs and the 2002 WHO report on global public goods advancing their foundational values and practical realization (driven by the more Western dignity-based democratic capitalist approach of improving health through wealth synergistically, meant to ultimately advance the values of individual freedom and the common good). Such goods manifested a common value hierarchy balancing individual freedoms with public goods that therefore ordered its distinctive Western political economic structure. In addition, as the prior chapters sought to analyze, the post-COVID 2020s era is pivoting to a more inclusive decolonization of such values as dignity and justice to revise the global political economic structure for the North and South. The UN's (2020) policy brief emphasized these public goods as key to the post-COVID health and political economic recovery, in addition to how these public goods cannot solely be produced through market economics (state centralized or more open). They need multilateral cooperative, coordinated, cross-sector, and collective actions often through public–private–academic partnerships across communities, institutions, and states. These cooperative initiatives range from vaccine R&D, pandemic surveillance, data security and interoperability, and responsible health AI standards. But the UN emphasized how such political economic structures are insufficient. They also require such global values underlying them as "solidarity" to fairly share the material goods (i.e., vaccines, food, and housing) and immaterial goods (i.e., freedom, rights, and duties) necessary for individual and collective flourishing. Citing "dignity" and "rights" in declarations and policies are not enough in this account. Rather, their substantive description and normative implications must be considered and then inform such derivative values as global solidarity, made concrete in global policy and programs which manifest inclusive, equitable, and efficient governance in the global public health ecosystem facilitating these global public goods. Solidarity, or understanding ourselves as members of the common human family with equal intrinsic value as such, implies the complementary moral value of local subsidiarity in which higher levels of the social hierarchy respect and support local cultures, agency, identity, and governance. Both operational values invoked by the UN assume and are derived from the deeper metaphysical value of individual human dignity (or integral and intrinsic value of the human person), which finds its fulfillment and fullest realization in the common good (encompassing the good of individuals freely acting through duty to advance the common good of their community, which in turn facilitates the individual goods needed for their fulfillment) (Monlezun 2023). Solidarity informs and defends the need to leverage the scope of the AI-powered global public health ecosystem (with its partners' resources and technologies to treat with equal regard every member of the human family internationally), while subsidiarity informs and defends its scale (right-sizing the application of that scope however big or small, global or local, for the needs of the people served).

There is broad awareness how democracies and autocracies can both devolve into totalitarianism—respectively soft and hard totalitarianism—in which both dignity and goods are diminished or denied for much of a population (Tocqueville 1840). The 19th-century French sociologist and political scientist, Alexis de Tocqueville, cautioned against the radical extremes of both (as he lived through both the French Revolution's bloody Republic and Napoleon's subsequent despotism). He argued that collective democratic rule of the many over the many (without sufficient institutional checks and balances) may eventually collapse into "a network of small, complicated rules," in which the powerful "democratic" ruling few with shrinking accountability and social trust increasingly control the weak many. The way democracies in general can (and America specifically did, at least at the time) avoid this fraught political economic fate is by nourishing its common integral values uniting the local community, or "habits of the heart" as he described (i.e., equality of opportunity, civil dialogue, meritocracy leadership, and collective progress toward the common good). Such substantive common values flow from a deeper minimum shared metaphysical vision, as with the 1776 US Declaration of Independence in which the American colonies first rose up against the supposedly imperial British monarch to declare what became the liberal democratic capitalist vision which generated America and its post-WWII liberal world order:

> We hold these truths to be self-evident, that all men are created equal, that they are endowed by their Creator with certain unalienable Rights, that among these are Life, Liberty and the pursuit of Happiness. That to secure these rights, Governments are instituted among Men, deriving their just powers from the consent of the governed...But when a long train of abuses and usurpations...reduce them under absolute Despotism, it is their right, it is their duty, to throw off such Government (US 1776).

Now in a pluralistic globalized modern world, is it possible for our global human community and its global public health ecosystem to generate a decolonized, dynamic, and self-corrective values foundation that allows effective, efficient, and equitable governance?

Can such common values allow a resilient and adaptive political economic framework? (Such as local globalism generally and its Personalist Liberalism specifically we will explore shortly). Can such a values-driven framework successfully maximize "managed strategic competition" and minimize the risks of catastrophic conflict among different political economic blocs such as the West and East, while enhancing cooperative collaboration between the North and South (Rudd 2022)? There are sustained signs these are global aspirations shared in different geopolitical blocs. While Xi's Belt and Road Initiative (BRI) for instance reportedly builds up developing nations, he urged private local companies through his featured domestic policy of "Common Prosperity" to "be rich and loving" by more fairly sharing their growth with the people in a "community of shared interests," a common "family" (Tian 2023). We will therefore shortly analyze emerging solutions to these value challenges from the perspective of the AI-powered global public health ecosystem. We will particularly assess if the growing international support for such a local globalism approach can pragmatically complement the comparative advantages of both dimensions (with local equity and global efficiency), including through more inclusive, just, ecological, and resilient value supply chains balancing local and global political economic demands through subsidiarity and solidarity values. Especially we will survey an approach represented with the 2023 simplified formulation of health's future as $H = AE^2$ (in which "H" or health at global scale can be shown to be generated by the product of efficient and responsible AI or "A" and equity or "E" squared; Monlezun 2023).

5.1.3 From background and breakdown to breakthrough: managed strategic (cooperative) competition

5.1.3.1 Background: health political economics

The previous four chapters historically and technically built up to the current epoch moment describing the evolution of health political economics within the larger global political economics. What we call China and India today, formed generally by Confucian, Buddhist, and Hindu values, traded back and forth in premodern times for the title of the largest nation and economy (as they collectively accounted for approximately half of the world's GDP from the 1st to 19th centuries; Lin and Rosenblatt 2012). Meanwhile, Western Europe emerged from the fall of the Greek and Roman empires to be formed by Judeo-Christian values until the other epoch dawn of the modern age in which the Scientific Revolution, Enlightenment, and Industrial Revolutions powered its eventual transition from its Imperial Age of empire conquest of much of the world to the post-WWII liberal world order built by the purported American "empire by invitation" rather than invasion (Ferguson 2005). By the dawn of the third millennium, the US alliance was humanity's most powerful empire, albeit one that largely denied this label and structure. It nonetheless globalized its classical liberal values of dignity, freedom, equality, democracy, free market economics, and digital industrialization, in addition to over 750 military installations in two of every three countries worldwide (institutionalizing this power through its multinational companies and nongovernment organizations including the UN, WHO, and World Bank made in its image and led by its allies). Then in the 2000s, the United States tried to remake communist China in its image by admitting it to this world order, only to find out by the late 2010s that its state centralized capitalism not only retained its Marxist−Leninist communism, but it also sought to progressively and explicitly challenge the United States for generating and leading the world order in its (Xi-dominated) image. We analyzed how global public health became a first for humanity, facilitating record levels of health, wealth, and equality the world over with sophisticated science, global justice, and cooperative collaboration diffusing through the public and private sectors and rich and poor communities. But particularly following the Great Recession, COVID, Russia's invasion, and other rising geopolitical tensions, there is growing international concern that sustainable AI-enabled global public health may be an unattainable common goal. It may even soon be collateral loss in this global competition.

As we have gradually led up to, there appears to be not only intensifying strategic West−East competition threatening to divide the world into similar value blocs of competing political economic paradigms. According to the Harvard and Stanford historian, Niall Ferguson, it may even be generating Cold War II (Ferguson 2022). Except this one seems increasingly fought principally over global AI, semiconductor, and economic dominance, while remaining riddled with persistent and interlinked armed conflicts, both proxy and open. According to Ferguson, there is the haunting historical specter of Pearl Harbor over Taiwan in the face of China's threat of force to retake it, particularly after the discussion of the 2022 US export controls attempting to temporarily cut China off from advanced semiconductors in Chapter 1. Such AI and digital technologies are more critical to today's daily survivability let alone growth of nations than the oil of the early 1900s. Japan prior to declaring war on the United States in 1941 launched a massive surprise bombing attack on America's Pearl Harbor in response to the United States blocking oil exports to Japan, which itself was a response to Japan's invasion of the Indo-China region. In the strike's aftermath, imperial Japan, Nazi Germany, and fascist Italy declared war on the United States, triggering the American entrance to the eventual victorious Chinese and British war alliance. By May 2023, Japan hosted the G7 (the intergovernmental forum of the world's largest advances economies that also are the largest among liberal democracies including the United States and United Kingdom). It did so in Hiroshima that had been decimated by the first wartime use of nuclear arms. By the G7 2023 summit, it was remade into the platform denouncing Russian imperialism and Chinese "economic coercion," while advocating for global rules-based cooperation by all nations on "trustworthy AI" standards, fair clean energy transition, free trade, and sustained development support (Irish and Murakami 2023). There, the G7 welcomed India, other Global South representatives, and Ukraine's Zelenskyy who after speaking with the largely nonaligned Arab League the day prior thanked in person India's Prime Minister, Narendra Modi, for India's support of democratic and UN rule of law defending states' sovereignty and borders (Wire 2023). Modi responded with reiterating India's continued pharmaceutical and humanitarian support for Ukraine, in addition to its political support to help end the war as promptly as possible with a just and durable peace, for in his words, "I don't consider it merely as a political or economic matter, but it is about human values." Such comments are particularly notable considering India is not only the most politically and economically influential Southern state by the early 2020s, but also the vanguard for nonaligned nations in the post-WWII period.

Such potentially era-defining events suggest an emerging three-part political economic structure for our globalized AI digital age in which the North's liberal democratic Western nations and more autocratic capitalist Eastern nations (particularly China and Russia) compete for greater power between the two blocs, in addition to greater influence and partnerships with the mostly nonaligned developing Global South hedging between them both (Monlezun 2023). The overarching "thin" world order over these competitive domains features a rules-based human security-driven multilateral world order (Bremmer and Kupchan 2023; Monlezun 2023). This political economic structure facilitates its underlying AI-driven global digital ecosystem, binding these blocs together technologically and economically. It also deepens the framework's foundational common human security values of integral sustainable development and self-determination as the necessary means to the end of wellbeing —individually, communally, and thus globally. In this framework, democratic and autocratic states cooperate for shared security and compete fairly for shared stability according to consensus-based rules rather than imperial power dynamics (while having strategic guardrails preventing and mitigating conflicts). Poverty, noncommunicable diseases (NCDs), pandemics, climate change, and conflicts in decreasing order of total mortality therefore became shared existential threats to this global human security framework of values-based health political economics—as the human person is the fundamental reality and common denominator of all political economic structures, digital technologies, and health ecosystems. And it appears there is global momentum advancing this architecture. India, China, Brazil, and Indonesia joined the 122 countries voting in a 2023 UN resolution to acknowledge the "aggression by the Russian Federation against Ukraine" violating its sovereignty and security (with only five votes against the declaration, including Russia, Belarus, Syria, North Korea, and Nicaragua; UN 2023). In addition, China brokered a historic "peace" deal normalizing diplomatic ties between Saudi Arabia and Iran in 2023, while expanding bilateral infrastructure and green energy−orientated raw mineral investment deals in Zimbabwe and throughout sub-Sahara Africa (Cloud and Ramzy 2023). Some Western critics argue the US and European deinvestment and deinvolvement in such areas to protest their states' human rights abuses are being filled by predatory Chinese debt-trap diplomacy and economic coercion. But they nonetheless offer attractive financial offers particularly to authoritarian leaning states by bypassing domestic human rights concerns for more pragmatic interest-based multilateralism. Such critics counter that short-term smaller economic wins undermine longer term political stability and sustainable and equitable economic growth by benefiting China first and local elites second, leaving their developing populations further behind. Chinese and their allies' proponents point to shared wins, minus the West's supposed ideological rhetoric of rights.

Western states generally have counter by highlighting collective resilience and security through AI-driven technological and integral sustainable development of the global public health ecosystem, in addition to a more ecological and inclusive global economy and supportive institutions as seen with the G7 above (Bremmer and Kupchan 2023). This "derisking" emphasizes the dual approach of engaging with China and other autocratic regimes in productive areas while hedging against their actions in others which undermine national and human security (Irish and Murakami 2023). This is done by on one hand emphasizing health collaboration especially in the global health priorities of poverty, NCDs, communicable diseases (CDs), and climate change. On the other hand, it includes in parallel targeted friend-shoring to strengthen diversified supply chain resilience away from excessive dependence on single points of supply chain failure or perceived economic coercion, that is, with China's technology and Russian energy firms. The related "China +1" policy seeks to diversify global supply chains through increasing economic collaboration with India, Vietnam, and other Global South nations that are both democratic and autocratic leaning, while attempting to preserve minimum standards for worker rights (Bremmer and Kupchan 2023). Yet the more extensive decoupling and less extensive deriskign approaches still both entail a growing fundamental risk to the global overarching political economics, especially for the embedded global health ecosystem by threatening to increasingly divide and so undermine the regulated technology and information flows required to empower health collaborations (Spence 2023). As the United States seeks to strengthen its political economic cooperation with its allies (i.e., with the high-profile Japanese and Dutch joining 2022 US export controls of advanced semiconductors to China), China is concurrently racing to shore up its technological, economic, and energy self-reliance. This regionalization (and in some ways deglobalization) translates into less efficient economic integration and multilateral and multinational cooperation. It in turn undercuts global responsiveness to recurrent shocks, from health (especially pandemics) to politics (conflicts especially driven by revisionist rogue state actors) to economics (inflation and recession) to technology (including generative AI and the absence of global standards of this explosive technology). Global societal cooperation and technological innovation and diffusion thus suffer—along with cooperative technological acceleration of such critical sectors as the global public health ecosystem, which requires a certain degree of consensus and funding for the global political economic structure to function (Spence 2023). Health's political economics up to this point therefore appear to be a mixed bag of successes and failures, promises and shortcomings at best, clouding future projections and solutions.

5.1.3.2 Breakdown: democratic versus autocratic capitalism

To plot a sustainable global path forward for health political economics, we will therefore pivot to a brief (and as balanced as possible) structural analysis of democracies and autocracies, their increasingly influential cooperative solution, and then its application for the AI-powered global public health ecosystem. The structural analysis will focus on efficient, sustainable, and collaborative dimensions:

1. *Efficient*: Chapter 1 considered empirically how the world was essentially capitalist by the 1990s, dominated by free market economics that were formalized by the 18th-century Scottish moral philosopher, Adam Smith (Sachs 1999). By the 21st century, China's

Peking University economist, Zhang Weiying, observed how "China's rapid economic development over the past four decades is a victory of Adam Smith's concept of the market," as its socialist and communist regime opened up in the 1980s with private property rights and market reforms, followed by a plummeting of extreme poverty from 88% in 1981 to less than 1% by 2021 (Zitelmann 2023). Since the 1980s, states have generally fallen on the more liberal democratic end of the political spectrum (shortened below simply as "democratic" in its general modern colloquial use) or illiberal democratic (or autocratic; Kotkin 2015). Both political regime types must maintain sufficient societal support to preserve power, typically by "proving" they provide superior public goods in national security, political stability, and economic prosperity (in descending order of societal "need") compared to alternative actors or regime types. Generally, democracies note their reportedly superior historic track record generating unprecedented health, wealth, and equality for humanity as discussed in Chapter 1 to the degree and duration their structural elements are adapted, compared to the more ancient autocratic formula of foreign imperialism and domestic suppression under centralized rulers. Democracies' short political economic pitch is that humanity's (and thus our health ecosystem's) future is democratic as it best represents and protects the person as the basic building block of any political structure, while it also is our present world order (without any state power predominating now nor in the foreseeable future) and recent past (with more global health, wealth, equality, and stability the more it is adopted). According to this argument, democracy at its core is freedom and equality along with cooperation and competition, held in balance by being rooted in human dignity and collectively aimed at the common good. The alternative is our long premodern and early modern imperial past in which strong men dominated the masses domestically and internationally through conquest, resolving disputes through conflict and power rather than consensus and values. Autocracies generally respond that democracies seek to impose their values and political economic structures on other peoples, especially in ways that destabilize their politics, undermine their economics, and erode their cultural identities. These questions are of course politically charged and difficult to measure let alone identify a "winner." So for what is most relevant for our health purposes here and what is pragmatically much more possible to quantify, we can see how the largest empirical head-to-head health comparison of 158 countries from 1995−2015 demonstrated that democracies over autocracies generate superior health ecosystem efficiency in greater population health, including with lower costs, corruption, and inequalities (with such estimates holding even after repeated robustness checks for endogeneity and diverse indicators for democracy and population health; Roessler and Schmitt 2021). The superior health benefit of democracies over autocracies were greater in higher income nations also (we will analyze the Bremmer J-curve to explain this shortly below in this section). These findings are additionally relevant for the larger political economic debate as the regime type that best secures the most critical public goods (namely health, without which other public goods are irrelevant and weakened) would presumably have the strongest case for being the superior regime type.

2. *Sustainable*: The Pew Center documented how democracies have continued to expand globally to include nearly 60% of nations following 20th-century decolonization, while autocracies have fallen to a historic low of 13% (with the remainder having mixed elements; Desilver 2019). The consistent consensus estimates on sustainability by political regime are reflected by the largest and longest study of its kind by an international team from India, Bangladesh, the United Kingdom, and the United States with Harvard University (Sen et al. 2017). It analyzed 125 nations from 1950–2010 and concluded that democracies outperform autocracies in the long-term (through higher per capita incomes and political regime stability), medium-term (preventing large growth collapses), and short-term (reducing volatility). The study did show that party-based autocracies (i.e., China's CCP rather than personalist, military, or monarchy autocracies) may produce superior medium term growth acceleration, though they do not reduce the size of deaccelerations after such high-risk growth is followed by implosion. It additionally appears that the political sustainability of the regime type is largely driven by its economic performance for its people (which is intrinsically tied to its defense capacities). The case example of these trends was the unprecedented explosion in China's economic growth after its 1990s free market reforms and 2000s entry into the US-led free trade world order, followed by its political influence expansion (through the BRI and institutional leadership in the UN, WHO, etc.) and increasingly assertive military buildup and threats against Taiwan and neighbors in the South China Sea. But there is growing global questioning by 2023 internally and externally about the CCP's ability to sustain growth let alone stability in the increasingly complex and globally interconnected state. Its debt-to-GDP has surged to over 295% (outpacing all other emerging markets combined), 60% of local governments risk exceeding debt ceilings, foreign direct investment has been sliced in half to less than 2% from the prior decade, GDP growth has been on a steady general decline since 2010, its population continues to rapidly age and retire without sufficient replacement workers, youth employment is ballooning (to over 20%), and domestic consumption remains less than 40% (about half of the United States and much less than what is required for stable domestic growth; Xie and Douglas 2023). The CCP accordingly is shifting its messaging to how it can preserve state security and identity (and deemphasizing its previous focus on sustaining economic growth and equality).

   Stephen Kotkin, the Pulitzer Prize finalist and Princeton University historian (studied at the CCP's school under Xi before he was elevated to the government's supreme position), argues that it is this sustainability that modern autocratic regimes assert is their primary advantage over democracies: unity through repressed dissent can stabilize a state in the short run, but it also reduces the self-corrective dynamism of collective intelligence required for countries to adapt to changing domestic and international shocks and challenges (Kotkin 2015). Structurally, this sustainability is pursued in the most successful and powerful current autocratic regime, Xi's China as a successor to Stalin's Soviet Union. It is a Marxist–Leninist political economic paradigm of participatory totalitarianism, centralized capitalism, illiberal modern nationalism, and coercive power expansion internationally (through financing, supply chain, and military power projection with disproportionate domestic benefit over partner benefits). It is ultimately focused on *regime* survival, even if it means sacrificing economics and its citizens for politics and the collective. But according to Kotkin's analysis, autocratic regimes lack mature democracies' self-corrective mechanisms, from free markets to elections to dissent and self-critique. They are ultimately focused on *state* survival (which thus allows the country to right its course when heading in the wrong direction), as politics and the individual complement economics and the collective, and vice versa. Maximizing individual good thus leads to maximizing the collective good in a positive sum game, in contrast to the autocratic zero-sum game. To illustrate this, we can remember the Soviet's Berlin Wall built ideologically and concretely to block the poorer Communist-run East Germans from fleeing to the richer self-governed West Berlin Germans.

These structural differences appear to translate empirically and historically as noted earlier into greater sustainability for democracies over autocracies, though with an important caveat about the maturity of democracies and autocracies. Bremmer's novel J-curve describes how states' sustainability generally falls along a slanted "J" representing stability (y-axis) and openness (x-axis; Bremmer, 2006). More mature and closed autocratic states on the far left of the curve can be initially stable by centralizing the people's power among a smaller group of elites and even an individual (as dissent is purged and prevented through censorship and propaganda). Yet the magnitude of this stability is less than the more mature and open advanced democracies on the far right of the curve. As autocratic regimes open by moving from left to right (as the Soviet Union did in the 1980s), they temporarily can become less stable as power begins to decentralize (at the lowest point on the "J" curve). Yet as power becomes more transparently and effectively shared through robust consensus-based democratic institutions (operating between and by the people and their leaders), openness and stability accelerate in parallel to greater heights than their autocratic alternatives. From left to right of the curve, state's structural transformation can be understood as the transition from anarchy to autocracy to immature democracy (mixed with autocratic elements) to mature democracy. These advanced democracies take longer to fall back to the lowest point compared to autocracies should they reverse course. The most competitive and adaptive capitalist states therefore generally are the most open, stable, and sustainable democracies (and thus regime type overall). Their people are free to correct in real-time and at scale with a complexity that even the most efficient autocratic regimes have not sustainably matched. In AI-driven health ecosystems, more open and stable democratic states generally have the more open and rapid data flows driving more effective and efficient AI development and governance, in turn driving more adaptive and competitive digital economies overtaking and staying ahead of foreign competitors (Monlezun 2023). Accordingly, the World Happiness Report by the UN's Sustainable Development Solutions Network consistently up to 2023 showed the global consensus how states' primary objective should be their people's happiness (as self-reported satisfaction with life or fulfillment of it, principally by sufficient health, wealth, and connectivity), and that empirically, the happiest states are mature democracies (Koop and Routley 2023).

3. *Cooperative*: Democracies appear to cooperate more durably, effectively, and extensively domestically (across private and public sectors) and internationally (with both democracies and autocracies; Mattes and Rodríguez 2014; Monlezun 2023). A multidecade global empirical analysis of the 10 Million International Dyadic Events dataset support how democracies globally cooperate and even collaborate to a greater degree of interdependence and institutional density (across more of the private–public sectors) with other states regardless of regime type. This advantage does appear to extend (though with less success) for mixed regimes in which party and military-based autocracies (in contrast to personality-based ones) feature greater democratic traits like greater transparency, accountability, and adaptability. Generally, democracies collaborate with different regimes and regime types (as sustainable partnerships with shared goals and mutual durable benefit), while autocracies generally are reduced to more limited cooperation (as temporary transactions for transient individual overlapping goals with mutual often shorter-term benefit). Otherwise, greater collaboration can accelerate greater state openness and thus undermine centralized autocratic power, which such regimes often seek to prevent and mitigate. And generally, there are greater structural barriers to public–private sector collaboration and cooperation within autocracies as unchecked power accumulation for instance among corporations and cultural groups are often perceived as threats to state power (Chin 2018; Yuan 2022). For example, China since 2010 consistently spends more on its inward facing domestic security than outward facing military security forces (with both surging forward much faster than its economy), especially as massive state investments in AI are accelerating its AI-powered digital mass surveillance, censorship, and detention infrastructure that is the most sophisticated and extensive in history. In addition, even state-aligned high-level Chinese figures are cautioning about the CCP's Great Tech Clampdown of 2020–2022 in which Xi's regime targeted the "golden goose" of China's technological growth. It did so using what internal leading figures describe as opaque, shifting, and even arbitrary fines, leader removals, and CCP leadership insertion into its technology corporations. Domestic and international short and long-term investments, workers, innovation, entrepreneurship, and collaboration are therefore drying up in China's technology sector, with internal and external analysts concerned these trends may therefore fry the "battery" charging the "EV" of China's growth, in exchange for redistributing that power back to the CCP rather than actually making its technology sector more accountable and responsible to the Chinese people (whose prosperity and opportunities are hurt as the technology sector hurts).

This collaborative distinction between both regimes is particularly relevant for digital regulation, especially the AI-powered internet enabling the global digital ecosystem and its subsidiary, the global public health ecosystem. Without digital connectivity, they cannot function technologically. But without their data, they cannot function practically. And competing regulatory frameworks, following their diverse political economic regimes, only complicate how they are allowed to grow, develop, and operate. There is a widespread cross-sector consensus that global cooperation of any meaningful kind in general requires cooperation in these digital regulatory frameworks specifically (Echikson 2022). Money, goods, and services only flow if their underlying data does. And how governments regulate the technology firms that facilitate this flow can either block its necessary flow or propagate harmful effects of its abuses if left unchecked. Among the dominant regulatory blocs, Europe is often critiqued for overregulating, the United States for underregulating, and China for weaponizing regulation (coercing foreign firms to give up their data and intellectual property, cracking down on domestic firms seen as starting to rival the CCP's power, and breaking international trade rules to supercharge its domestic firms to overtake global competitors). These collaborative challenges additionally are complicated by China's unique approach to digital regulation as its existing laws require all Chinese companies to hand over their data to the CCP, including its domestic technology firms that bank health, biomedical, genetic, financial, and demographic data even from people in other countries (see Article 7 of China's National Intelligence Law and Article 28 of its Cybersecurity Law; Goujon 2023). Proponents argue doing so protects the Chinese people and the fair competitiveness of their companies. Multinational critics assert that China weaponizes "data security" to imperialistically expand its digital totalitarianism domestically and internationally (including in mandated data localization, restricted cross-border data flows, forced transfer of source code, and practically unlimited state surveillance). This progressively antagonistic competition (framed as a democratic vs. authoritarian) in the very digital infrastructure undergirding the global human ecosystem (which enables its constitutive health ecosystem) therefore threatens our shared capacity for any substantive modern cooperation.

5.1.3.3 Managed strategic cooperative competition: (digital) sovereignty versus imperialism

The US–China multidomain global relationship is becoming the critical test of whether democracies or autocracies can work better with others now and in the foreseeable future, while each trade blame for why the breakdown of collaboration and cooperation is threatening to fracture into greater competition and conflict (from health to technology to development; Goujon 2023; Rudd 2022). Further, this regime tension is straining collaboration and cooperation for the rest of the world's nations, as others generally try to resist the pull to anchor themselves in one camp or another amid the inherent dependencies of the world on both of these top global powers. Both nations are increasingly engaged in digital indigenization policies, protectionist industrial policies (state-directed and preferential domestic investments), export controls (limiting domestic technologies for foreign consumption), outbound investment screening (reducing domestic private equity in foreign countries), and aggressive cybersecurity. Following China's multiyear zero-COVID policy and growing international resistance to its alleged economic and technological coercion, the amount of foreign direct investment has flatlined, and its backers have shrunk to mostly industry partners while the United States is expanding its alliance of technological, political, and economic partners (leaving China to respond with its own retaliatory measures and doubling down on its BRI networked nations).

And data is the deadlock. The minimum global cooperation and integration of technological and political economics for the AI-powered global human and health ecosystems are progressively ensnared in entrenched battle lines over digital sovereignty versus imperialism, transcending the basic distinction of democracies versus autocracies. According to public, private, and academic analysts domestically and internationally, China may generally be characterized as pursuing a more imperial approach (maximizing societal censorship and information control) in contrast to the United States and Europe prioritizing a more sovereign approach (maximizing individual agency and information access; ANU, 2023; CFR, 2023; Cho, 2020; Rudd, 2022; SCCEI, 2023; Yang, 2022; Yu-Hsin Lin and Milhaupt, 2021). Some critics describe the dichotomy in terms of China's "digital totalitarianism" within its borders including with its Social Credit System and outside those borders through its coercive attempts to confiscate foreign firms' technologies, algorithms, and data (including for non-Chinese citizens). Such elements are becoming flash points as critics allege the Social Credit System is not just a domestic authoritarian template, but also represents an imperialistic trajectory extending China's technological power the world over to control the Big Data that powers the world's economy. Officially, the credit system, for instance, is meant to be an AI-accelerated, data-driven approach to comprehensively and extensively rank Chinese citizens and corporations according to their "trustworthiness" or "social creditworthiness." Notably, English-based media reporting has often misrepresented this system. But generally it is officially intended to incentivize citizens and companies to reliably contribute to the common good through rewards and punishments (including state restriction of individuals sending their children to private schools, traveling by plane, taking certain jobs, and receiving loans, while companies can be fined or have their leadership replaced or augmented by CCP members). Caution has been raised nonetheless as empirical analyses by the City University of Hong Kong and Stanford University, for instance, suggest the corporate dimension of the score system may be trending toward "surveillance state capitalism" (Yu-Hsin Lin and Milhaupt 2021). The first publicly available scores from Zhejiang Province demonstrated that Chinese corporations showing greater political allegiance and support of the CCP (through corporate governance and donations to CCP-preferred policies) receive higher scores—not firms that demonstrate greater economic prosperity and transparency. The Australian government additionally raised concerns about China's alleged exporting of digital imperialism, as with its "global registry of Uighurs" reportedly used to coerce family members globally into providing personal information for tighter social control, expanding its BRI's "digital Silk Road" (and Chinese technology companies' surveillance on BRI built infrastructure through other nations), and exporting its mass surveillance technology intentionally to regimes generally characterized as repressive autocracies, including in Zimbabwe and Venezuela (ANU 2023).

The four major dimensions in which collaboration opportunities risk becoming increasingly antagonistic competition are the same global policy priorities China appears to have set in the Xi era: global health, development, digital governance, and climate change (CFR 2023, Monlezun 2023). The cultural value paradigms of the Chinese *zhongguo* ("Middle Kingdom") and American exceptionalism appear to fundamentally stifle or at least challenge effective political economic cooperation in these areas. China has long described itself as the civilization center of the world (as the largest economy for 18 of the last 20 centuries minus the two latest, thus expecting tribute from the rest of the world supposedly trailing it in cultural and scientific sophistication and political economic power). Similarly, the United States from its earliest days according to de Tocqueville saw its unique historical identity (Protestant Christianity-shaped, capitalist framed, liberal democratic operated, technologically driven, and geographically secure) as propelling it to supposedly generate unique positive impact globally for freedom, prosperity, and equality—unlike past imperial empires from which it arguably saw itself as the definitive break from, to instead achieve the highest evolution of governance regimes and thus of human societies (Ferguson 2005). So, the two states collide. Xi's China increasingly counters the perceived US-born and led rules-based international order by its own global health policies (criticized for their opaque, transactional nature), digital governance (criticized for its reported censorship and control locally and globally through AI digital technologies, principally as means of state power rather than societal tools for the people's good), development (with the BRI lacking transparency, accountability, and adherence to environmental and safety standards), and climate change (mostly focused on improving Chinese market share of green energy while still exporting BRI coal factories, producing over two times America's carbon dioxide emissions). The United States says China's BRI specifically, like its global policies generally, are fundamentally tools meant to extend China's power at the expense rather than development of others (i.e., using its own companies, workers, and capital to build infrastructure and thus market shares and often controlling stakes in other nations, which cannot afford or proportionally benefit from this infrastructure), unlike, for instance, the West's focus on soliciting local aid and development requests from and co-designing programs with mostly Southern partners to allow mutual consensus-based benefit as durable allies rather than simply as transactional business partners. China instead says the United States hypocritically preaches rights while trouncing them for its own interests. Yet the most clear, empirical, immediate, and pervasive global challenge in this cooperation devolving into competition is likely in its digital domain. If China restricts internet and information access to its own people (among the most populous on the planet) and pushes its digital governance model to other countries, while the United States and its Western and Southern allies champion a more open model, how can data (and thus cooperative AI-powered global public health) flow past this new Great Wall of great power competition?

China's nonaligned movement historically invoked principles that Mao himself adopted from the UN Charter, beginning with sovereignty (implying territorial integrity, within which a states' people collectively assert their self-rule and self-determination of their cultural values, embodied by their political economic structures sufficiently free of external undue influence; Ferguson 2005). The Eurasia Groups thus highlights AI digital technologies as "weapons of mass disruption," spurring the era's overriding global political economic challenges (Bremmer and Kupchan 2023). These are especially concentrated in their potential for progressive destabilization of global power imbalances, international relations, and domestic cohesion. All of these are critical requirements for the collective generation and sustainment of the global public health ecosystem. And still the four abovesaid primary global policy dimensions for our existential crises require US and China collaboration to succeed for humanity, not just their own countries.

The hope for cooperation appears to be dimming, however. Expressing China's near-term expectations for its relationships with the United States and other "major countries," Xi's 2022 report to the 20th CCP Congress (as its 5-year strategic plan) notably replaced "cooperation" (合) with the toned-down target of "positive interaction" (良性互动) to advance "peaceful coexistence, overall stability, and balanced development" internationally (Lin et al. 2022). "National security" (安全) was Xi's most common phrase in his 2-hour report at 91 mentions (nearly double the mentions in the prior 5-year report, with development in the context of the BRI mentioned only twice). National security is explicitly asserted as the "bedrock of national rejuvenation" with the "unification" of Taiwan as its "natural requirement." Reunification is the capstone to this rejuvenation, Xi's primary ideologically grounded grand vision in political economics, meant to restore the greatness of Chinese civilization that stretches back over five millennia to its purported rightful historic place as the world's Middle Kingdom. "Cooperation" and "diversity" therefore appears to be advocated from both the Chinese and American views of the world, but only when the world predominantly runs according to their own vision of it.

Thus, we turn to what may be a breakthrough in the otherwise seeming linear trend from cooperation breakdown to escalating conflict—the sovereign values-rooted political economic strategy of "managed strategic competition." It is influentially defined and defended for this relationship by the former Australian prime minister and current ambassador to the United States, Kevin Rudd, who is fluent in Chinese (AND repeatedly credited as a constructive diplomat by CCP officials), trained by Oxford University, and one of the premier Chinese analysts (according to Henry Kissinger, the Nobel Prizing winning Cold War architect and former US Secretary of State and National Security Advisor; Rudd 2022). Like Kissinger did for US−Soviet relations in the 20th century, Rudd attempts to advocate and facilitate for US−China relations in the 21st century. Managed strategic competition works to avoid globally catastrophic conflict between the world's digital technology and political economic superpowers—who can make or break the global human and public health ecosystems. It seeks to do so by fostering collaboration in shared interests (like the abovesaid four dimensions starting with global health), while placing strategic guard rails on their core competitive interests (particularly in AI digital technologies providing disproportionate force multiplying power for their economies and militaries to dominate this new global digital era). This "engagement and hedge" or "guarded trust" approach seeks to ultimately optimize productive competition, in parallel with constraining their full-spectrum multidomain ideological great power struggle within minimum safety parameters, required for mutual self-survival and preservation of their sovereignty, identity, and security (and thus the security and stability of the world and its diverse nations). This begins by understanding, identifying, communicating, and respecting each other's core interests. This process then generates interest-specific cooperation however thin to shared existential threats (like conflict deescalation, pandemics, NCDs, climate change, poverty, and AI's disruptive societal effects). Yet hurdles are daunting. Through CCP official speeches and position papers, and his conversations with

the foundational global conception of human dignity, protected in human security, fostered in appropriately financed integral sustainable development at scale, safeguarded in a sovereignty-based multipolar world order, and accelerated by responsible AI and interoperable data architectures that empower an effective, efficient, and equitable global public health ecosystem, which may in turn generate humanity's sustainable development and survival. Formally, it seeks to accomplish this by refining early modern classical liberalism with late modern pluralist personalism, rooted in ancient realist Aristotelian metaphysics (doing for political economics what the Personalist Social Contract does for ethics; Monlezun 2023). Historically, it defines and defends the classical liberalism which produced the UN's 1948 *UDHR* and resultant modern international law and rules-based global order, uniting the world's 193 nations through their ratification of the UN Charter as derived from the *UDHR*, while generating, guiding, and governing the resultant related global institutions since. It shows how human dignity (and the derivative values of freedom, rights, and duties) in addition to national sovereignty (and the derivative values of the common good, security, and self-determination) are common denominators across our pluralistic states, value frameworks, and belief systems. But it also develops this vision to account for the historically underrepresented and marginalized voices (including non-Western) by emphasizing our common capacity of human experience, in its unique concrete context of each person, fulfilled in community through a commitment to the common good (collectively safeguarding and constituting the individual good). When this internal content is applied externally, it substantively defines and defends the suprastructure or the institutional layer of the existential global order of rules not rulers (as seen with the UN and WHO most prominently but also related organizational, government, business, academic, and cultural networks and interest-specific coalitions, manifesting our shared awareness of our common humanity, home, and future which in turn generates and manifests our institutions). These include hard and soft institutions, with the former including the UN, WHO, and other organizations with often comprehensive membership, mechanisms, and longitudinal strategic goals. The latter include interest-focused coalitions like the 86 countries from the Global North and South that united in the US-led Global Coalition to Defeat ISIS, enabling often broader consensus from more diverse actors through more limited and short-term goals. More specifically, this top structural layer is a network of overlapping global orders, including security, political, economic, cultural, and digital (driven by American and Chinese companies and militaries primarily seeking to get to the latest qualitative advantage over competitors for enhanced influence capacities and user engagement, particularly through products, platforms, and services faster than laws and regulations can keep pace). Personalist Liberalism shows how it facilitates the cooperation, collaboration, and managed competition among and between democracies and autocracies (in the state-level political economic structure) and these overlapping orders over them (where certain countries, companies, and value blocs dominate over others). And it demonstrates how both layers are anchored in the substructure or foundational layer of shared values, common to and embodied in diverse states and belief systems in the form of human dignity and state sovereignty—required for and fulfilled by human security as our unifying common good, but articulated in measurable and empirical terms. Notably, it emphasizes these "integral values" common to diverse peoples, cultures, and belief systems.

Meanwhile, it avoids the more polarizing "ideological values" (those separated from underlying moral systems that otherwise would allow rational debate and civil resolution among them). These are especially predominant in the West and are often critiqued externally and internally for dividing populations for or against gender categorization, abortion, imposed religiously affiliated or unaffiliated belief systems, nationalism rather than patriotism, and so on. Echoing the Tocqueville-like warning about totalitarianism, either in its decentralized Western democratic "soft" version or its centralized Eastern autocratic "hard" version, the foundational stability of integral values may thus be required for the structural integrity of the abovesaid layers by avoiding the extremes of both ends, where durable resolution is rare at best if possible at all (Ryan 2012).

These institutional (suprastructure), state (structure), and value layers (substructure) articulate how our global human and embedded global health ecosystem already exists and works, but with sufficient detail and depth so we can resolve disagreements and ambiguity about our ultimate objectives, and thus the strategies and operations to get us there. Further, it shows how the micro dimension of human disease and macro dimension of human security in our era's AI digital globalization permeate these layers. Pragmatically, Personalist Liberalism seeks to therefore preserve a minimum complementary balance by retaining the comparative advantages of autocratic led collectivism (equality of outcome) and democratic led individualism (equality of opportunity), while seeking to prevent, reduce, and mitigate excessive tensions between the two and gross violations of dignity and sovereignty within them. As AI technologically is rapidly transforming the global public health ecosystem with scope, scale, and speed, Personalist Liberalism seeks to make its societal context intelligible in those domains as well through the confluence of nontechnological factors that frame, influence, and to some extent even determine them. It chiefly does this by its unique essential demonstration of "ecosystem interoperability" at its heart, uniting partners, optimizing collaboration, and resolving disagreements. This structural interoperability is conceptual convertibility of local (neighborhood, regional, and national) security and global (international) security in the dual dimensions of human security. The person central to the global human and health ecosystems is metaphysically and existentially both individual and communal, simultaneously requiring local goods (i.e., health, work, relationships, etc.) and global goods (i.e., protection from pandemics, climate change, conflicts, etc.). Both dimensions of security are already joined in reality. Personalist Liberalism therefore joins them conceptually and operationally, putting them to work for the necessary political economics to sustain and grow the global human, health, and public health ecosystems. Personalist Liberalism therefore force multiplies the dynamic complementariness of local globalism. It does so instead of prioritizing self-sabotaging narrow nationalism that prioritizes a domestic audience so radically that it ultimately undermines them by unplugging them from the global human community (with which they are intrinsically interconnected in reality) and the global digitalized economy (on which their own supply chains and diffusion of innovation at least in part depend). But it also avoids the self-sabotaging superficial globalism the prioritizes the international audience (of government, corporate, and institutional elites) so radically that it undermines their stable grip on power by eroding popular support for their governance (especially through a loss of livable job security and culture identity). Accordingly, the derivative values or ethical principles of solidarity and subsidiarity above (described by the WHO and diverse institutions and states) underlying this political economic framework are additionally convertible to allow the rightsizing of policies to advance this ecosystem. Therefore, Personalist Liberalism describes what security as self-determination and flourishing looks like (and how it can be achieved) with scope, speed, and scale.

5.2.1.2 Deployed for global public health

Personalist Liberalism is therefore the first known globally comprehensive political economic framework applied to health in our digitalizing world. As such it may explain and guide the societal factors, policies, and governance driving the maturation of the AI-empowered global public health ecosystem, operationalized as a development-driven human security-based cooperative competition between democracies and autocracies (Monlezun 2023). We will analyze the specific operational advances in health political economics from this perspective by first considering the general strategic domains in its deployment for (1) health determinants, (2) institutionalizing interoperability, and (3) the debt to development transition.

1. *Health determinants*: This chapter opened with how political economics is the metadeterminant of health determinants, as individually it drives lifelong health behaviors that children learn early (including diet, exercise, relationships, and risk avoidance) and societally it structurally enables or discourages healthy behaviors and the provision of medical care and public health (Labonté and Ruckert 2019). In our three-layer Personalist Liberalism framework, we will analyze in greater depth the value determinants in Chapter 6, but we will include the state (especially traditional political economics) and institutional (global intergovernment and corporate) determinants here. To understand the last two levels though, let us briefly describe the value determinants of health that frame the other levels. Given the rich diversity of cultures and belief systems, there is a wide range of definitions, rights, and duties for health. Across these different domains, there can be different consensus definitions for the minimum accepted level of well-being (according to the previously noted WHO definition negatively as the absence of disease, disability, and debility and positively as the presence of integral physical, mental, and social healthy functioning), and an even greater range across individuals within those domains. In addition, there is a large spectrum describing what individual duties we have to care for ourselves (such as through healthy behaviors) and contribute to the well-being of others (including through taxes for medical care and public health). Therefore, reform of healthcare and global health fundamentally requires a recovery of what we mean by health and public duties to it. Further, the global debt crisis challenging high-income countries (HICs) and low- and middle-income countries (LMICs) place historic pressure on governments to distinguish between health needs and wants, thus enabling codification in law and policy what "essential health services" will be prioritized, provided, and funded. Diverse political economic regimes are distinguished structurally by how they manage limited societal resources for collective wellbeing (generally considered their primary objective), and individually by their performance in doing so.

Generally, liberal democratic regimes prioritize greater individual freedom, free markets, and decentralized power (i.e., through fair elections, transparent institutions, and free media). In contrast, illiberal autocratic regimes prioritize greater societal equality, state-controlled markets, and centralized power (i.e., through an absence or questionable degree of free elections, state political hierarchy, and state-controlled media). Above these regimes at the institutional global sovereign order, we analyzed in the finance and data chapters how the WHO is seeking to accelerate the AI digitalization of developing regions through public-private-academic and North–South partnerships (codesigned by local communities and empowered by international resources).

But how can limited ecosystem resources and cooperation in and between the institutional and state levels of political economics drive the highest value impact on global public health? The different dimensions of health determinants provide a powerful consensus-based analytic approach to make measurable progress toward it, including (1) social, (2) political, (3) economic, (4) commercial, and (5) digital determinants of health. The WHO defines the (1) social determinants of health as the "non-medical factors that influence health outcomes," including cultural (values), societal (norms and policies), and political economic "forces and systems" along with the daily living conditions shaped by them (WHO 2023a). They exacerbate or alleviate socioeconomic inequities directly and indirectly by improving or worsening health, with greater or worse socioeconomics integrally linked to individual and community well-being or its decline. These conditions include childhood development, education, social inclusion, conflict, healthcare access, and security (in jobs, food, and housing). As the broadest determinant of health, the WHO notes empirically how they drive more health outcomes than even health behaviors or healthcare, including up to 55% of such outcomes (depending on the specific outcome and related determinant).

The (2) political determinants of health were explored earlier in how different regime types and their performance shape how well societal and economic resources are coordinated to hurt or help peoples' wellbeing. As noted with the abovesaid emblematic Roessler and Schmitt (2021) study and the Sen et al. (2017) study, democratic regimes generally outperform autocratic regimes in greater political sustainability and stability over time as prerequisites for their additional superior efficient and equitable delivery of population health and related public goods. Yet North–South politics also are at play as with the poignant example of the COVID-19 lockdowns, which northern HICs broadly adopted serially until effective mRNA-based vaccines were available largely within just a year of the pandemic (with concurrent unprecedented fiscal stimulus to prop up locked down and slowed economies). Meanwhile, southern LMICs attempted to follow suit according to the supposed global health consensus on "best practices" at the time, despite being unable largely to implement lockdowns, sustain the economic suppression (domestically and internationally for exports), fiscally bail out their struggling industries, and wait the extended time before vaccines began trickling down from HICs. Further, growing scientific public health consensus including from such representative studies as from John Hopkins University (including a metaanalysis of 18,590 initially screened studies), the WHO's COVID-19 special envoy's updated state guidance, and the G7's 2021 Carbis Bay Health Declaration (promoting vaccines instead of lockdowns) ultimately highlighted the general questionable net health benefit (negligible to no short-term COVID mortality reduction in exchange for significantly worsened long-term poverty and healthcare access-related mortality) all the way up to clear net harm of lockdowns globally, with disproportionate damage for LMICs (Herby et al. 2022; Jones and Hameiri 2022; Gómez and Monlezun 2023, p. 8; Eyawo et al. 2021). Specifically, Jones and Hameiri argued in their 2022 study in *International Affairs*, the world leading academic publication in international relations edited by the United Kingdom's Chatham House, showed how the North–South political determinants of health illustrate the "failure of global health governance" for COVID-19. This was epitomized by the excessive reliance on a WHO-led "neoliberal" global governance model in which local governance and capacities were hollowed out and transferred to neoliberalism "meta-governance": the WHO and related powerful institutions wielded centralized power defining and distributing "best practice" policies to states, which then sought to implement these one-size-fits-all rules. Personalist Liberalism therefore offers an alternative framework as noted earlier to balance the efficiency of global resources and expertise with the effectiveness and ethics of local-driven priorities and policy implementation across the North and South along with democracies and autocracies (i.e., through the global public health ecosystem facilitating a bottom-up approach, allowing real-time AI-accelerated edge computing to identify and respond to local health needs, complemented by a top-down approach of international institutional guidance and coordination of partners and resources).

Although powerful, it is programmatically difficult and ethically questionable to conceptualize and measure social determinants and their related political determinants of health. A broad range of factors must be identified, massive data collected, and health officials often arbitrarily required to prioritize the most "relevant" and/or "actionable" determinants for their interventions meant to address them (Freudenberg 2023). Economic, commercial, and digital determinants of health may advance a more quantifiable, precise, and transparent complement as part of a larger health determinant framework by leveraging a WoW or whole-of-world approach (for improving global health through understanding the right "pressure points" in their societal and political economic context). We considered in the finance chapter how the (3) economic determinants of health generally can accelerate sustainable and sufficient funding for the global public health ecosystem through supply chains (especially AI, digital products, semiconductors, other computing components, and more traditional global public health products and services), public–private partnerships, and efficient business models. The (4) commercial determinants of health are an emergent perspective on understanding and potentially improving global wellbeing in ways that the abovesaid determinants of health have not thus far. The commercial determinants may be the most precise and effective pressure points to empirically improve health as they clearly define commercial actors (businesses) as global health's primary causative agents (worsening or improving diverse health challenges), their means of influence (influencing science, technology, production, marketing, and politics), the widespread consensus on needed reforms (to refine their relationship with and thus enhance the benefit for the public sectors, including regionalization as a national security hedge against the risks of excessive hyperglobalization, in addition to more equitable but still fair societal sharing of economic growth without hampering business competitiveness).

These commercial determinants of health in turn are largely fueled and framed by the primary driver of today's (digital) global economy—AI, along with its enabling digital technologies, particularly its foundational building block of semiconductors—which therefore shape the derivative (5) digital determinants of health that connect all the abovesaid health determinants. Socially, politically, economically, and commercially, we have progressively explored how the AI digital transformation of our world and its global public health ecosystem are deepening our interconnectedness, lowering costs, and boosting performance through data-driven efficiencies. Chapter 1 emphasized why and how the WHO's global digital health strategy, influentially shaping this ecosystem's evolution, details the roadmap to achieving global health through the primary means of AI digital technologies united with (by accelerating the realization of) an SDG-based health strategy (WHO 2021). The primary objective for these technologies is to advance the "digital determinants of health." They are identified as digital literacy and technological access (computing, broadband, internet, and edge devices) as health increasingly is shaped, advanced, and financed digitally with AI force multiplying this process. The critical challenge to scaling such efforts that address these digital determinants is how best to bridge political economic divides between competing regimes and blocs. As this chapter discussed earlier, democracies largely birthed the social media and internet advances that initially accelerated the global digital ecosystem with its interconnectedness, but increasingly is now accelerating its fragmentation through misinformation-based societal polarization and demonization (by an "enrage to engage" operating model of AI algorithmization of user engagement, hyping fear and anger against the "other" in a radicalizing echo chamber of manipulated behaviors). Concurrently, autocracies are utilizing such technologies to boost their domestic censorship and foreign power projection (undermining democracies and exporting surveillance and suppression digital technologies to other autocracies) that further fray the ecosystem's cohesion and its related digital determinants of health. The 2020 Broadband Commission cited in Chapter 4 on data architecture therefore emphasized "consent-driven" health AI, standards, regulations, and collaboration (Broadband 2020). This is meant to *democratize* data and so *develop* global health through minimum ecosystem and thus data interoperability, rather than *divide* data and *dominate* people through insufficient safeguards against misinformation, discrimination, fraud, surveillance, censorship, and internet balkanization (i.e., autocratic restriction on domestic access to the free flow of information). The WHO's (2021) report above highlighted this consent-driven approach treating "digital technologies as digital public goods," meaning that the digital determinants of health are also societal duties for communities and states to individually and collectively advance human security as global wellbeing at scale. Personalist Liberalism defines and defends the *why* behind this (promoting human security, stability, and sustainability including mitigating conflict amid competing political economic regimes), while elaborating on the *how* its implementation can optimally work (through local capacity development and values safeguarded and empowered by global networks' resources and coordination).

2. *Institutionalizing interoperability* is the primary means structurally to effectively address health determinants at scale, by making this interoperability a defining and enduring feature embedded in equitable cooperation and managed competition in the global public health ecosystem. Central to this interoperability is the common end identified by history's first and most substantive consensus of the world's peoples, as articulated by the UN's Charter: "the dignity and worth of the human person," which entails "equal" and "fundamental human rights" especially freedom among all peoples (UN 1945). This dignity intrinsically and integrally binds us together to promote the common good, in which our individual dignity is fulfilled, and which serves as the main object of collective justice. In this shared moral vision, justice is the primary enabler and foundation of "international peace and security," which is the primary "purpose" of the world's first substantive political economic collaboration (the UN coordinating collective intergovernment development of the global population). Personal dignity as the primary foundational individual value therefore generates its primary foundational communal value expressed as the "principle of sovereign equality" of all countries. Profit is the central organizing principle theoretically for a business, uniting its diverse stakeholders in an ecosystem of shared strategy, data, architecture, and AI tools to realize that common end. Dignity is realized in the common good (safeguarded by security) and is therefore the central organizing principle for our global human ecosystem (and its derivative global public health ecosystem). It is embodied by what Personalist Liberalism describes as the three-level political economic framework above, and it is enabled by the interoperability allowing its diverse stakeholders at each level to cooperate, manage competition, and reduce conflict. Dignity, sovereignty, and security thus structurally unite the global human (and public health) ecosystem(s). And (health) AI technologies digitally unite, energize, and animate the ecosystem(s).

The key features of this Personalist Liberalism approach institutionalizing interoperability in the global ecosystem include its (1) ultimate aim, (2) intermediary aim (3) strategic paradigm, (4) micro-institutional structure, (5) and operating protocols, derivative from its essential principles outlined in Section 5.2.1.1. The 2023 World Economic Forum's Global Risks Report (drawn from over 1200 organizational, government, business, and academic experts and supplemented by over 12,000 business leaders from 121 countries) highlights the global consensus on how reducing poverty and mitigating climate change are respectively the top short-term (2-year) and long-term (10-year) critical objectives for our world (WEC 2023). Worsening living costs increase vulnerability to the next most severe short-term risks: extreme weather, societal polarization, and political economic confrontation (particularly investment screening, sanctions, trade wars, inflation, stagnation, and cyberattacks precipitating armed conflicts and involuntary mass migration). Failing to mitigate and adapt to adverse climate change is seen as the quickly approaching beyond-the-horizon threat which will compound the above near-term risks. Personalist Liberalism therefore (1) ultimately prioritizes human security as the aggregate local globalism aim by strengthening the synergistic relationship of community capacities and global networks (of resources, experts, supply chains, institutions, organizations, and governments). The (2) intermediary or process aim toward this human security at scale is human resilience. It balances individuals and societal vulnerability to risks which are generated and worsened by the power oscillation between distributed networks and centralized hierarchies (as individuals and institutions within and between democracies and autocracies vie for societal influence). Generally, this resilience seeks to avoid hard imperialism (i.e., a Russian autocrat's 2022 full-scale invasion of Ukraine's democracy based on "historic" colonial claims to it) and soft imperialism (i.e., certain US or EU-dominated global institutions tying certain foreign aid for Southern countries to alleged ideological rather than integral values like family planning mandates which contrast with local values desiring larger families), both of which undermine local self-determination and capacities to actualize it. Such resilience in the global sovereign cooperative order discourages undue influence from Western hypocrisy, Eastern autocracy, and Southern instability (i.e., of debt crises ballooning into bankruptcies or recurrent government violence maintaining power or overturning current regime's power). The (3) strategic paradigm to advance political economic resilience and achieve human security is the Chinese Sun Tzu-inspired "strategic empathy" noted in the finance chapter, rather than the rampant "strategic narcissism" of viewing another's latent drivers and constraints (particularly revealed during pattern breaks, i.e., crises revealing other's priorities through costly choices) from one's own perspective rather than the other's (and thus missing what actually motivates others; Store 2014).

For this strategic paradigm to realize its intermediary and ultimate aims, the (4) microinstitutional structure of institutional interoperability applies to both nations and networks. Within developing countries prior to becoming advanced mature economies, "micro-institutional foundations of capitalism" from China to Russia to India manifest as the sector structures (i.e., how digital technologies or manufacturing operate), institutional organization (i.e., governance and ownership), and state intervention (i.e., state investment and protectionism). States' elites prioritize different sector's strategic values (i.e., Xi's prioritization of AI and semiconductors) and then seek to internally develop them and internationally integrate them with the global digitalizing economy, proportional to their assigned strategic value (Hsueh 2022). These microinstitutional factors determine how much states intervene in certain sectors, who owns what property rights, and how much political, economic, and even military power will be deployed to protect those sectors' strategic value. Such value can be elevated to different degrees of core national security interests (all the way to being seen as vital interests for state survival). Personalist Liberalism informs the lines that are drawn to demarcate areas of collaboration, cooperation, and competition (managed strategically to avoid conflict on those core national security interests). Aside from these "hard micro-institutions," the "soft micro-institutions" can be seen in societal self-organization. It is influenced by such dominant expressions as digital social networks, distinguished according to their typically private digital platforms (i.e., Facebook friend networks and X/Twitter or TikTok influencers and their followers). History's political economic "breakpoints" can be understood from the perspective of power shifts in these social networks between "old power hierarchies" and "new social networks" (Ferguson 2018). Examples include the US-accelerated post-WWII decolonization of the Global South from old European empires. The imperial hard power-based world order generally gave way to a more democratic soft power-based world order of the latter 20th century. Popular will, self-determination, and diplomacy sought to increasingly determine domestic and foreign policy, instead of prior periods' military might, colonial pressure, and conflict. Social networks within and across states have exerted increasing influence on national and international political economics especially since the dawn of the 21st century. This trend accelerated with the internet's digital platforms amplifying these social networks, which progressively were powerfully harnessed by populist leaders from the 2010s onward to polarize and marginalize other groups. There is a growing multisector global push to counter this digital decay of social networks into unsocial networks by recovering their underlying foundational value hierarchy. This is meant to order otherwise excessively decentralized networks appropriately and transparently by appealing to local values (i.e., freedom and identity) and global values (i.e., security and justice) to guide relationships in such networks.

Digitalization and globalization trends in microinstitutional structures within and across states bring stakeholders within the global human and public health ecosystems closer together (enabling cooperation but also risking conflict if competition is insufficiently managed). They also advance the interoperability that maximizes the former and minimizes the latter. The (5) operating protocols that put this interoperability into action within Personalist Liberalism are dynamic fitting or calibrated cooperation: right-sizing the breadth, depth, and pace of institutional and interstate relationships according to the degree of compatibility in values, political economics, and benefits shared among stakeholders. Cooperation in international relations generally is minimal, thin, or thick, depending on whether it is implied policy, explicit policy, or collective action (Graefrath and Jahn 2023). Minimal cooperation helps explain China's 2023 Iran−Saudi Arabian diplomatic resumption, predicated upon greater economic activity with China and decreased political reliance on the United States. Thin cooperation can be seen between pre-Xi China and the United States declining to explicitly attempt use military force to change the status quo of democratic Taiwan governing itself separate from communist China (with this policy since repudiated explicitly by Xi, who asserted the right to use force to take it back as the basis for his unprecedented third term as the state's supreme leader, replacing the CCP's prior "social contract" of minimal cooperation with the people centered on economic prosperity with a new thin cooperation of nationalist unity and military power manifested chiefly by retaking Taiwan; Schuman 2022). The 1980s minimal cooperation between communistVietnam and the democratic United States avoiding repeat conflict gave way to the 1990s thin cooperation of graduated diplomatic resumption, which in turn became the thick cooperation manifested by their 2000 Bilateral Trade Agreement (accelerating Vietnam's ascension to the World Trade Organization and global economic integration, which increased bilateral profit by 1200% to $20 billion by 2011, and enforced minimum bilateral adherence to fair and open trade, worker safety rights, and intellectual property protection; US−Vietnam 2000). This more durable partnership model of calibrated cooperation rather than tenuous transactions seeks to respect states' different value and political economic structures, while strengthening the convergent consensus for enduring relationships that empower institutionalized interoperability, in addition to enhancing the responsiveness of relationships to dynamic external and internal factors to sustain efficient cooperation. Managed strategic competition can therefore be operationalized in all three domains, such as with implied US−China policies to avoid nuclear exchange, explicit policies to reduce mutual miscalculations and misunderstandings through improved diplomacy and dialogue, and shared actions to cooperate on shared existential threats (chiefly including global public health challenges like poverty, pandemics, climate change, excessive arms proliferation, and political economic confrontation especially with AI digital technologies).

3. *Debt to development*: This is the final strategic domain for which we will analyze Personalist Liberalism's application to health political economics. Institutionalizing interoperability to improve global well-being by a more comprehensive understanding of health determinants additionally requires collective progress from debt to development. The prior chapters (particularly for finance and development) assessed the evolution of our post-WWII late modern world in which early modern imperial mercantilism gave way to liberal democratic capitalism, as colonial European powers could no longer subjugate American, Asian, African, and Middle Eastern colonies through political expansionist foreign policies and economic protectionist domestic policies. The mid to late 1900s therefore saw the US-led world order marked by hyperglobalization, decolonization, industrialization, and digitalization. This then produced unprecedented diffusion of development in humanity's health, wealth, and equality. Yet post-2000s, the structural challenges in the US-led liberal world order increasingly manifested as exploding debt crises (as developing economies increasingly struggled to industrialize, digitalize, and integrate with the global economy that is largely driven by advanced democratic countries). By then, global overindebtedness meant that global underinvestment in public health manifested as developed countries borrowing too much at enviable rates, leaving too little capital at too high rates for developing counties. They were increasingly caught in seeming perpetual development cycles, but not sustainable growth out of the poverty-disease cycles (plagued by costly health, energy, food, and conflicts). Prior to the COVID-19 pandemic battering emerging markets, China's Cheung Kong Graduate School of Business expressed broader domestic worries that the nation may not overtake the United States, let alone escape the lower-value add manufacturing and state investment-dependent "middle-income trap" to reach diversified high-value add service and consumption-based high-income status (like past developing but now developed markets like Japan, South Korea, and Taiwan; Shek 2019). Not only are the odds generally against

emerging markets to escape the trap (as over 85% since 1960 have been unable to make the leap out of it). But also, China as the fastest developing country features prominent domestic figures cautioning about the dimming chances of current and future developing markets to escape. As the growth of the hypergloblized international economy of the 1990s–2010s slows, so do the pathways for countries to develop into mature economies —especially as this transition typically is a prerequisite for sustainable politics locally and globally as the pressures on them mount from worsening public health, world debt, climate change, and conflicts. Seeing those storm clouds brewing, the UN's 1987 Brundtland Report formalized the concept of "sustainable development" to call for humanity to broaden our "spheres of cooperation" for "sustainable human progress and human survival," "based on policies that sustain and expand the environmental resource base," and so preserve our "common future" collectively needed and shared justly (UNWCE 1987). The report outlined the "pathway" to realize the prior year's global consensus in the landmark 1986 UN General Assembly declaration asserting that "the right to development is an inalienable human right," manifested integrally individually and communally (in the multiple dimensions of political economics, society, and culture), and "in which all human rights and fundamental freedoms can be fully realized." The process of "decolonization" was not enough for people to be free *from* old imperial powers, they had to be empowered to be free *for* their "full realization" as "person[s]" in the global huma family, initially outlined in the global moral vision of the 1948 *UDHR* and political economic vision of the 1945 charter.

The critical debt-to-development priority for global political economic cooperation generally and the global public health ecosystem specifically includes (1) debt restructuring, (2) affordable clean energy transition, and (3) affordable AI digital transformation to advance the existing SDG operational framework. The American Public Health Association, the largest public health professional organization which also hosts the largest annual meeting for such professionals in the world, adopted policy number 20222 to join outspoken advocates at intergovernmental institutions (including the International Monetary Fund [IMF], World Bank, and G20), government agencies, businesses, universities, and faith-based community organizations to strongly advocate for (1) debt restructuring (APHA 2022). It highlighted how crushing debt not only means 64 countries spend magnitudes more on foreign debt payments than their public health or healthcare systems. But countries also regardless of wealth level are struggling to recover from the economic shock of COVID-19, equitably expand current essential public health and healthcare services, and prepare for the inevitable future pandemics and global health challenges. Such advocates therefore call for canceling debt for countries in the most intense debt distress, extend debt relief for all indebted LMICs, diversify affordable debt options (including through regional development banks and emergency reserve funds), advance debt restructuring (legally reorganizing payments through short-term delays and longer term more affordable schedules), and engineer sustainable debt relief (avoiding excessive austerity programs or deinvestment from essential domestic health capacities, especially in health). Consider the compounding challenges of financial pressures piling on our overindebted world: prolonged prepandemic low interest rates and slow growth (increasing debt and risky bets), the pandemic's lockdowns and massive Global North bailout of their economies (worsening their deficits and then inflation, triggering their central banks particularly in the United States to rapidly raise interest rates to control it, in turn increasing developing countries' dollar-denominated debt and output contractions), Russia's full-scale invasion of Ukraine (crushing global energy and food supplies), and China's economic slowdown (with its aging population, worsening geoeconomic confrontation with the West, increasing protectionist policies, decreasing manufacturing on which the world depends, and questionable capacity to continue bailing out failing BRI investments in developing countries; IMF 2022; Chan and Dimitrijevic 2023; CEPR 2022). Global debt hit a global record by 2023 of $300 trillion, or 349% of global GDP (meaning we borrow about three times as much as we make). Governments' debt-to-GDP exploded 76% from the 2010s up to 2022, unleashing an estimated $3 trillion more in global interest payments by then. Accordingly, there is growing institutional and intergovernmental pressure noted earlier to restructure debt by generating only productive new debt (that grows economies sustainably), forgive unproductive debt (holding them back), and reduce overconsumption and spending (that would prompt new debt).

But to get to development, the growing debt threat from (2) unaffordable clean energy transitions are additionally plaguing the global economy, particularly in LMICs already facing the above headwinds from existing structural over-indebtedness (Tongia 2022; World Bank 2023). While trying to dig their way out of debt, developing countries are additionally facing what the World Bank describes as the "triple penalty" of the clean energy transition or trilemma: having to choose among sustainability, security, and affordability, though all three are simultaneously needed. Unsustainable fossil fuels are cheaper but more destructive for an alarmingly fragile global ecological ecosystem. Conflicts and autocrats regularly challenge global energy security (as seen with Russia withholding oil and gas to Europe in 2022 to pressure them into withholding humanitarian and defensive aid to Ukraine). And developing countries receive the smallest green energy investments, generate the lowest carbon emissions, and yet face shared pressure championed by the Global North to similarly reduce emissions (despite needing affordable often fossil fuel energy to catch up to developed nations who already produced the majority of modern greenhouse gases, while China produces over twice as much carbon emissions as the second top emitter, the United States, and over 90% more than the average from the next top ten country emitters, thus dwarfing any Southern efforts to reduce emissions without China and the United States also reducing). A 2021 UN report highlighted the importance for instance of nuclear energy technologically —accelerating the excessively slow global progress toward carbon neutrality—and political economic cooperation between the North and South in energy infrastructure and investments (UN 2021). Hospitals, public health services, affordable agriculture and other food sources, medicines, medical devices, and AI digital technologies all run on energy. Overwhelming existing structural debt and excessive new energy debt thus can freeze any significant development in the global health ecosystem if left unaddressed. The World Bank cautions how "the poverty trap is becoming an energy trap that is becoming a climate trap"

(World Bank 2023). This doom spiral is collectively also becoming a disease and dedevelopment trap, requiring effective and equitable political economic cooperation to salvage the needed sustainable progress of the global human and health ecosystems out of it. The World Bank thus advocates for a "power transition virtuous cycle" in which public–private partnerships generate, optimize, and scale innovation, infrastructure, and investments globally. Doing so streamlines affordable pricing, sufficient capacities, and reasonable regulations to bridge from fossil fuels to cleaner fossil fuels like liquefied natural gas before ultimately reaching clean, carbon neutral energy sources (including nuclear and renewables like wind, water, geothermal, and solar). And finally, (3) affordable AI digital transformation is increasingly key for accelerating this structural and energy debt to development process. As Chapters 2, 3, and 4 respectively on finance, development, and data highlighted, AI's strategic and concrete use cases are expanding to demonstrate enhanced technical efficiencies driving enhanced capacity efficiencies in public–private–academic partnerships. Health AI advances better governance and thus provision of public goods with less resources, by leveraging global resources for local autonomy directing those resources where they are most needed.

5.2.2 Advances: health AI uses cases in cooperative political economics

Now with an overview of the theories, concepts, and trends complete, we can next analyze leading concrete AI use cases advancing the necessary cooperative political economics for the global public health ecosystem, adapting to our shared global opportunities and challenges (by maximizing synergistic partnerships and minimizing destructive conflicts).

5.2.2.1 Health development with deterrence and defense guardrails

Personalist Liberalism applied to the political economics of this ecosystem help explain the evolution of our world's dominant global "3-D" cooperative framework of *development, *deterrence, and *defense. The traditional three pillars of modern foreign policy or international relations (diplomacy, deterrence, and defense) are adapted in the account by Personalist Liberalism for our existing world order. In it the UN and influential like-minded public–private partnerships (particularly in the West) advocate and facilitate in the top structural institutional level of our global political economics a "development-driven human security-based cooperative competition between democracies and autocracies" described earlier. Historically, modern states have applied diplomacy to prevent misunderstandings, deterrence to prevent conflict, and defense to end it promptly. Chapter 1 explored how concurrent with this trend, "development" was progressively conceptualized, deployed, and supercharged post-WWII by the UN to avert war by building domestic capacities for prosperity, equity, and thus peace (as the United States and Soviet Union prior to the 1990s competed for "medical diplomacy" and development aid to developing countries, especially to expand their spheres of influence). Post-2000s, development increasingly featured a more transparent and multipolar international dimension in addition to a domestic dimension. This occurred through ecosystem capacity building (decolonized North–South public–private partnerships) and local governance (accelerating equitable benefit of the globalizing and AI digitalizing political economics, avoiding nationalist populist backlash against perceived disproportionate elitist/globalist benefit). Now deterrence and defense are similarly being revamped to adapt to the post-COVID world of intensified US–China strategic competition. There is growing shared concern about Taiwan being a flashpoint for great power conflict, in addition to growing awareness of defense inadequacies revealed by Russia's 2022 full-scale invasion of Ukraine and its weaponization of energy, food, and migrants against the West and South. Such refined deterrence and defense appear to increasingly serve as the guardrails in the managed strategic competition of competing great powers and affiliated power blocs.

"Deterrence" is an ancient concept updated for modern times during the Cold War by the Nobel Prize-winning American economist, Thomas Schelling, who focused on nuclear war deterrence and the derivative sobering strategy of "mutually assured destruction" (Schelling 1981). Through game theory, Schelling influentially shaped what became the modern foreign policy orthodoxy to preserve the status quo in international relations, chiefly by dissuading states from unprovoked threats or attacks on internationally recognized borders and sovereignty. Essentially, deterrence is when a state through its own actions (direct deterrence) or in concert with its allies (extended deterrence) dissuades an opponent or competitor from a course of action. It does so by credibly communicating to the opponent that the benefit of an attacking action and the probability of achieving it are sufficiently outweighed by the cost and probability of producing that cost inflicted on the attacker by the deterring actor. It typically operates through denial (preventing the attacker from reaping the benefits of an attack) and retaliation (inducing the attacker to cease the attack because of excessive costs inflicted on them after the attack is begun). Generally, ancient and early modern history (including imperial Europe, China, Japan, etc.) is the story of wars waged by powerful autocratic leaders to expand territory and resources, often explicitly "justified" to preserve national security (and at least implicitly the survivability of their regimes). But late modern history post-WWII from the UN Charter onward is the story of wars averted through democracies promoting diplomacy, deterrence, and defense (by powerful institutions and alliances inducing often autocratic leaders from resurrecting the specter of colonial-style conflict as the old status quo). The above noted 2023 UN General Assembly Resolution condemning Putin's Russian invasion of Ukraine—affirmed by China, India, and much of the Global South—is diplomacy. It also includes the purported closed-door discussions by China, India, and the West dissuading Putin from following through with his nuclear weapon threats against Ukraine and the West. It extends to the June 2023 African peace delegation led by South African President Cyril Ramaphosa to Russia urging Putin to stop the war and return Ukrainian children (even amid the delegation being forced to take shelter in Kyiv while Russian missiles struck Ukraine's capital during their diplomatic visit; Radford 2023). More multilateral diplomacy additionally includes the Saudi Arabia-convened coalition meeting in August 2023 assembling 42 countries—including China, India, the United States, Brazil, Japan, Egypt, and South Africa, while Russia was not invited—that expressed their consensus on continuing discussions for facilitating a durable peace in Ukraine, predicated on a UN-style respect for territorial integrity and national sovereignty, implicitly rebuking Russia's forceful seizure of Ukrainian lands and peoples (Ebrahim 2023). The US−European strengthening of Ukraine's defense (after the West's widely perceived failed deterrence by denial) is deterrence by retaliation. And the United States attempts to preemptively bolster Taiwan's defenses (as a "porcupine" model similar to Israel through asymmetric defense capacities, while strengthening the economic mutual benefit, supply chain resilience, and global technological interdependence of its critical semiconductor manufacturing) is meant to be an integrated deterrence by denial.

Applied by Personalist Liberalism for the global public health ecosystem, the human security-based SDGs are meant to be a shared operational grand strategy in which development facilitates global cooperation as a lattice of shared global interests (like global health threats, climate change, and poverty reduction) and mutual local benefits (reducing the above through improved domestic capacities). And it is this development cooperation that is bounded by defense and deterrence (alliance, military, and political economic) guardrails to manage the inherent, inevitable, and indefinite strategic competition of great powers (particularly the United States and China) and power blocs (particularly aligned democratic and autocratic states). The durable pragmatism of this approach is reflected in the entrenched policies of the greater powers already as "integrated strategic deterrence." The 2022 US National Security Strategy explicitly anchors itself in this development-based diplomacy and deterrence backed by a robust defense (Krishna et al. 2023; White House 2023). This approach is highlighted by the Indo-Pacific Economic Framework for Prosperity, a novel multilateral development framework for the regional economic integration of India, the United States, Japan, South Korea, the Philippines, and Vietnam among 14 nations that account currently for 40% of global GDP. It is on track to be the majority of global GDP in the near term by cooperatively aiming to advance a structural economic transformation through values-driven politics, making this transition supposedly fair, resilient, clean, and (AI-enhanced digitally) connected. The National Security Strategy also highlights the trilateral AUKUS alliance (of Australia, UK, and United States) as a network regional security architecture. It emphasizes its 2023 defense industrial partnership building domestic production and sharing nuclear-powered submarines through the alliance to protect freedom of navigation on the seas (including its focus on protecting the multidecade status quo of acknowledging the self-governing democratic Taiwan as officially part of autocratic China without permitting any side to use force to change this, while also protecting the world's economic dependence on Taiwan's semiconductors that a Chinese provoked conflict would devastate; Townshend 2023). Similarly, China's academic and government publications increasingly advance its own conceptual evolution and practical operationalization of integrated deterrence by unifying conflict spectrum (hot to gray to cold wars), domains (land, sea, air, cyber, and space militarily, but also diplomatic, economic, scientific, technological, and information nonmilitarily), theaters (globally and regionally), alliances (focused on joint interoperability, capacity development, and cooperation in diplomatic, economic, and deterrence), and political economic power (translating the above government-driven efforts with public−private partners; Chase and Chan 2016; White House 2023, p. 22). China's take on this integrated deterrence shares striking echoes and even identical elements with that of the United States. Although America operates much more through and with alliances, China is notably with its BRI expanding such network efforts.

AI digitalization is accelerating this integrated deterrence in ways that seek to preserve military force for defense rather than offense while ensuring effective deterrence against unprovoked aggression (both of which endanger the health development central to the global public health ecosystem's primary mission of global well-being despite divided power blocs of states). This is in parallel with AI's digitalization of defense, especially as the US–China AI arms race is rapidly advancing more autonomous, efficient, and lethal fighter jets, drone swarms, command-and-control systems (including nuclear war decision making), hacking, and disinformation (including deepfakes digitally altering images, audio, and videos often to make people appear to say or do that which they did not; Hirsh 2023). There is growing international worry therefore about the disruptive, unpredictable, and (potentially unforeseen and unmanageable) destructive elements of AI, undermining responsible force (failing to prevent accidental wars amid proponents of rogue AI war applications), societal trust (manipulating societal support for war or violence against states or other communities), and truthful communication (curtailing or preventing it across governments, institutions, and communities). Consider the US Air Force chief of AI operations who reported the results of a simulated test in June 2023 that an AI-enabled drone was trained to eliminate surface-to-air missiles with a human-in-the-loop giving the final "go/no go": realizing the human operator was hampering its mission with "no-go" decisions, the AI program appeared to have eliminated the human and then continued on to its targets unhindered (RAS 2023). Such elements undermine responsible defense and effective deterrence, particularly with the latter through misunderstanding, miscalculation, and mismatching one's own capacities to objectives. To reduce such undesirable AI applications and futures, there is a growing uptake particular in the United States and its allies of an AI-accelerated Bayesian approach for managed strategic calculation in a way that applies Bayesian analytics for defense (like the finance chapter explored for clinical trials; Combe et al. 2023). It does so through its foundational principle of Bayes' Theorem which is arguably the most crucial principle for probability theory and AI. It essentially represents mathematically how we learn by regularly updating our beliefs about reality as we get more information, progressively enabling us to more effectively choose means to achieve our desired ends. Formally, Bayesian probability theory in statistics predicts future events (conditional posterior probability) based on past and present information (weighted by the confidence of their accuracy). In defense, Bayesian AI applications demonstrate the strategic military, scientific, and political economic pivot to an AI data science-driven approach to risk management and deterrence paradigms, shifting from understanding and calculating "risk as isolated, discrete, and deterministic to Bayesian integrated, interdependent, adaptive." If deterrence substantively rests on a cost-benefit calculation, AI appears already to be helping us reach more timely and precise insights, empowering us to make faster and better decisions while adapting in real-time to new data coming in from diverse sources and perspectives (even when it is incomplete or "messy").

Concretely, the integrated deterrent of SpaceX's Starlink (low latency low earth orbit broadband internet system) serves as what may be the world's largest AI-powered neural network and edge computing architecture spanning 11,000 satellites in constellation (Jayanti 2023; Zecchin et al. 2022). Through DL, machine learning (ML), and reinforcement learning (guiding rocket launches, avoiding space collisions, and coordinating data sharing and cybersecurity), Starlink provides agile and resilient digital connectivity powering digital telecommunications networks (faster and with more data access than traditional fiber-based internet, especially for remote locations or disaster situations). Although an exhaustive detail of the AI methodology is not public, there is growing evidence that it may feature a robust Bayesian learning boosting DL's capacity to drive such reliable and robust wireless digital communication (avoiding traditional analytics' disadvantages of limited speed and prediction accuracy, in addition to DL's limited ability to handle uncertainty, misspecification, and outliers inherent in real-time communication data). Ukraine requested this private service via X (formerly known as Twitter) directly to Musk—he approved it within 12 hours, shipped the terminals within 2 days, and enabled over 150,000 citizens within 3 months of Russia's full-scale invasion to use it to preserve critical civil, defense, political, and economic digital functions through this public—private partnership. Starlink became one of the first high profile AI digital technologies that was successfully and widely deployed to force multiply population resilience capacities, from defense with Ukraine's drones and command and control chains, to deterrence with its civilian infrastructure demonstrating the futility of Russia's regular bombardments, to development with Starlink enabling Microsoft's cloud computing to preserve government and health services. By unifying development with its deterrence and defense guardrails, integrated deterrence may be considered as the whole-of-government (WoG)-driven, defense-originated, political economic translation of the WoW-driven, society-originated, human security-based development paradigm the related chapter previously explored.

5.2.2.2 WHO-coordinated cooperative medical diplomacy as multilateral development

Despite rising political economic tensions, there remains promising durable partnerships in development by the United States and China in multilateral cooperative medical diplomacy, which nonetheless retain elements of managed strategic competition as both sides seek to expand their soft power through it especially in the Global South (Bouey 2019). Such areas span drug design, production, resilient supply chains, pandemics (i.e., SARS-CoV-1 and influenza), NCDs, CDs (including HIV), biomedical research capacity building, workforce education (including student and scholar exchanges and conferences), multilateral organization collaborations (including with the WHO, World Bank, and IMF), and regulatory interoperability (i.e., United States and China FDAs). Yet as cooperative medical diplomacy deepens in global health, the AI digitalization of this ecosystem may either worsen or improve the overall bilateral relationship central to security, economic, and scientific progress for the world. AI and its Big Data are increasingly becoming essential, pervasive, and integrated with global health efforts. Accordingly, they potentially accelerate the derisking or even decoupling since both nations describe AI and its related digital technologies as "paradigm-shifting technologies" that are "national security priorities" (Sullivan and Deese 2021, p. 66). The better the cooperation, the better the technologies become, the more pressure builds to restrict them from perceived competitors. But to pull out AI digital technologies from US−China bilateral and cooperative development efforts would likely be to pull out effectiveness and efficiency from those efforts.

Yet progress continues in the meantime. There are synergistic advances using AI digital linkages of SDGs with precision medicine at an individual level that is then scaled up regionally and nationally to enhance precision public health, which can then be exported through the global public health ecosystem, optimized by cross-learning from similar programs, and then personalized for local communities in other nations (Kwon et al. 2021). Specifically, the above team quantified intervenable deficits in local communities' SDGs through the Social Deprivation Index (spanning education, employment, and housing) and paired them with individual-level electronic health record (EHR) medical data to facilitate greater AI empowered and digitally enabled cooperation between public health and medical sectors for population health. Greater cooperation in this multilateral and multinational development accelerated by AI thus provides greater opportunities to bridge political economic divides (and risks of exacerbating underlying tensions among strategic competitors and value blocs). Although there is increased political jostling for influence within it, the WHO is emerging as potentially the coordinating institution best positioned at the center of the global public health ecosystem (to effectively facilitate strategic managed competition, reorientating multinational medical diplomacy back principally to global well-being and away from predominantly expanding national soft power; WHO 2023b). Reinforced by the diplomacy momentum as the UN's primary health body, and the explicit consensus of the world's nations accordingly, the WHO highlights its role "providing leadership on global health matters, shaping the health research agenda, setting norms and standards, articulating evidence-based policy options, providing technical support to countries and monitoring and assessing health trends." Its main operational pillars are cooperative equity and efficiency since "health is a shared responsibility," unifying our world to advance together "equitable access to essential care and collective defense against transnational threats." The WHO over the last two decades appears to have double-downed on its dominant position as the coordinator of cooperative integrated deterrence against insufficient responses to acute and chronic health threats (including the breakdown of cooperation amid strategic competitors like the United States and China). As Chapters 2 and 4 respectively on finance and data assessed, the WHO emphasizes its efforts to coordinate the progressive investments and programs with the United States, China, and the broader multinational support of promoting UHC (with agile AI-accelerated financing and more cost-effective population health for essential health services and innovations, including the WHO Pandemic Hub for AI-enhanced prevention, detection, and mitigation of global infectious threats).

5.2.2.3 Democratizing artificial intelligence: deep medicine, ChatGPT, and large language models

AI is not only digitalizing the global health ecosystem (in both its public health and medical dimensions), but also AI itself is generally becoming democratized—and thus those ecosystems by extension (Rubeis et al. 2022). The most advanced, pervasive, and globalized AI health uses are developed by and in free market democracies for domestic and international use. As this regime's hallmark is more free information flows, the AI made in its image is thus opening up more of the overarching global digital ecosystem, while freeing it up for more people from democracies and autocracies. The American physician-scientist, Eric Topol, is credited with charting and pioneering this influential trend as one of the world's most cited medical researchers and the National Institute of Health (NIH) colead for the "All of Us Program" or Precision Medicine Initiative Cohort (the largest diverse integrated dataset in history, uniting -omics, clinical, lifestyle, and environmental data particularly from underserved and minority communities; Topol 2019). He details this trend in his seminal 2019 book, *"Deep Medicine: How artificial intelligence can make healthcare human again."* Topol describes how AI's medical digitalization may progressively empower each patient—as a unique person and health consumer—to finally "own" her/his own health data and decisions, equal with physicians through the democratization of that decision-making process with the shared goal of the optimal wellbeing of each patient. This process is the clinical application of what Chapter 1 introduced with DL or "deep learning," the technological trend enabling AI to process and analyze data more akin to the human brain, including understanding complex patterns in sounds, images, and text (and even better replicating subsequent human-like behavior applying such understanding to different tasks). In this account, deep medicine gives way to its ultimate strategic goal of "deep empathy." In it, the relationship of healthcare professionals is enriched and humanized through AI's technical empowerment of healthcare data's use and related work processes (particularly mechanical and time-consuming tasks). AI health democratization has expanded not only through these technical means of patient empowerment, but also through expanding its producers, development, access, and governance (through democratic consensus-based definition and defense of public goods and equitable means of achieving them). All of Us is a WoG and emerging whole-of-society private—public—academic partnership manifesting this AI democratization process. Its researchers from the Broad Institute (research collaborative with Harvard University and Massachusetts Institute of Technology) utilize the NIH's deidentified patient data with Microsoft's cloud computing-based Terra platform (an open-source secure and scalable data architecture for globally accessible data storage, AI/ML algorithm analytics, and interoperable collaboration among ecosystem partners). Terra thus empowers partners equitable access to such sophisticated Big Data capacities for their own priorities their communities require, regardless of partners' local data storage and analytic capacities (Townes-Whitley and Moore 2019). Both the NIH (the world's largest biomedical researcher funder) and Microsoft (the world's largest software maker) justify such partnerships as needed to "democratize" healthcare, as their research studies and software products run most of health advances and their prerequisite digital capacities, carrying forward this digital democratization by embedded design. Yet given the greater profit potential in medicine and more free and open democratic states predominantly driving its evolution (particularly in developed nations), the democratization of global health into "deep health" (spanning higher income democratic and autocratic developed countries) means developing countries lag behind accessing it and its benefits.

Open AI's ChatGPT may be changing that. Such free and widely available internet-based large language models (as introduced in Chapter 1) became in the first 6 months of launch what may be the most widely adapted, applied, and influential sophisticated AI method across states and sectors globally (Parray et al. 2023; Economist 2023). It already appears to outperform traditional large EHR-based clinical prediction models, telehealth for under-served patients, infectious disease surveillance, personalized community health education, and NLP-based drug discovery by integrating an unprecedented volume, variety, and velocity of scientific literature, chemical datasets (including toxicity), -omics datasets, traditional news, social media, and the massive spectrum of internet resources. It is thus largely credited with bringing the AI revolution to the masses. But much less explored is how ChatGPT as the most dominant large language model was first and since predominantly trained on English speaking digital sources, since those are the most widely available sources. Accordingly, our most powerful and pervasive AI is democratic at its core, with the related latent values and assumptions explored in this chapter's opening. This suggests the foreseeable trajectory for health AI will fundamentally feature a more open, free, and globalized structure prioritizing individual agency and national sovereignty.

5.2.2.4 Digital supply chain resilience: artificial intelligence—augmented microchip manufacturing + diversification

Digital supply chain resilience is a key deterrent guardrail and resilience requirement for human security—based development, especially given global vulnerabilities that COVID-19 and Russia revealed about global health, local public health, and healthcare system capacities still struggling to respond to population health needs. The threat of China's invasion (or extended blockade) of Taiwan further highlights such vulnerabilities given the growing awareness of our global dependence on Taiwan's advanced semiconductors running our digital world. Developing countries have limited options to address such vulnerabilities directly. Even the most digitally advanced developed countries have no clear answer, despite blowout government spending attempts by the United States and its Western allies to shore up domestic manufacturing and friend-shoring supply chains in case of China compromising them by conflict with its alleged colony/territory (Agrawal 2023). In 1991, the UN Security Council (with Russia and China declining to veto) invoked the UN Charter to back a US-led coalition of 39 countries from the Global South and East joined with the West which successfully drove Iraq out of Kuwait following Saddam Hussein's invasion of the latter—morally and politically threatening the modern right of national sovereignty and the pragmatic need for the world's oil access (which Iraq at the time controlled 20% of after the invasion; UVA 2023). If China successfully invades and holds an intact Taiwan, it will control 90% of the world's advanced chips, and practically 100% of the global digital economy on which modern economies and states depend (with significantly less likelihood the world would unite to successfully repulse it, let alone have a UN Security Council resolution condemning the invasion, since China and its allied Russia both are permanent Council members). Therefore, both in green energy explored earlier and in digital supply chains described here, there is an international push for greater supply chain resilience as enhanced deterrence and sustainability for global stability and development. Aside from the abovesaid political economic countermeasures, there was a 2023 technical breakthrough in the fabrication process with human—AI teams preserving quality while halving the cost of microchip design (instead of the current dependence on small numbers of highly trained but costly engineers manually required for it; Wang and Huang 2023). Smarter and smarter AI increasingly runs and creates iteratively more powerful and efficient digital technologies. This in turn accelerates the democratization and diversification of the global digital economy's most critical nonrenewable resource, while suggesting a successful template for enhanced global stability through reductions in excessive reliance on choke points in supply chains that are especially vulnerable to unpredictable political economic crises.

5.2.2.5 Liquified natural gas, nuclear, and commercial fusion as sustainable artificial intelligence energy

Cooperative and digitalized political economics still ultimately requires affordable energy to power everything, including the production and purchase of affordable food and health services required to power people who constitute the global ecosystem. The intergovernmental organization, the International Energy Agency whose member and associated countries represent 75% of global energy demand, notes how nuclear power and hydropower together generate three quarters of low-carbon energy generation globally (IEA 2019; ANS 2023). The former has reduced carbon emissions by 60 gigatonnes in the last five decades, though developed countries' investments in it has dried up while developed countries face capital restrictions to ramp them up. But these trends began reversing after Russia's 2022 invasion of Ukraine and subsequent weaponization of oil, catalyzing renewed global investment in nuclear power—even in Japan which had been deliberately attempting to phase out nuclear completely after the 2011 Fukushima accident. Additionally, the UN Environment Programme notes how liquified natural gas (LNG) as a "cleaner" fossil fuel (producing less air pollutants) may be an effective energy bridge from "dirtier" fossil fuels like coal and oil to cleaner renewable energy sources, given their cheaper cost and widespread availability, while also serving as a backup for renewables (UNEP 2023). Over 20 new LNG terminals alone from Germany to China were built in the first year after Russia's war, with LNG already replacing coal as the primary generating source for electricity in many nations (while the significant price drop in solar, wind, and other renewable sources becomes significant and widespread enough for wider adoption). Finally, Helion Energy (back by the founder of OpenAI), signed the first commercial fusion energy contract with Microsoft in 2023 to provide electricity from fusion by 2028, or pay financial penalties; Microsoft plans to scale up such clean energy production through their global AI and data network for "unlimited clean [carbon free] energy" to power it, after Microsoft already scaled OpenAI's AI through its platforms earlier in the year following ChatGPT's launch (Hiller 2023). Harnessing this energy which powers our sun, Microsoft is leveraging its position not only as one of the world's dominant AI and quantum computing players but also as among the largest software producers and power-purchasers for its vast data centers, pressuring the rest of the global digital ecosystem to follow suit pairing cleaner energy with responsible AI (as the company repeatedly predicts AI, quantum, and clean energy particularly fusion power are the key disruptive innovations of our era that is framing our near future).

5.2.3 Global public health ecosystem: newer rules-based order of integral values versus older ruler-based world order of ideological values

This big chapter tried to pull together the big ideas of the preceding chapters to show how political economics is the societal dimension that complements its digital dimension of the data architecture. Together they account for the structural framework of the global public health ecosystem. This framework operationalizes the ecosystem's design, built around integral sustainable development and its related financing. Chapter 6 will consider the inhabitants (culture and demographics) and its foundation (human/national security and ethics) for our common home, before concluding Chapter 7 and the book on how this ecosystem concretely operates now and in our common tomorrow. Before getting there, let us recap how this chapter analyzed the role of political economics as the meta-determinant of health determinants, and explain how humanity organizes itself and operates (according to a foundation of common values supporting our economics and how those economics are politically governed). In our capitalized world, we considered the empirical evidence suggesting how the competing political regime of (liberal) democracies appear to outperform (illiberal democratic) autocracies by more effectively, sustainably, and cooperatively providing public goods for the greatest number of a population. We then moved on to the political economic model of Personalist Liberalism. We spent the last few chapters building up to this model to consider how it may structurally enable the needed integration, interoperability, and institutionalization of the AI-powered global public health ecosystem. It seeks to account for and facilitate this transformation by comprehensively and effectively targeting global public health determinants, advancing the needed structural cooperation among diverse stakeholders and political economic regimes (democratic, autocratic, Northern, and Southern states), and facilitating the transition from debt to development. From this perspective, we considered the health AI advances in development-focused political economics (with deterrence and defense guardrails), WHO-facilitated coordination of consensus-based multilateral development, democratization of health AI and data, digital supply chain resilience, and affordable energy transition. Ultimately, political economic regimes risk falling if they fail to sufficiently secure equitable public goods. Doing so typically requires raw materials, supply chains, and structural societal factors, including self-determination, sovereignty, development, deterrence, defense, digital capacities, food, and energy. We particularly focused on integrated deterrence as the WoG-driven (minimal political economic) translation of the WoW-driven approach (of maximal human security-based development). As the United States is the largest funder of global public health and AI advances, and China is its primary multidomain challenger, such guardrails are key to sustaining global development by maximizing global cooperation and minimizing global conflict.

This now sets us up for Chapter 6 to consider the cultures and values animating this political economic framework so we can apply it to the concrete AI advances in the global public health ecosystem's evolution—innovation in individuality, strength in unity, and sustainability in their union, grounded in the common (not simply public) good. Aside from the top-down perspective in this chapter, we will next consider the bottom-up one. We will pivot to considering how the local level may avoid Hobbesian hard totalitarianism of (near) absolute state control and the Rousseauian soft totalitarianism of listless democratic control (in which the public lose unifying transcendent values and thus become vulnerable to manipulative elitist and autocratic consolidation of power unrestrained by those higher and intrinsic values). Instead, we will consider in our pluralistic local health ecosystems how the Aristotelian personalist community of the common good recognizes that unlike Hobbes and Rousseau, the state is not artificial but rather existentially and essentially human. In this argument, the human person belongs to and is understood only in community as a unique member of the community—they are not solely an individual or lost in the collective. This means personal dignity and the communal common good are operationalized in the ethical principles of subsidiarity and solidarity that can animate the responsible and sustainable political economics that Personalist Liberalism sought to help analyze in this chapter. Accordingly, we will shift from ideological and even imperial values (wielded by rulers who traditionally have ruled humanity) to integral values (codified into consensus-based rules for a better tomorrow). We will therefore analyze the multicultural, pluralistic, but still convergent principles showing that just peace requires just power (fair not simply power to govern society). This cumulatively builds to how just political economics are rooted in real shared values of human security, national sovereignty, and global sustainability—necessities that we and our global public health ecosystem existentially need for us to have a common future.

References

Agrawal, R. 2023. "Why Taiwan Has a Lock on the World's Chip Market." Foreign Policy. Accessed June 17, 2023. https://foreignpolicy.com/2023/06/14/taiwan-microchips-semiconductors-tsmc/.

Anderson, J., Rainie, L., and Vogels, E.A. 2021. "Experts Say the 'New Normal' in 2025 Will Be Far More Tech-Driven, Presenting More Big Challenges." Pew Research Center. Accessed May 11, 2023. https://www.pewresearch.org/internet/2021/02/18/experts-say-the-new-normal-in-2025-will-be-far-more-tech-driven-presenting-more-big-challenges/.

ANS. 2023. "Countries Change Nuclear Policies in Response to Ukraine War." American Nuclear Society Newswire. Accessed June 18, 2023. https://www.ans.org/news/article-4623/countries-change-nuclear-policies-in-response-to-ukraine-war/.

ANU. 2023. "How China Is on the Verge of Totalitarianism 2.0." Accessed May 8, 2023. https://nsc.crawford.anu.edu.au/department-news/13026/how-china-verge-totalitarianism-20.

APHA. 2022. "A Call to Expand International Debt Relief for All Developing Countries to Increase Access to Public Resources for Health Care." American Public Health Association. Accessed June 5, 2023. https://

apha.org/Policies-and-Advocacy/Public-Health-Policy-Statements/Policy-Database/2023/01/18/Expand-International-Debt-Relief.

Birn, A.E., Pillay, Y., and T.H. Holtz. 2017. *Textbook of Global Health*, 4th edition Oxford: Oxford University Press.

Bollyky, T.J., Castro, E., Aravkin, A.Y., Bhangdia, K., Dalos, J., and E.N. Hulland, et al., 2023. "Assessing COVID-19 Pandemic Policies and Behaviours and Their Economic and Educational Trade-Offs Across US States from Jan 1, 2020, to July 31, 2022." *Lancet* 401 (10385): 1341–1360.

Bouey, J. 2019. "Implications of U.S.–China Collaborations on Global Health Issues." RAND Corporation. Accessed May 13, 2023. https://www.rand.org/content/dam/rand/pubs/testimonies/CT500/CT516/RAND_CT516.pdf.

Bremmer, I. 2006. *The J Curve: A new way to understand why nations rise and fall*. New York: Simon & Schuster.

Bremmer, I. and Kupchan, C. 2023. "Top Risks 2023." Eurasia Group. Accessed May 8, 2023. https://www.eurasiagroup.net/issues/top-risks-2023.

Broadband. 2020. "Reimaging Global Health Through Artificial Intelligence: The Roadmap to AI Maturity." Broadband Commission for Sustainable Development. Accessed April 21, 2023. https://www.broadband-commission.org/wp-content/uploads/2021/02/WGAIinHealth_Report2020.pdf.

CEPR. 2022. "Will US Rate Hikes Harm Developing Countries?" Center for Economic and Policy Research. Accessed May 8, 2023. https://cepr.net/will-us-rate-hikes-harm-developing-countries/.

CFR. 2023. "China's Approach to Global Governance." Council on Foreign Relations. Accessed May 2, 2023. https://www.cfr.org/china-global-governance/.

Chan, T. and Dimitrijevic, A., 2023. "Global debt leverage." S&P Global. Accessed June 8, 2023. https://www.spglobal.com/en/research-insights/featured/special-editorial/look-forward/global-debt-leverage-is-a-great-reset-coming.

Chase, M.S. and Chan. A. 2016. "China's Evolving Approach to 'Integrated Strategic Deterrence'." RAND Corporation. Accessed June 9, 2023. https://www.rand.org/pubs/research_reports/RR1366.html.

Chin, J. 2018. "China Spends More on Domestic Security as Xi's Powers Grow." *The Wall Street Journal*. Accessed May 26, 2023. https://www.wsj.com/articles/china-spends-more-on-domestic-security-as-xis-powers-grow-1520358522.

Cho, E. 2020. "The Social Credit System." Princeton University Journal of Public & International Affairs. Accessed May 8, 2023. https://jpia.princeton.edu/news/social-credit-system-not-just-another-chinese-idiosyncrasy.

Cloud, D.S. and Ramzy, A., 2023. "China-Brokered Deal Between Iran, Saudi Arabia Marks a New Middle East." *The Wall Street Journal*. Accessed May 8, 2023. https://www.wsj.com/articles/china-brokered-deal-between-iran-saudi-arabia-marks-a-new-middle-east-d1eaf94e.

Cochrane, S. 2023. *The Fiscal Theory of the Price Level*. Princeton, NJ: Princeton University Press.

Combe, P.C., Jensen, B., and Bogart, A. 2023. "Rethinking Risk in Greater Power Competition." The Center for Strategic and International Studies. Accessed May 11, 2023. https://www.csis.org/analysis/rethinking-risk-great-power-competition.

Cutler, D. 2020. "The World's Costliest Health Care." Harvard University Magazine. Accessed March 14, 2023. https://www.hsph.harvard.edu/news/hsph-in-the-news/understanding-why-health-care-costs-in-the-u-s-are-so-high/.

Desilver, D. 2019. "Despite Global Concerns About Democracy, More Than Half of Countries Are Democratic." Pew Research Center. Accessed May 25, 2023. https://www.pewresearch.org/short-reads/2019/05/14/more-than-half-of-countries-are-democratic/.

Ebrahim, N. 2023. "China Praises Ukraine Talks in Saudi That Russia Said Were 'Doomed to Fail'." CNN. Accessed September 24, 2023. https://www.cnn.com/2023/08/07/middleeast/saudi-arabia-ukraine-talks-china-mime-intl/index.html.

Echikson, B. 2022. "Europe Overregulates, US Abdicates—and China May Win the Race for Tech Supremacy." Center for European Policy Analysis. Accessed May 27, 2023. https://cepa.org/article/europe-overregulates-us-abdicates-in-race-for-tech-supremacy/.

Economist. 2023. "Large, Creative AI Models Will Transform Lives and Labour Markets." *The Economist.* Accessed May 8, 2023. https://www.economist.com/interactive/science-and-technology/2023/04/22/large-creative-ai-models-will-transform-how-we-live-and-work.

Eyawo, O., Viens, A.M., and U.C. Ugoji. 2021. "Lockdowns and Low- and Middle-Income Countries: Building a Feasible, Effective, and Ethical COVID-19 Response Strategy." *Globalization and Health* 17 (1): 13.

Fang, S., Li, X., and A.Y. Liu. 2022. "Chinese Public Opinion About US−China Relations from Trump to Biden." *The Chinese Journal of International Politics* 15 (1): 27−46.

Ferguson, N. 2005. *Colossus: The Rise and Fall of the American Empire.* New York: Penguin Books.

Ferguson, N. 2018. *The Square and the Tower: Networks and Power, from the Freemasons to Facebook.* New York: Penguin Press.

Ferguson, N. 2022. "How Cold War II could turn into World War III." Bloomberg. Accessed May 22, 2023. https://www.bloomberg.com/opinion/articles/2022-10-23/cold-war-2-with-china-and-russia-is-becoming-ww3-niall-ferguson.

Freudenberg, N. 2023. "Framing Commercial Determinants of Health: An Assessment of Potential for Guiding More Effective Responses to the Public Health Crises of the 21st Century." *The Milbank Quarterly* 101 (S1): 83−98.

Gan. 2021. "14 Countries and WHO Chief Accuse China of Withholding Data from Pandemic Origins Investigation." CNN. Accessed May 8, 2023. https://www.cnn.com/2021/03/31/asia/who-report-criticism-intl-hnk/index.html.

Gómez, A.G., and D.J. Monlezun. 2023. "Ethical Challenges in COVID-19 Biomedical Research, Vaccination, and Therapy." In *Bioethics During the COVID-19 Pandemic,* edited by A.G. Gómez.

Goujon, R. 2023. "China and the U.S. are Struggling over Data Security: A Breaking Point May Be Near." Barron's. May 8, 2023. https://www.barrons.com/articles/us-china-data-security-db49e68a.

Graefrath, M., and M. Jahn. 2023. "Conceptualizing Interstate Cooperation." *International Theory* 15 (1): 24−52.

Herby, J., Jonung, L., and Hanke, S.H. 2022. "A Literature Review and Metaanalysis of the Effects of Lockdowns on COVID_19 Mortality." John Hopkins University Studies in Applied Economics. Accessed July 1, 2023. https://sites.krieger.jhu.edu/iae/files/2022/01/A-Literature-Review-and-Meta-Analysis-of-the-Effects-of-Lockdowns-on-COVID-19-Mortality.pdf.

Hiller, J. 2023. "Microsoft Bets that Fusion Power is Closer Than Many Think." *The Wall Street Journal.* Accessed May 11, 2023. https://www.wsj.com/articles/microsoft-bets-that-fusion-power-is-closer-than-many-think-cb1b09dc.

Hirsh, M. 2023. "How AI Will Revolutionize Warfare." Foreign Policy. Accessed May 8, 2023. https://foreignpolicy.com/2023/04/11/ai-arms-race-artificial-intelligence-chatgpt-military-technology/.

Hsueh, R. 2022. *Micro-Institutional Foundations of Capitalism.* Cambridge: Cambridge, University Press.

IEA. 2019. "Nuclear Power in a Clean Energy System." International Energy Association. Accessed June 18, 2023. https://www.iea.org/reports/nuclear-power-in-a-clean-energy-system.

IMF. 2022. "IMF Annual Report: Crisis upon Crisis." International Monetary Fund. Accessed June 8, 2023. https://www.imf.org/external/pubs/ft/ar/2022/english/.

Irish, J. and Murakami, S. 2023. "Ukraine's Zelenskiy Courts 'Global South' at G7 Summit." Reuters. Accessed May 22, 2023. https://www.reuters.com/world/g7-aims-bridge-vast-gap-with-emerging-markets-awaits-zelenskiy-2023-05-19/.

Jayanti, A. 2023. "Starlink and the Russia−Ukraine War." Harvard University Kennedy School. Accessed May 11, 2023. https://www.belfercenter.org/publication/starlink-and-russia-ukraine-war-case-commercial-technology-and-public-purpose.

Jones, L., Hameiri. 2022. "Explaining the Failure of Global Health Governance During COVID-19." *International Affairs* 98 (6): 2057−2076.

Kadakia, K.T., Beckman, A.L., and H.M. Krumholz. 2023. "A Prescription for the US FDA for the Regulation of Health Misinformation." *Nature Medicine* 29 (3): 525−527.

Koop, A. and Routley, N. 2023. "Mapped: The World's Happiest Countries in 2023." Visual Capitalist. Accessed March 26, 2023. https://www.visualcapitalist.com/worlds-happiest-countries-2023/.

Kotkin, S. 2015. *Stalin: Paradoxes of Power, 1878−1928*. New York, NY: Penguin Books.

Krishna, J., Butani, M., Singh, K., Gupta, A., 2023. Can IPEF be a Watershed Moment for U.S.−India? The Center for Strategic and International Studies. Accessed June 11, 2023. https://www.csis.org/analysis/experts-react-can-ipef-be-watershed-moment-us-india.

Kwon, I.G., Kim, S.H., and D. Martin. 2021. "Integrating Social Determinants of Health to Precision Medicine Through Digital Transformation." *International Journal of Environmental Research and Public Health* 18 (9): 5018.

Labonté, R., and A. Ruckert. 2019. *Health equity in a globalizing era: Past challenges, future prospects*. Oxford: Oxford University Press.

Lahart, J. 2022. "Globalization Isn't Unraveling: It's Changing." *The Wall Street Journal*. Accessed May 10, 2023. https://www.wsj.com/articles/globalization-isnt-unraveling-its-changing-11650015032.

Lawrence, L. 2023. "FDA Commissioner on Regulating New Digital Health Tools." STAT News. Accessed May 12, 2023. https://www.statnews.com/2023/05/09/fda-ai-digital-health-care/.

Lin., B., Hart, B., Funaiole, M.P., and Lu, S. 2022. "China's 20th Party Congress Report." Center for Strategic and International Studies. Accessed June 18, 2023. https://www.csis.org/analysis/chinas-20th-party-congress-report-doubling-down-face-external-threats.

Lin, J., and D. Rosenblatt. 2012. "Shifting Patterns of Economic Growth and Rethinking Development." *Journal of Economic Policy Reform* 15 (3): 1−24.

Lusigi, A. 2022. "Shaping Our Future in a World of Transformation." United Nations Development Programme. Accessed May 10, 2023. https://www.undp.org/ghana/blog/shaping-our-future-world-transformation.

Maizland, L. 2022. "China's Repression of Uyghurs in Xinjiang." Council on Foreign Relations. Accessed May 17, 2023. https://www.cfr.org/backgrounder/china-xinjiang-uyghurs-muslims-repression-genocide-human-rights.

Mallapaty, S. 2023. "WHO Abandons Plans for Crucial Second Phase of COVID-Origins Investigation." *Nature*. Accessed May 11, 2023. https://www.nature.com/articles/d41586-023-00283-y.

Mattes, M., and M. Rodríguez. 2014. "Autocracies and international cooperation." *International Studies Quarterly* 58 (3): 527−538.

Mattis, J. 2018. "Secretary Mattis Remarks on the National Defense Strategy in Conversation with the United States Institute for Peace." United States Department of Defense. Accessed May 8, 2023. https://www.defense.gov/News/Transcripts/Transcript/Article/1678512/secretary-mattis-remarks-on-the-national-defense-strategy-in-conversation-with/.

Miller, C. 2022. *Chip War: The Fight for the World's Most Critical Technology*. New York: Simon & Schuster (Scribner Books).

Monlezun, D.J. 2023. *The Thinking Healthcare System: Artificial Intelligence and Human Equity*. New York: Elsevier.

Parray, A.A., Inam, Z.M., Ramonfaur, D., Haider, S.S., Mistry, S.K., and A.K. Pandya. 2023. "ChatGPT and global public health." *Global Transitions* 5, 50−54.

Porter, M.E., Lee, T.H. 2013. "The Strategy that will Fix Health Care." *Harvard Business Review*. Accessed May 10, 2023. https://hbr.org/2013/10/the-strategy-that-will-fix-health-care.

Radford, A. 2023. "Ukraine War Must End, South African President Ramaphosa Tells Putin." *BBC*. Accessed June 19, 2023. https://www.bbc.com/news/world-europe-65940655.

RAS. 2023. "Highlights from the RAeS Future Combat Air & Space Capabilities Summit." Royal Aeronautical Society. Accessed June 15, 2023. https://www.aerosociety.com/news/highlights-from-the-raes-future-combat-air-space-capabilities-summit/.

Roessler, M., and J. Schmitt. 2021. "Health System Efficiency and Democracy: A Public Choice Perspective." *PloS One* 16 (9): e0256737.

Rubeis, G., Dubbala, K., and I. Metzler. 2022. "Democratizing' Artificial Intelligence in Medicine and Healthcare: Mapping the Uses of an Elusive Term." *Frontiers in Genetics* 13902542.

Rudd, K. 2022. *The Avoidable War. The Dangers of Catastrophic Conflict Between the US and Xi Jinping's China*. New York: Public Affairs.

Ryan, A. 2012. *The Making of Modern Liberalism*. Princeton, NJ: Princeton University Press.

Sachs, J. 1999. "Twentieth-Century Political Economy: A Brief History of Global Capitalism." *Oxford University Review of Economic Policy* 15 (4): 90−101.

Sauer, P. 2023. "Putin Recycles Old Grievances on Victory Day as Russian Army Battered in Ukraine." *The Guardian*. Accessed May 17, 2023. https://www.theguardian.com/world/2023/may/09/putin-recycles-old-grievances-on-victory-day-as-russian-army-battered-in-ukraine.

SCCEI. "China's Corporate Social Credit System and Its Implications." Stanfard University Center on China's Economy and Institutions. https://sccei.fsi.stanford.edu/china-briefs/chinas-corporate-social-credit-system-and-its-implications (accessed 28 May 2023).

Schelling, T. 1981. *The Strategy of Conflict*. Cambridge, MA: Harvard University Press (1960).

Schuman, M. 2022. "What Xi Jinping's Third Term Means for the World." Atlantic Council. Accessed June 4, 2023. https://www.atlanticcouncil.org/in-depth-research-reports/issue-brief/what-xi-jinpings-third-term-means-for-the-world.

Sen, K., Pritchett, L., Kar, S., Raihan, S., 2017. Democracy Versus Dictatorship? The Political Determinants of Growth Episodes. Harvard University Kennedy School. Accessed May 25, 2023. https://www.hks.harvard.edu/publications/democracy-versus-dictatorship-political-determinants-growth-episodes.

Sharkey, C.M., and K.M.K. Fodouop. 2022. "AI and the Regulatory Paradigm Shift at the FDA." *Duke Law Journal* 72 (November): 86−112.

Shek, C. 2019. "Aiming for the Top: Can China Escape the Middle Income Trap?" Cheung Kong Graduate School of Business. Accessed June 5, 2023. https://english.ckgsb.edu.cn/knowledges/china-middle-income-trap/.

Spence, M. 2023. "Destructive Decoupling." Council on Foreign Relations. Accessed May 31, 2023. https://www.cfr.org/article/destructive-decoupling.

Stewart, P. and Ali, I. 2018. "How Mattis is Trying to Keep U.S.−China Tensions from Boiling Over." Reuters. Accessed May 14, 2023. https://www.reuters.com/article/us-usa-china-mattis-insight/how-mattis-is-trying-to-keep-u-s-china-tensions-from-boiling-over-idUSKCN1NE0FF.

Store, Z. 2014. *A Sense of the Enemy: The High Stakes History of Reading Your Rival's Mind*. Oxford: Oxford University Press.

Sullivan, J. and Deese, B. 2021. "Building Resilient Supply Chains, Revitalizing American Manufacturing, and Fostering Broad-Based Growth." The US White House. Accessed February 10, 2023. https://www.whitehouse.gov/wp-content/uploads/2021/06/100-day-supply-chain-review-report.pdf.

Tian, Y.L. 2023. "China's Xi Urges Private Firms to 'Be Rich and Loving' in Pursuit of Prosperity For All." Reuters. Accessed May 21, 2023. https://www.reuters.com/world/china/chinas-xi-urges-private-firms-be-rich-loving-pursuit-prosperity-all-2023-03-06/.

Tocqueville, A., 1840. Democracy in America. Mansfield, H.C., Winthrop, D. (Trans.). Chicago, IL: University of Chicago (2002).

Tongia. 2022. "It is Unfair to Push Poor Countries to Reach Zero Carbon Emissions Too Early." The Brookings Institute. Accessed June 9, 2023. https://www.brookings.edu/blog/planetpolicy/2022/10/26/it-is-unfair-to-push-poor-countries-to-reach-zero-carbon-emissions-too-early/.

Topol, E. 2019. *Deep Medicine: How Artificial Intelligence Can Make Healthcare Human Again.* New York: Basic Books.

Townes-Whitley, T. and Moore, G. 2019. "Partnering with the NIH to Advance Biomedical Research." Microsoft. Accessed June 16, 2023. https://blogs.microsoft.com/blog/2021/07/20/partnering-with-the-nih-to-advance-biomedical-research/.

Townshend, A. 2023. "The AUKUS Submarine Deal Highlights a Tectonic Shift in the U.S.—Australia Alliance."Accessed June 11, 2023. Carnegie Endowment for International Peace. https://carnegieendowment.org/2023/03/27/aukus-submarine-deal-highlights-tectonic-shift-in-u.s.-australia-alliance-pub-89383.

UN. 1945. "Charter." United Nations. Accessed May 8, 2023. https://www.un.org/en/about-us/un-charter/full-text.

UN. 2020. "The Importance of Investing in Global Public Goods for Health." United Nations. Accessed May 8, 2023. https://www.un.org/development/desa/dpad/wp-content/uploads/sites/45/publication/PB_83.pdf.

UN. 2021. "Global Climate Objectives Fall Short Without Nuclear Power in the Mix: UNECE." United Nations. Accessed May 8, 2023. https://news.un.org/en/story/2021/08/1097572.

UN. 2023. "Cooperation Between the United Nations and the Council of Europe: Resolution 77/284 adopted by the General Assembly." United Nations. Accessed May 8, 2023. https://digitallibrary.un.org/record/4009707?ln = en.

UN EP. 2023. "Is Natural Gas Really the Bridge Fuel the World Needs?" Accessed June 18, 2023. https://www.unep.org/news-and-stories/story/natural-gas-really-bridge-fuel-world-needs.

UN WCE. 1987. "Report of the World Commission on Environment and Development: Our Common Future." United Nations World Commission on Environment and Development. Accessed April 5, 2023. https://sustainabledevelopment.un.org/content/documents/5987our-common-future.pdf.

US. 1776. "Declaration of Independence." United States of America National Archives. Accessed May 20, 2023. https://www.archives.gov/founding-docs/declaration-transcript.

US—Vietnam. 2000. "United States and Vietnam Bilateral Trade Agreement." Accessed June 4, 2023. https://vn.usembassy.gov/our-relationship/policy-history/bilateral-trade-agreement/.

UVA. 2023. *The Gulf War.* Miller Center: University of VirginiaAccessed June 17, 2023. https://millercenter.org/statecraftmovie/gulf-war.

Wang, Y.L., and M.C. Huang. 2023. "Human—AI Team Halves Cost of Designing Step in Microchip Fabrication." *Nature* 616 (7958): 667—668.

WEC. 2023. "The Global Risks Report 2023: 18th Edition." World Economic Forum. Accessed June 2, 2023. https://www3.weforum.org/docs/WEF_Global_Risks_Report_2023.pdf.

White House. 2023. "National Security Strategy." The United States White House. Accessed June 11, 2023. https://www.whitehouse.gov/wp-content/uploads/2022/10/Biden-Harris-Administrations-National-Security-Strategy-10.2022.pdf.

WHO. 2002. "Global Public Goods for Health." World Health Organization. Accessed May 19, 2023. https://apps.who.int/iris/bitstream/handle/10665/42518/9241590106.pdf.

WHO. 2021. "Global Strategy on Digital Health 2020—2025." World Health Organization. Accessed June 11, 2023. https://www.who.int/docs/default-source/documents/gs4dhdaa2a9f352b0445bafbc79ca799dce4d.pdf.

WHO. 2023a. "Social Determinants of Health. World Health Organization." Accessed June 11, 2022. https://www.who.int/health-topics/social-determinants-of-health#tab = tab_1.

WHO. 2023b. "WHO Agenda, Reform, and Role in Public Health." World Health Organization. Accessed June 11, 2022. https://www.un.org/youthenvoy/2013/09/who-world-health-organisation/#:~:text = WHO%20is%20the%20directing%20and.within%20the%20United%20Nations%20system.

Wike, R., Silver, L., Fetterolf, J., Huang, C., Austin, S., Clancy, L. et al., 2022. "Social Media Seen as Mostly Good for Democracy Across Many Nations." Pew Research Center. Accessed May 17, 2023. https://www.pewresearch.org/global/2022/12/06/social-media-seen-as-mostly-good-for-democracy-across-many-nations-but-u-s-is-a-major-outlier/.

Wire. 2023. "Nobody Knows Agony of War More Than You: Modi to Zelenskyy." *The Wire*. Accessed May 22, 2023. https://thewire.in/diplomacy/ukraine-india-modi-zelenskyy-meet-g7.

World Bank. 2023. "Breaking Down Barriers to Clean Energy Transition." The World Bank. Accessed June 9, 2023. https://www.worldbank.org/en/news/feature/2023/05/16/breaking-down-barriers-to-clean-energy-transition.

WSJ Editorial Board. 2021. "The Woke Chinese Community Party." *The Wall Street Journal*. Accessed May 17, 2023. https://www.wsj.com/articles/the-woke-chinese-communist-party-11615153949?mod = article_inline.

Xie, S.Y. and Douglas, J. 2023. "China's Fading Recovery Reveals Deeper Economic Struggles." *The Wall Street Journal*. Accessed May 30, 2023. https://www.wsj.com/articles/chinas-fading-recovery-reveals-deeper-economic-struggles-31f4097b.

Yang, Z. 2022. "China Just Announced a New Social Credit Law." MIT Technology Review. Accessed May 28, 2023. https://www.technologyreview.com/2022/11/22/1063605/china-announced-a-new-social-credit-law-what-does-it-mean/.

Yu-Hsin Lin, L. and Milhaupt, C.J. 2021. "China's Corporate Social Credit System: The Dawn of Surveillance State Capitalism?" *The China Quarterly*. Accessed May 28, 2023. https://papers.ssrn.com/sol3/papers.cfm?abstract_id = 3933134.

Yuan, L. 2022. "As Beijing Takes control, Chinese Tech Companies Lose Jobs and Hope." *The New York Times*. Accessed May 26, 2023. https://www.nytimes.com/2022/01/05/technology/china-tech-internet-crackdown-layoffs.html.

Zecchin, M., Park, S., Simeone, O., Kountouris, M., and Gesbert, D. 2022. "Robust Bayesian Learning For Reliable Wireless AI. arXiv 220700300."

Zitelmann, R. 2023. "Adam Smith's Solution to Poverty."Accessed June 16, 2023. https://www.wsj.com/articles/adam-smiths-solution-to-poverty-economic-growth-300-years-wages-8274f904.

6

Foundations and families: artificial intelligence ethics of demographic, multicultural, and security shifts

6.1 Foundations and their families

Our earlier analyses of the digitally enabled health political economic framework of the global public health ecosystem (driven by its development financed design) sets us up to consider the foundation upon which it rests: the national and human security ethics, governing the ecosystem caring for the global human family. We will do so from the perspective of our diverse demographics and multiculturalism, shaping and shaped by local families. Given the significant ground this penultimate chapter must cover, we will focus on the dominant demographic, cultural, and security impacts on the global ethics embodying the common values most relevant for the key artificial intelligence (AI) trends and use cases, which in turn drive the ecosystem's current and evolving form. The earlier chapters largely focused on the top-down approach of structures embodying the ecosystem, which generally set the norms and limits of stakeholder and individual actions. This one will focus on the bottom-up approach of the human spirit animating it, which generally defines what kinds of actions are taken according to how we treat each other within that ecosystem. We will particularly focus on the personal elements in this discussion routinely omitted from global public health, but required for a decolonized, inclusive, and comprehensive understanding of our collective actions that bring the ecosystem to life. We will additionally consider how we can more effectively act toward the shared end of our common well-being and thus good, accelerated by the AI digitalization of this ecosystem. Ultimately, an ecosystem is lifeless without the lives of its inhabitants living and working together. And it is in this human ecosystem of persons in which we will explore the embedded and emergent ethics (in its demographic, cultural, and security dimensions and contexts), describing how we interact and how should interact with our coinhabitants in this common home to generate a mutually desired common future. AI is made better by being an interdisciplinary and intersector tool (drawing from the advances in health, mathematics, computer science, business, ethics, etc.). Similarly, our treatment of health AI ethics requires a certain breadth of comprehensive analysis that draws from metaphysics (the study of being), anthropology (the study of human cultures and behaviors), biology (how humans are made and kept well), mathematics (how AI facilitates the above), and other complementary fields (from which we will focus on only the most relevant elements and depth to them) to hopefully address effectively the related challenges in the global public health ecosystem).

Responsible Artificial Intelligence Re-engineering the Global Public Health Ecosystem. DOI: https://doi.org/10.1016/B978-0-443-21597-1.00006-8

6.2 North to South demographics

What is more imminent and real than concepts and paradigms are concrete persons. It is the person who you can see, touch, and hear, and who creates concepts, paradigms, and their related institutions that you cannot experience directly. To understand the cultural and security elements of the AI ethics for our global public health ecosystem, let us examine then the current and emergent demographics for it. Chapter 1 introduced how our millennia old humanity may be at a demographic inflection point—our peak and fall are set to occur by the end of this century, according to the United Nations (UN) and other supportive consensus-based datasets and analyses (Cilluffo and Ruiz 2019; Monlezun 2023). Global population aging—with a demographic decline or even collapse in the Global North and a surge in the South—is widely expected to change the face and operations of global public health. Its demographic, cultural, and power center of gravity are therefore expected to shift or at least be more balanced with the south, particularly to Africa and India and away from China, the United States, and Europe, as capital and innovation follows population "flows." Africa is the only region expected to have sustained growth through this century, quadrupling to 4.3 billion. Asia is projected to peak at 5.3 billion shortly after 2050 and be surpassed by Africa near the dawn of the 22nd century, as all other regions remain relatively static or declining (most sharply in Europe followed by Latin America). There is some estimated growth however modest in North America, but mostly from migration that should keep the United States approximately the fourth most populous country by 2100 (434 million), behind Nigeria (733 million), China (1065 million), and India (1450 million).

Aging populations in our increasingly globalized world (with greater consumption of cheaper but unhealthier foods and growing societal isolation) are thus facing seismic demographic North–South shifts. These compounded challenges are facilitating explosive rises in noncommunicable disease (NCD) incidence and the related death and disability rates especially for low- and middle-income countries (LMICs)—at a rate over three times faster than wealthier nations had to adjust to them (Bollyky and Shendruk 2017). Over the next quarter century, African LMICs followed by Southeast Asian nations are projected to have the largest spike in NCD disease burden, despite having the lowest ranked health system capacities to address them (along with the worst ranked WHO quality metrics spanning hospital beds, physicians per 1000 people, and total health expenditures). Meanwhile, North American and western European high-income countries (HICs) have the lowest projected NCD rises and the best ranked healthcare systems. For instance, Rwanda, Ethiopia, and Tanzania, respectively, are expected to lead the world in NCD increases of 31.8%, 31.5%, and 28.3% (despite ranking among the worst nations by health system capacity index). Yet the Netherlands, Germany, and Denmark should have the lowest NCD rises (at 1.0%, 1.4%, and 1.4%, respectively), while their healthcare systems are in the top 10 globally.

Poor populations are generally getting bigger, sicker, and more unaffordable to treat—at the same time their governments generally are expected to increasingly struggle to keep up with the global political economic challenges Chapter 5 discussed (from unaffordable debt, energy, and food) limiting local health sector investments required to reverse these trends. Yet there are clear wins still possible for affordable and scalable global public health solutions, including reducing tobacco use, household air pollution, and barriers to local primary care and essential health services, concurrently with expanding local–global and North–South public–private partner-ships (in finance and AI-enhanced digital capacities) and lower cost lay community health work-ers (which Chapters 1 and 2 highlighted). Following ChatGPT's launch in 2022, generative AI and large language models triggered a flurry of media reports and scientific literature publica-tions grappling with their societal implications, including with such global health adoptions within the demographic shifts noted earlier (van Heerden et al. 2023). Physician shortages are felt particularly acutely in the Global South dealing with the worsening mental health crisis as one of the more difficult to address global health challenges. Yet there are growing and scalable AI use cases for psychiatric prediction models for earlier diagnosis, treatment pathways, remote sensors, optimizing therapy sessions (through natural language processing–monitoring of ses-sions transcript), telehealth, and personalized chatbots paired with community health workers to extend limited physician resources for larger underserved populations.

6.3 Decolonization unity in global development: from multicultural diversity to biodiversity

We explored the historic and technical evolution of our human ecosystem encompassing the global public health ecosystem as 20th-century decolonization developed into 21st-century diversification. Old colonial empires, decimated by World War II (WWII), retreated. New nations advanced under the US-accelerated industrialized, capitalized, liberalized, and digi-talized rules-based international order, facilitated and articulated by the UN. But what comes after this decolonization? France, one of the most influential centuries-long nation-empires (which served as a founding architect of the UN and birthed many of the seminal Enlightenment thinkers inspiring the United States), still launched an unsuccessful attempt in the 1940s to retain its prewar global power structure (Duranti et al. 2020, pp. 54–78).
From Vietnam to Africa, those efforts faltered diplomatically and militarily as the UN concur-rently gained momentum promoting the global right to national self-determination, secured through individual rights at scale. This post-WWII modern state strove to shake off its colo-nial past, end its mid-20th-century abuses of its remaining African colonies (particularly in Morocco, Algeria, and Tunisia), and ultimately embraced a global future of human security through development that the UN advocated with political breadth and philosophical depth (more in Section 6.5). The old empire receded to reveal vibrant diverse cultures under its frayed imperial flag. Young states found their voices and joined global supply chains, multi-national institutions, and international development cooperatives, particularly in global pub-lic health as its ecosystem took shape. By 2015, the world's nations collectively ratified the *2030 Agenda for Sustainable Development* affirming a global citizenship in a multicultural world (complementing not contradicting national citizenship), bound by the "shared respon-sibility" to justly and jointly protect the common good framing a new power structure of the world order: "We acknowledge the natural and cultural diversity of the world and recognize that all cultures and civilizations can contribute to, and are crucial enablers of, sustainable development" (UN, 2015). Decolonization was thus accelerated under the global banner of

multicultural development. It in turn increasingly set the strategic agenda and operational framework for the global public health ecosystem. To prevent this ecosystem-facilitated development from becoming modern colonialism under a different name, it thus must remain anchored in a respect and reliance on the diverse local cultures on the ground. Such political economic trends therefore shaped the emergence and integration of the AI digital revolution which grew up within it, reflected in the AI ethical principles and instruments of the global institutions and power players we explored throughout this book (particularly as emblematically articulated by the WHO with the recurrent themes of autonomy, inclusivity, and transparency; WHO 2021a). In the next section, we will explore the content of multiculturalism worldwide that embodies our global public health ecosystem, and the way it shapes the emergent ethical framework of its future.

But before we get there, we must dig deeper to explore how an effective AI-enabled global public health ecosystem is only that if it is culturally diverse (to inclusively represent and be run by the world's peoples, rather than the elitist few over the weaker many), while also nourishing the biodiversity required for it. Listed as the 15th goal among the UN's sustainable development goals (SDGs), the grand strategic framework for the WHO's health agenda, "biodiversity" refers to the variety of planetary life on which our global human ecosystem integrally depends to survive (for medicines, food, economics, and climate change mitigation; UN 2015; WHO 2015). Consider the semiconductor global supply chain we earlier explored: remove just one node (Taiwan), and the global digital economy collapses. In the ecological "supply chain," remove the wrong or too many species and the global ecosystem is endangered (not simply those species). Accordingly, there are growing efforts to pair AI with global development efforts to nourish biodiversity. A 2022 *Nature* study demonstrated that a reinforcement learning−based approach to prioritizing conservation areas (balancing biodiversity cost−benefit trade-offs) outperformed older methods in more affordably, effectively, and reliably saving more species (Silvestro et al. 2022). Meanwhile, there are a myriad of AI use cases demonstrating proven affordable effectiveness and scalability, including supercomputer-powered geographic information systems (mapping species' movement in real time in response to resource limitations and climate change), blockchain-augmented marine sensors (doing the above but for ocean life), forest-based acoustic sensors (for early warning for nature officials protecting endangered species from illegal poachers and deforestation), wireless robotic jellyfish drone swarms (for marine cleanup), and financing schemes with enhanced cost−benefit analytics (informing sustainable forest and land management practices and carbon sequestration for public−private partnerships; Shine 2023).

6.4 Global/human security (not just national security)

Who makes up the world and how their worldviews shape them in turn translates into a convergent vision of security, the necessary minimum floor for mutual survival to reach toward the existential ceiling of human development and thus flourishing. Chapter 1 described how the modern consensus understanding of "human security" was introduced in the UN's 1948 *Universal Declaration of Human Rights (UDHR)* as the most intrinsic right of each human person after life and liberty (Cummings et al., 2018; UNDP, 1994). It was refined in the 1994 *Human Development Report* as "freedom from fear…and want" before being codified in the UN's 2012 General Resolution 66/291. Post-WWII, security principally was about states using force and the threat of it to safeguard its borders and sovereignty from collective external threats. But post−Cold War, security expanded to also describe what governments, institutions, communities, and the individual did through development to safeguard the personal goods needed for personal flourishing, which internal not just external threats endangered. Human security therefore was formalized as the strategic sum of freedoms: from poverty, hunger, disease, disability, violence, ecological damage, cultural imperialism, and political oppression. These seven conceptual elements became the 15 concrete goals in the operational framework of the UN's 2015 SDGs (eliminating poverty and hunger, optimizing well-being, protecting biodiversity and mitigating climate change, fostering cultural diversity and institutionalized civil protections, etc.). During this time, the WHO through its Egyptian-led Eastern Mediterranean regional office, expanded the consensus conception of health security within global health—informed by its Islamic perspective and unique culture—to be an integral component of human security ultimately, an expansion which it justified pragmatically and by "values…deeply rooted in the culture," defended by "justice and equity as essential determinants of human security at national, regional, and global levels" (WHO 2002). The 2012 UN Resolution embraced this framework by declaring that "improving global health" requires "comprehensive strategies" empowered by the "human security approach" (UN 2012a, p. 13). The UN General Assembly adopted the 2018 General Resolution on "Information and communication technologies for sustainable development" (73/218) which fine-tuned this global health and human security link by not only recognizing the reality of the growing global digitalization of the health ecosystem. But it also highlighted the need for comprehensive digital strategies specifically to accelerate the realization of health through security and security through health in our AI age. Thus the WHO launched its first "Global strategy on digital health" in 2020, endorsed by the 73rd World Health Assembly (WHA73 [28]), to guide states in translating lofty global concepts into concrete local wins (WHO 2021b). In the short-term (less than 2 years), medium term (2−4 years), and long-term (over 4 years), the WHO advised national health systems with interlinked public health agencies to respectively catalyze security-based development through AI-enabled digital technologies promoting innovation, building capacities to deploy them (with secure global health data sharing according to WHO-informed regulations and standards), and formalizing a global governance structure for the above (as a unified global regulation, benchmark, and certification framework to facilitate individual safety, interoperable effectiveness, and societal equity). Yet at the advent of the 2020s, COVID-19 spotlighted the failures of global health and international cooperation on global crises specifically and existential threats more generally—or at least their inadequate progress toward their eventual sufficient effectiveness. Concurrently, more powerful and versatile AI became increasingly accessible for more stakeholders and their use cases delivering more proven and scalable value for them. Collectively, influential voices underscore AI's unique value proposition in the interlinked global health and human security challenge at the intersection of these historic trends.

Chatham House underscored how the solution to effective, equitable, efficient "comprehensive strategies" that the UN called for above may be technical, not conceptual or political (Cummings et al. 2018). There is already global consensus, however superficial, about the interdependent relationships of health AI (in security and development) and the need to cooperatively leverage them for global and local benefit. The bigger the strategic vision, the more complete and thus efficacious it may be (but also the more complex and difficult to execute, as it pulls in greater numbers and diversity of stakeholders, along with their varied primary motives, constraints, perspectives, and resources). Yet as AI becomes more sophisticated, it may make this problem simpler by offering unprecedented value understanding the global human ecosystem (and thus its global public health ecosystem), identifying optimal cooperative areas and terms (along with conflicts to avoid), and enabling more personalized and real-time adaptive solutions for the ecosystem to prioritize (focused on better prediction, prevention, and mitigation of challenges to human security). If the adage holds that no plan survives contact with reality, then what if AI enables a better plan by better understanding its complex reality? Chatham thus reinforces how AI's main contribution to human and thus health security will be its ability to accelerate answers to their barriers that can be quantified: find, coordinate, and leverage ecosystem partners to predict and manage threats (by translating data into insights, insights into plans, and plans into empowerment that adapts with the real situation on the ground). Yet this does not solve the paradoxical problem about what if AI makes human security–based development for global health *too* successful? Chapter 5 emphasized how the world's dominant political economic powers and AI developers (the United States and China) see AI as a crucial national security priority and thus a primary area of competition (which can enable victory over competitors and adversaries). If it is concurrently becoming *one* of if not *the* crucial enabler of human security in the global public health ecosystem and of national security in global great power competition, does the faster success in one domain accelerate the point of conflict in the other? We will now explore how global health AI ethics and their policy translations may address (and even advance solutions to) these problems, in addition to their implications for countries globally even outside the abovesaid parties.

6.5 Global health artificial intelligence ethics beyond democracies versus autocracies

6.5.1 Beyond democracies versus autocracies

Chapter 5 explored how Personalist Liberalism proposes a comprehensive and substantive political economics framework for the sustainable and equitable AI transformation of the global public health ecosystem. By avoiding extremes and false binary choices, it is a *both/and* framework rather than *either/or*. It seeks to show how the Global West *and* East, the North *and* South, democracies *and* autocracies, human security *and* national security, localism *and* globalism, healthcare *and* public health, artificial intelligence *and* personal care can both be leveraged for synergistic cooperation in a global ecosystem that is dynamically greater than the sum of its parts, through orientating these traditional ends of their conceptual spectrums to a third dimension that points ultimately to the common good (metaphysically, conceptually, and practically ordering them effectively for global benefit). But political economics alone is not enough to solve these tensions and their related challenges for the global ecosystem. Therefore, we turn to the global ethics embedded in this political economics framework, shifting from the overarching Personalist Liberalism to its underlying Personalist Social Contract ethics in this section. In doing so, Personalist Liberalism may thus serve as the strategic bridge between national security and human security, central to the effective AI-enabled global public health ecosystem bridging the United States and China, in addition to the related major political economic and technical competitors and power players on the world stage. To show how these pairs can progress toward the common good as their common end (ethically and thus practically, not just strategically), it may thus provide the most substantive reinforcement to the necessary strategic guardrails of managed strategic competition in our AI age. Rather than testing boundaries by bouncing off them, this ethics may help keep competitors and cooperators on the same road by showing how they can move together in the same direction, and thus how the ecosystem can be held together and grow together with its constitutive stakeholders, sectors, and belief systems. This vision proposes that the dominant narrative of our emergent future is not democracy versus autocracy, but security versus vulnerability, and thus how together we can reach the former as the means to the ultimate end of humanity's common good, realized in the global well-being for which the AI-empowered global public health ecosystem exists. The United States talks about preserving the current world order. China talks about seeking harmony instead of hegemony. How can these two sides of the same coin be welded together as complementary pairs in an integral whole? Ethics may show us answers to these deeper questions, allowing us to build on a global AI ethics of human security to generate sustainable global cooperation in regulation and innovation for shared governance (crucial for the interoperability and effectiveness of the ecosystem to collectively advance toward equitable global well-being).

6.5.2 Ethical roadblocks to regulations and innovations

We will first analyze ethical roadblocks to such cooperation and promising early answers to them, in both their strengths and shortcomings (which will then set us up to analyze how the Personalist Social Contract ethics may uniquely maximize the former and minimize the latter). These roadblocks center on AI (1) risks, (2) consensus constraints, (3) principle proliferation, and (4) interoperable enforcement:

1. *AI risks*: There is no clear comprehensive response to the scale, speed, and complexity of global AI risks, especially in global health. This reality was grimly highlighted by The Center for AI Safety's 2023 "Statement on AI Risk," a seminal global multisector declaration signed by the "godfathers of AI" including Geoffrey Hinton and Yoshua Bengio, along with the CEOs of Google DeepMind and OpenAI (among the world's top AI centers) and other leading UN, government, academic, and corporate leaders

internationally (particularly in China and the United States; Vallance, 2023). They assert that "mitigating the risk of extinction from AI should be a global priority alongside other societal-scale risks such as pandemics and nuclear war." Critics counter that AI is societally disruptive, but not existential. Nonetheless, there is growing multinational and multisector concerns that laws and regulations cannot keep up with the widespread, rapid, and unprecedented technical evolution of AI. These risks appear concentrated in their already exhibited roles in weaponization (i.e. propaganda, chemical, biologic, and nuclear), destabilization (through social media misinformation), centralization (few actors enforcing "narrow views" on the many through "pervasive surveillance and oppressive censorship"), enfeeblement (worsening isolation from people and excessive dependency on tech undermining global human security and resilience), and superintelligence (the farthest threat but most difficult to counter; Vallance 2023; Bremmer and Kupchan 2023; Monlezun 2022). COVID provided potentially the first high-profile global demonstration of the societal extent and power of AI misinformation politically, ethically, and scientifically. It helped stoke divisions (through subgroup profiling and polarization), false dichotomies (policies and financing caring for "us" versus "them" according to such above artificial or arbitrary lines), and shoddy evidence (lacking biological plausibility and statistical confidence). Yet there is no clear solution to combatting AI-accelerated misinformation. Social media algorithms amplify polarizing posts and news reports that can be worsened by deepfakes, bots, and computer algorithms mimicking human users. Consider the politically tense incident of a US federal judge in July 2023 ruling that President Biden's administration violated citizens' First Amendment rights by unconstitutionally coercing social media companies to censor their COVID-related posts that questioned government policies in what the judge asserted "involves the most massive attack against free speech in United States' history" (Myers and McCabe 2023). Where should the line be drawn between countering misinformation and censoring dissenting views? Such challenges appear to be only mounting, fueled by the powerful though perplexing societal impact of generative AI. ChatGPT by 2023 already could produce research paper abstracts that scientists were not consistently able to identify as done by AI—and there is no clear global regulation or enforcing mechanisms to make the AI programmers declare them as such (Else 2023). "Science" alone cannot be an effective final arbiter of societal disagreements.

2. *Consensus constraints*: We previously explored the broad critique that COVID accentuated the fundamental failure in the global public health ecosystem—faulty ethics, not just effectiveness. A weak consensus on values undermined strong societal responses, as the technology was there, but not the shared moral vision of how to use it (that otherwise could inform the necessary global political and economic structures to operationalize that shared values-driven strategy). From the critiques especially in the Global South explored in Chapter 1, there are growing voices that argue we owe to each other more than just what we choose to owe—because our societal duties to each other are existentially intrinsic to our essential humanity, not dependent on our volitional will. A physician has a duty to sick patients, even when they are tired and may not want to care for them. The

solution, so this line of critique goes which the Personalist Social Contract will consider, is recovery of rather than revolution from our common humanity with its intrinsic interdependencies, shared vulnerabilities, and unifying common good. This solution requires a comprehensive ecosystem approach that more accurately reflects our complex global human society (multidimensional, multisector, and multicultural), bound by political economic guardrails, and anchored in and animated by a common ethical foundation in which we understand we cannot survive or succeed alone. We belong to each other and are most uniquely and fully ourselves as an existential gift to each other. The *Lancet* COVID-19 Commission, partnering with leading academics and the UN Sustainable Development Solutions Network, articulated the existence and impact of constraints to such ethical consensus for global public health in an extended but influential passage:

The COVID-19 crisis has exposed major weaknesses in the UN-based multilateral system, resulting from excessive nationalism, tensions among the major powers, chronic underfinancing of global public goods including the UN system itself, lack of flexibility of intellectual property regimes to ensure that global public goods are available to all, lack of adequate sustainable development financing for LMICs, and the erosion of political support for multilateral solutions by the major powers. Despite major efforts to stimulate recovery and a just transition to sustainable development, the lack of ambition in the global response to COVID-19 is like that of other pressing global challenges, such as the climate emergency; the loss of global biodiversity; the pollution of air, land, and water; the persistence of extreme poverty in the midst of plenty; and the large-scale displacement of people as a result of conflicts, poverty, and environmental stress. In this light, our most basic recommendation is the strengthening of multilateralism in all crucial dimensions: political, cultural, institutional, and financial [italics added]…We encourage member states to enrich their deliberations and decisions with the voices of civil society, the private sector, local governments, parliaments, academia, and young people, among others. We note the timeliness of recommitting to the Universal Declaration of Human Rights, the UN's moral charter *[italics added], as we celebrate its 75th anniversary in 2023 (Sachs et al. 2022).*

A multidimensional, multisector, ecosystem-based approach to understanding and solving global health problems begins with the unifying moral vision that gives life to the institutions and policies meant to solve them. If the ethical consensus is lacking, so will the foundation be lacking for the derivative AI-enabled political economic and development framework, required for the healthy functioning of the global public health ecosystem. As Chapter 1 introduced and the *UDHR* declared (with endorsement by the world's diverse nations and belief systems since), the "recognition of the inherent dignity and of the equal and inalienable rights of all members of the human family is the foundation of freedom, justice and peace in the world" (UN 1948). This moral vision begins with personal dignity and protected through human rights at scale globally, which in turn generates peace through justice. How can we recover this consensus and thus embed and animate our AI-enabled global public health ecosystem with it? (Because its modern COVID stress test shows it is missing in action). The high-level principles noted earlier including from the WHO, European Union, United States, and Microsoft manifest the broad belief AI ethics is needed. But there is no clear substance, convergence, or applicability (at scale, speed, and specificity) for the underlying moral vision that can sustain them, nor the practical framework to operationalize them.

3. *Principle proliferation*: A 2021 Oxford University analysis of the first high profile frameworks for AI ethical principles demonstrated significant convergence on beneficence, nonmaleficence, justice, autonomy, and explicability, which follows the seminal Beauchamp and Childress four US bioethical principles (Floridi and Cowls 2019). These were identical except for adding explicability to express both epistemological intelligibility (showing how AI algorithms work) and ethical accountability (showing who is responsible for it). Yet the analysis noted the trade-off between consensus and usability, as generally the more general and superficial the global principles and related ethical frameworks are then the less applicable and effective they are guiding concrete local actions. Accordingly, there is a widespread decentralized proliferation of AI ethical frameworks as governments, companies, institutions, public health agencies, and healthcare systems are often left to define and deploy their own frameworks. This limits their interoperability, standardization, scale (up of best practices), and effectiveness (resolving disagreements among and within them).

4. *Interoperable enforcement*: In addition, having consensus frameworks and enforcing them are entirely separate challenges. As the landmark Oxford analysis of AI for human development demonstrated in the Chapter 5, "AI $\times$ SDGs cannot be inconsistent with ethical frameworks guiding the design and evaluation of any kind of AI" (Cowls et al. 2021). Yet there are persistent and substantive global political economic disagreements about resource allocations (who gets what) and distributive justice (who does the giving). They in turn reveal fundamental disagreements on the underlying ethical values and mechanisms to operationalize them; therefore, they require more substantive ethical foundations. If two competing public health agencies both claim they are owed a certain amount of government funding, the government as a third party invokes the established laws and/or policies to resolve the debate. And yet if there is no clear ethical third party or standard to resolve disagreements in the content or the application of competing AI ethical frameworks, then the global public health ecosystem faces fundamental headwinds to advance the derivative interoperable digital and political economic frameworks required for its policies and programs to effectively align stakeholder interests, efficiently coordinate resources, and generate equitable results.

6.5.3 WHO artificial intelligence ethics

The WHO provides potentially the highest profile and most influential ethical standards and frameworks both for AI and the global public health ecosystem to address such significant challenges. The WHO's 2021 six core AI principles for global health are autonomy, well-being, sustainability, accountability, transparency (intelligible explainability), and equitable inclusivity (WHO 2021a, 2023). They track generally in line with the consensus principles noted earlier and have progressively been invoked for WHO guidance on AI health developments, including its 2023 recommendations for ChatGPT and generative AI by teasing out the more specific implications of the abovementioned abstract principles. Yet the principles, similar to the larger Western tradition of principalism (focused generally on minimizing metaphysics and the person and emphasizing abstract principles for autonomous agents) lack a logical hierarchy, pluralism approach (resolving disagreements of competing ethical frameworks particularly non-Western), (realist) metaphysical foundation, and larger philosophical and anthropological accounts that can resolve disagreements among competing principles and their concrete applications. For instance, what if it is unsafe and unequal to accelerate the health preferences of autonomous agents in the richer North through greater deliberate use of nonessential health services for them instead of using those resources for essential health services for the poorer South? The WHO 2021 Digital Transformation Toolkit appears to invoke the *UDHR* tradition that emphasizes human dignity as its central ethical concept (inferring a deeper realist metaphysical account of the human person), in addition to its derivative principalism concepts of beneficence, nonmaleficence, and justice like above by Beauchamp and Childress to inform responsible AI for public health (García Saisó and D'Agostino 2021). Instead of going deeper, the UN Secretary-General's 2020 "Roadmap for digital cooperation" goes further to guide principle implementation in eight focus area recommendations identified by the High-Level Panel on Digital Cooperation: advancing equitable and efficient connectivity, digital public goods, digital inclusion, digital capacity building, digital human rights, digital trust and security, critical infrastructure, and global digital cooperation (UN 2020). The WHO ethical framework published the following year was meant to elaborate on this ethical foundation. Yet the abovesaid challenges persist in both substance and application, in a pluralistic world that still requires sufficient consensus for interoperable cooperation in security and development. Telling an AI algorithm to "be nice" is not exactly sufficient guidance for global health, especially what "nice" means is debatable, as is how to teach it to be so, and even what "it" is.

6.5.4 Metaphysical Turing Test: artificial intelligence existentialism separating man from machine?

Chapter 2 introduced Alan Turing's landmark 1950 description of AI as intelligent machines, and his now canonical (though controversial) standard for it in the Turing test. This "imitation game" is "won" by the AI that can consistently trick human interrogators through written communication into believing that it is another human. There is no widespread agreement that any AI has ever beaten the Turing Test such that it can "think" as we do. Chris Saad in 2023 proposed a refined version in the "AI Classification Framework" to better capture the eight domains (or cognitive capacities) of intelligence first described by the Harvard psychologist, Howard Gardner: the logical-mathematical, linguistic-verbal, visual-spatial, musical-rhythmic, bodily-kinesthetic, interpersonal, intrapersonal, and existential

(Orf 2023). Even ChatGPT—with its fourth iteration released in March 2023 as arguably the most powerful AI model—at best demonstrates average performance in the first two domains only. In the last three domains where ethical deliberations and decisions especially reside, it is not clear how AI can learn to become "ethical" (which is all the more important as its other capacities grow) because doing so would first require a computer to know itself, including the essence of what makes a computer a computer (i.e., machinery) and what makes a person a person (i.e., humanity). The philosophical subdiscipline of ethics (logically determining what actions should or should not be done by persons to other beings particular other persons) derives from its foundational subdiscipline of metaphysics (systematically determining the structure, relationships, and content of being and thus reality, including who the human person is in the first place and what is owed to them). If there is nothing real (or no real difference between human beings or other types of beings like a tree or a stone), then it is unclear if there is anything that should or should not be prescribed or prohibited. To solve our AI ethical challenges for the global public health ecosystem, we may therefore need to shore up our current superficial or nominalist metaphysics. We may even need a "metaphysical Turing test" to guide the development and identify the emergence of responsible health AI.

The historical trajectory that brought us to this contemporary need is the fundamental paradox in modern metaphysics and ethics. Generally, we have analyzed how the West's political economic paradigm of liberal democratic capitalism dominates late modernity, springing from its early modern roots in the religious and cultural values of Catholic Christian Europe (and its ancient agnostic Greek philosophy of Aristotle, refined by Aquinas in dialogue with an early version of secularism, Judaism, and Islam; Monlezun 2022). This realist Thomistic-Aristotelian metaphysical foundation argues that it can be logically demonstrated convincingly to reasonable audiences that reality (being as such) does exist and we can know it (including the existence of goodness itself). We subjectively experience this objective reality which then informs how we come to know and desire the good (in general and in its particular forms, such as good actions toward others in ethics and good tools in technology). But increasingly in the late modern age, a Western nominalist metaphysics developed that paradoxically argues there is no reality or way to know it if it does exist, and so all philosophy (and ethics) is subjective and shifting, and all societal governance whether economics or politics is ruled simply by power (through force or the majority, not by justice or logic). And yet a scientism within this tradition also sprang up that asserts the only "truth" of reality is from science, thus restricting human knowledge to the material dimension alone. Yet it still expects to have normative immaterial values (like justice and beneficence) that everyone must follow. Saying objectively that there is no objective truth (except for science) is what classical philosophy described as a circular logical fallacy—it self-contradicts and so refutes itself (while additionally committing the categorical error of trying to use one discipline such as science to disprove another such as philosophy). We cannot concurrently say that human dignity is a foundational universal moral value that can resolve disagreements within and across belief systems, while we also say that there is no objective truth or existence of dignity (or that the plurality of belief systems means there is no system or value more logical or robust than another). Ultimately, digital interoperability of the global public health ecosystem therefore foundationally require metaphysical and ethical interoperability, consisting of a basic breadth and depth of a real, substantive, and shared moral vision that unites us all through our common humanity. As the AI Classification Framework suggests, AI existentialism is unable now (and in the near and long-term foreseeable future) to separate man from machine.

We thus may need a metaphysical Turing Test which the Personalist Social Contract in the next section may be able to provide. We will seek to logically, experientially, multiculturally, and pluralistically demonstrate across states and belief systems what may really distinguish man from machine: love, as the origin and fulfillment of personal dignity, in which we become most fully and uniquely ourselves through an integral gift of ourselves to another person for the good of the other as other. Human life is fulfilled in love, which is justice that matures into peace societally. The healthy and thus good human community is when such individual ethical or just actions occur at sufficient scale, collectively giving rise to the common good that defines the content of this justice. We will briefly explore how the derivative personalism of Aristotelian realism (grounding the Personalist Social Contract) instead of modern nominalism's logical absurdity may recover a "real" ethics from otherwise volitional "ethics," existing only as rhetoric or politics under another name —insubstantial, shifting, and subservient to the strongest power rather than the strongest logic. And in doing so, Personalist Social Contract ethics may resurrect a human and thus global AI ethics from the common metaphysics of humanity uniting us all in our diversity. This personal ethics seeks to thus refine dominant modern ethics that appears to rely (solely) on what its critics assert is dehumanizing monolithic Western ideological colonialism and excessively rigid technical fixation that is excessively insular, slow, and abstract (focused on constructed principles to guide acts separated from the reality of the acting person, while largely excluding nonsecular values and voices). Human vulnerability that gives rise to personal love, not cognition that gives way to choice, is the metaphysical distinction that this test turns on.

6.6 Personalist Social Contract artificial intelligence ethics: at scale, speed, and specificity

The Personalist Social Contract as the embedded ethical framework within Personalist Liberalism seeks to address the AI challenges of AI risks, consensus constraints, principle proliferation, and interoperable enforcement by expanding and enriching the AI ethical discourse for the global public health ecosystem (Monlezun 2022, 2023; Monlezun et al. 2022). These strengths are meant to translate to ethical solutions at the scale, speed, and specificity that the current dominant Western principle−focused frameworks may lack. It does so by analyzing the questions that emerge from our real, lived, global, but still local experience of daily life: what is the common humanity, home, good, and future that bind us together? (The questions that Aristotle wrestled with millennia ago by questioning the orthodoxy of his age). The answers then inform and sustain how we become an integrally healthy and whole community (as unique persons in a shared community), rather than simply focusing on choices (which can prohibitively and artificially dehumanize and truncate effective dialogue, debate, and decisions in the global ecosystem, while blurring the line between the integral person who chooses an intermediate good pursuant to the common and highest good, instead, i.e., simply an AI algorithm that selects means to an objective stripped of its personal and communal context in which cognition evolves and choices happen). The imminent reality globally across diverse societies, states, cultures, and belief systems is that our human condition revolves around our vulnerabilities—we need each other to survive and thrive. None of us create ourselves nor can survive especially our earliest years without others, nor understand its intelligible meaning. Care for the most vulnerable and the pursuit of meaning pervades cultures the world over. We each seek a common end (as unique fulfillment, a deep abiding sense of well-being that goes beyond simple happiness and satiation of basic needs and desires). And it requires others to be realized. In this Aristotelian line of thinking, our experiences not just reason additionally show us we need purpose for prosperity and peace as the safeguards of human security—a meaning behind our existence—as they are means to our common end and good. This contrasts with their inverse of pleasure, power, and prestige that confuse means with ends, and so drive existential and societal isolation. When we conflate such intermediate ends as our ultimate ends, at the expense of ourselves and others, we generally experience the loss of our uniqueness—and if severe and scaled enough, even our humanity. The Personalist Social Contract therefore grounds modern personalism (bridging diverse secular and nonsecular belief systems) in Aristotelian realism as a form of communitarianism, rather than radical individualism (losing the community) or collectivism (losing the individual). It recognizes the need for our ethics to reflect our real lived experiences: relational (in which we belong to each other as members of the global human family) not simply algorithmic (in which autonomous faceless agents comply with "ethical" principles, a required checklist criteria of AI-like models mindlessly following their programming). We will now explore this framework's logical and practical defense and its content and deployment for the AI global public health ecosystem to understand how it may multi-culturally fill the gaps in the ecosystem's human security–focused ethical foundation.

6.6.1 Multidimension defense

The logical and practice defense for the Personalist Social Contract has been more extensively detailed (including by the book bearing its name). Therefore, we will focus on an over-view here on the dimensions that are most relevant for our focus on the AI-enabled global public health ecosystem (Monlezun 2022, 2023; Monlezun et al. 2022): (1) metaphysically, (2) existentially, (3) logically, (4) ethically, (5) practically, (6) technically, (7) digitally, (8) algorithmically, (9) historically, (1) societally, and (11) politically and economically.

1. *Metaphysical dimension*: It starts with our concrete, lived reality and reasons backwards to the Aristotelian realism that can then be understood as logically defensible, experientially compatible, and pluralistically convergent.

2. *Existential dimension*: Its anchors itself in the practical unique experiences of the common reality of our existence (logically, systematically, and multiculturally analyzed) to help resolve theoretical disagreements. Concepts, institutions, frameworks, and so on, are less real (metaphysically) than the concrete people who articulate them to explain the given reality in which we find ourselves. This framework considers how we are more fully ourselves when we conform ourselves to reality, rather than trying to force reality to conform to us.

3. *Logical dimension*: It defends the same realist metaphysical foundation that makes normative ethics and empirical science possible. It reasons through systematic formal logic from the foundation to those frameworks by showing how material and immaterial reality is intelligible. This then allows us to reason from perceptible and sensible particulars (i.e., seeing someone acting justly or an apple tree in front of us) to universals (i.e., just actions to justice itself or a falling apple to gravity itself). This progression of reason allows us to identify, articulate, and understand together the moral laws informing how to justly treat other persons appropriately as persons, especially as metaphysical ends rather than means, in addition to scientific "laws" informing how to make technologies and products to effectively achieve material ends for the common good.

4. *Ethical dimension*: It seeks to avoid ideological imperialism or colonization by focusing on common values embedded in our diverse cultures and belief systems, while respecting nuances in their expression. This diversity includes the contours of varying overlapping and convergent definitions of health and societal duties to it (because there is a general global consensus about what well-being essentially is, though how it looks in one person, community, and culture versus another can vary, though within a defined range).

5. *Practical dimension*: It expresses and defends the already substantive global consensus on agile, concrete, embedded ethical principles of responsible AI created by responsible acting persons (clarifying responsible to whom, for what, how, and why). Practically for responsible AI to move by design and at the speed and scale of current global ecosystem operations, the conceptions must already be present in the data scientists, policymakers, and leaders developing them. The Personalist Social Contract therefore practically puts ethical guard rails on that development by orientating it toward our multicultural humanity's common good. Instead of this global interoperable ethics (syncing diverse belief systems together like the hull of a ship keeping it afloat), a patchwork ethics cannot successfully mix and match its varying frameworks to patch a sinking ship in time. The Rawlsian modern social contract (described below) tried to fix the problem of fairness in pluralism where common rules are required for collective survival amid diverse individual beliefs. The Personalist Social Contract tries in turn to fix Rawls by anchoring its static social contract of "voting agents" in a more defensible and imminent Aristotelian metaphysical foundation. It therefore seeks to transform Rawls' contract into a living social communion of acting persons (including those who think differently than Rawls), thus resolving its inherent logical contradictions and

decolonizing its ideological Western bias (since philosophy without metaphysics becomes ideology, in turn becoming political economic weapons expanding the power of the few over the many). The Personalist Social Contract proposes the AI ethical foundation for the global public health ecosystem, or what the UN and the Vatican's 2023 workshops on the "The Fraternal Economy of Integral and Sustainable Development" describe as their goal: seeking "the institutional and ethical basis of a new economic framework fit for the challenges of the 21st century" (PASS 2023).

6. *Technical dimension*: It facilitates the metaphysical and thus ethical substructure for data architecture and political economic frameworks that are required for ecosystem interoperability in global public health. It does so by highlighting the ecosystem's embedded common values (generating and animating the myriad of actions and acting stakeholders in the ecosystem) that are orientated to the common good (which in turn can align those actions to build just structures toward this shared ultimate aim, realized in justice by giving to each what is due to them with the resources and relationships proper to each acting person and their relationships with others).

7. *Digital dimension*: It articulates and defends successful data security as derivative of human dignity to decolonize global data architecture, enabling a person-centered architecture built and sustained by solidarity.

8. *Algorithmical dimension*: It is designed and deployed through a novel related computational ethical mechanism—AI-driven Computational Ethics and policy analysis (AiCE)—translating its substance and structure into existing AI algorithms for more rapid and versatile deployment in responsible AI ethics.

9. *Historical dimension*: It provides the first comprehensive defense of a decolonial global AI ethics (which the next section on its content and on its relationship to Ubuntu summarizes).

10. *Societal dimension*: It guides a just centralized social hierarchy balanced with decentralized social networks, allowing global coordinators (like the WHO) and local enablers (like community public health agencies, healthcare systems, community organizations, and churches) to facilitate stable cooperation, advanced by dynamic innovation from the centralized and decentralized networks, respectively. The person and justice (as the end or object of ethics uniting human communities or dividing them by injustice or unethical actions) are already inherent in the global and local dimensions of these social networks that constitute our societies and thus our global human community. Earlier we analyzed how the world's nations are united through their ratification of the shared moral vision of the *UDHR* recognizing that peace is secured through justice—generated by respect for human dignity and thus equal derivative rights—for "all members of the human *family* (emphasis added)" (UN 1948). In 2012, the UN Secretary-General quoted the Nobel Laureate and Catholic religious sister known for her work for the world's poor, Therese of Calcutta, who expressed the multicultural belief that "if we have no peace, it is because we have forgotten that we belong to each other" (UN 2012b). The Personalist Social Contract recognizes that we are born into local families and so also to the global human family. The closer to our

local home, the more intense our duties are to them. Yet duty is common through the entire gradient of the global family (balancing solidarity and subsidiarity described below). Help and hurt throughout any of the network therefore also propagates throughout the global human and so public health ecosystems. In this line of argument, we belong to each other as interconnected members of the common human community bound by metaphysical relations to each other, rather than being disembodied and volitionally chosen artificial constructions or agents of transactional associations. We belong to each other, even when we do not "choose" to acknowledge or act upon it. Metaphysical being and thus ethical justice (fulfilled in love among persons as the only proper and just action toward another person) binds us together (as does the damage caused by unjust actions in which we use other persons as means to our ends, rather than at the same time as ends in and of themselves, which we will explore concisely below). The ecosystem—because of the living persons constituting it—therefore is living, breathing, and connected. It is therefore most social and resilient when metaphysical unity is embraced through ethical unity, in justice done at scale among persons globally.

11. *Political economic dimension*: It enables realization of effective and sustainable governance through operative ethical use of the tools of politics and economics. They are not sufficient alone to respect and protect humanity, and the derivative duties of developing and deploying responsible health AI and just operations of the global public health ecosystem. And neither is a responsible ecosystem's politics and economics survivable without such a robust ethical foundation, upon which it rests and which instills it with the self-corrective mechanisms to trim its inevitable unethical excesses. Combatting AI misinformation for instance, which can undermine and even undo states and institutions, is not possible without objectively identifying, demonstrating, and uniting populations around what true information is (tasks that political economics and AI alone are insufficient to accomplish as they are practical tools, not the philosophical foundation that can show the reality for which those tools are means to advance just ends).

6.6.2 Structure and content

The following briefly summarizes the Personalist Social Contract within Personalist Liberalism and then applies it to the AI-powered global public health ecosystem by considering its multicultural and pluralistic (1) history, (2) structure, (3) value, (4) content, and (5) application in terms of its moral interoperability (with a more detailed description and defense deferred to the following references to keep this book's focus on the abovesaid ecosystem; Benchaita 2023; Monlezun 2022, 2023; Monlezun et al. 2022; UNESCO 2020):

1. *History*: The world's first high-level multicultural and multisector global consensus on AI ethics including for health was formalized by the 2020 Rome Call for Ethics. This public–private partnership declaration was initially signed by Microsoft, IBM, the UN, and the Vatican. It was joined in 2023 by the Islamic United Arab Emirates' Abu Dhabi Forum for Peace and the Jewish Chief Rabbinate of Israel's Commission for Interfaith

Relations, supported by the related Global University Summit spanning 42 universities on five continents. The Rome Call—which at the same ceremony awarded the world's top doctoral dissertation distinction to the Personalist Social Contract as a comprehensive metaphysically grounded AI ethics framework that articulated and defended its consensus principles as derivative from the UN's *UDHR*—then set the stage for other high-level AI ethical principles including from the WHO.

2. *Structure*: The Personalist Social Contract is a unique pluralist integration of modern ethics (with a utilitarian-based Rawlsian social contract, bounded by Kantian deontology and augmented by feminist, ecological, deconstructionist, and Marxist ethics) with classical ethics (Thomistic Aristotelian virtue ethics, expressed as Norris Clarke's Strong Thomistic Personalism, refined by William Carlo's *esse*/essence distinction). Using less technical philosophical terms, this means that the framework starts with the most popular and robust framework of modern moral political and ethical philosophy from the Harvard professor, John Rawls, and his social contract theory of political liberalism, featuring a Western liberal democratic vision of "justice as political not metaphysical." Rawls argues that diverse peoples and belief systems, for reasons inherent to their "reasonable" belief systems, generate overlapping consensus about ethical principles of fairness. They are then codified into laws which balance the competing political goods of equality and liberty. All citizens of such a society have equal protected rights. Any social or economic inequalities are only permitted if they are tied to positions all have equal opportunities to attain, and such inequalities maximize the benefit of the less advantaged citizens. But the Personalist Social Contract embraces such genuine insights, while replacing Rawls' Western modern nominalism metaphysical foundation with a classical global Aristotelian realist one to preserve those insights. This is meant to avoid the former's inevitable cultural bias and logical contradictions (to instead argue for objective knowable truths unifying diverse belief systems; these include the existence of justice and normative ethical actions humans as members of the global human community have intrinsic moral duties to uphold, even without the threat of punishment or incentive from authorities such as governments). This version of personalism's logically explicated concrete reality of the human person replaces the modern abstract constructed conception of universal reason as the justification for its foundation to reach its ethical conclusions about what justice is and how it is knowable and enforceable. Truth of the objective common good as the object of justice in the Personalist Social Contract is its metaphysical source and arbitrating rather than arbitrary standard, in contrast to the power of shifting common agreement in the Rawlsian social contract. *Political* Liberalism and its *overlapping* consensus (which can turn with the political winds redefining subjectively asserted "goods" as a ship adrift on the ocean) is transformed into *Personalist* Liberalism and its *convergent* consensus (which is grounded in the metaphysical reality of human persons logically understanding the objective goods "given" by reality, which can be subjectively experienced like a mountain peak from which paths from diverse starting points can nonetheless reach together, coming closer to each other as they come closer to the peak). As such, the Personalist Social Contract substantively and uniquely

articulates and defends the foundational Aristotelian metaphysical concepts (i.e., communitarian human nature and its derivative reality of dignity and resultant rights) housed in a Rawlsian-like social contact framework of the *UDHR*.

From this metaphysical foundation arise its main structural pillars from which it is logically, experientially, and pluralistically derived:

a. *Metaphysical principles*: The Personalist Social Contract develops what the *UDHR* introduces by understanding the inherently linked objective (communicable) and subjective (noncommunicable) dimensions of each human person, seen as a unique member of the global human family in which the individual good is fulfilled in the common good (through justice operationalized as love), which concurrently safeguards the individual good at scale. Accordingly, it provides a novel detailed defense of the multicultural (realist) metaphysics underlying, operationalizing, and unifying the world's diverse religiously unaffiliated (or secular) and affiliated (nonsecular) belief systems, while explicating this consensus from the canonical and landmarks texts of those systems, in their own languages and contexts. The metaphysics of humanity (with its essential feature of dignity and the derivative features of rights and duties, freedom and equality, justice and peace) elaborates a common but underexplored three-dimensional conception of human dignity inherent in the world's diverse belief systems and cultures. The three metaphysical and therefore personal dimensions of the individual human being are their "existential origin, moral order, and goodness orientation." We have equal intrinsic value as we come into existence as members of the global human family. That value reaches or actualizes its full potential as we act ethically or justly by progressively aiming more and more freely and consistently toward the common and ultimate good. We increasingly become what we do (good or evil). As justice in this metaphysical vision is giving to each what is their due, the only just response to another person is love (recognizing them as an end unto themselves and thus never solely as a means). Love therefore is freely willing the good or end of the other as other. It is manifested by giving oneself as a gift in love, because persons are distinguished from other beings by our potential to give and receive another person by recognizing that each person deserves ultimately to be loved uniquely and unconditionally. Notably, love metaphysically as a mode of being is a universal. But it is always local in its action (proportional to the relationship type and concrete context of persons). Thus I can serve my patients and forgive my children (as they do me), but I cannot serve my computer or forgive my hammer. In addition, the closer someone is metaphysically to me the more intense my duty is to them (family then local community then global community), as expressed in the below ethical principle of subsidiarity.

b. *Theoretical principle*: Its main feature is human dignity, including its definition and defense of respect for personal dignity and communal cultures. The latter refers to the relational and collective pursuit of the common and ultimate good or goodness itself that characterizes humanity's most essential, personal, and communal act, realized in love that unites the person and community to and in love. In this framework, diversity is good not for its own sake but for the sake of the good, through which it is differentiated as varying paths pursuing it together, made clearer through the collective wisdom or progressive knowledge of it. Having different medical specialties like cardiology and pulmonology is only good clinically if the diversity of medical knowledge enables more complete and truthful understanding of health and how to achieve it for patients.

c. *Practical principles*: These are solidarity and subsidiarity, described in Chapter 5 on political economics.

d. *Ethical principle*: This is the Wojtylan Personalist Norm in this framework, modifying Kant's second categorical imperative by raising his minimalist and constructivist Western Enlightenment principle to the global personal dimension. Kant as the prerunner to Rawls (who tried to save Kant's philosophy as among the most formidable and influential of the Western early modern Enlightenment thinkers) argued that we must treat other persons as ends rather than merely means. The Personalist Norm integrated within the Personalist Social Contract shows how the way to treat someone as an end is to love them, as it is the most personal, just, and person-respecting act one person can do to another. Using them merely as a means violates their dignity, utilizing the other as a means or tool rather than respecting the person as an end or good. Persons are unique goods unto themselves, unlike other beings like generic tools that are good insofar as they achieve a higher good. The Personalist Social Contract traces the *reasoning* inherent in the world's diverse belief systems below to the "Golden *Rule*" as it is popularly expressed: do to others what you want them to do to you. We may get away with unethical actions for a time by escaping punishment. But as game theory shows empirically, our individual good is maximized when we contribute to the collective good for others' benefit and not just our own, more than if we solely pursued our individual good including at the expense of others. The Personalist Social Contract shows how the subtleties, nuances, and diversity in and across Buddhism, Christianity, Confucianism, Daoism, Hinduism, Islam, Judaism, and nonreligiously affiliated secularism including agnosticism emerge from the common metaphysical foundation above and substantively converge on this shared ethical principle (empowering more durable, detailed, and decisive dialogue for ethical decisions rather than simple, shifting, superficial overlapping consensus; see Phramaha 2012; Paul 1995; Tsai 2005; Hansen 2022; Nadkarni 2013; Hayatli 2009; Rothenberg 2017; Rawls 2005).

e. *Operative principle*: The Personalist Social Contract has been operationalized particularly in AI health ethics by integrating it within AiCE noted earlier rather than simply as a stand-alone ethical framework. In AiCE, clinical AI-augmented causal inference and cost effectiveness analyses generate results that are used as inputs in ethical and policy analysis, conducted according to the Personalist Social Contract to ultimately generate real-time, adaptive, precise policy recommendations for clinical care, population health, public health, and global public health (i.e., see the above text; Monlezun et al. 2022).

3. *Value*: Elaborating on what Chapter 1 introduced, the unique value proposition of the Personalist Social Contract is that it *effectively* makes substantive classical ethical solutions intelligible, compelling, and unifying to a multicultural and pluralistic modernity, while *efficiently* integrating at speed, scale, and specificity this consensus for AI global health ethics in a way that alternatives do not. It delivers this value through its (1) practical, (2) political, and (3) philosophical advantages compared to competing alternatives. (1) Practically, the basic pillars of the Personalist Social Contract are historically formulated in and makes philosophically intelligible modernity's dominant ethics: human dignity–based rights and duties, captured paradigmatically by the *UDHR*, the consensus foundation of its politically derivative institutions like the UN, WHO, and modern international law. The UN is the first and most successful globally cooperative intergovernment institution with an unprecedented track record reducing conflicts worldwide. But its future is undermined without reclaiming its substantive origin in its unifying global moral vision stretching across borders and belief systems (a vision that the Personalist Social Contract uniquely unpacks, defends, and develops for 21st-century audiences and challenges). (2) Politically, this framework deepens, strengthens, and accelerates the cooperative convergence of states globally through the substantive moral convergence of its belief systems to prevent common catastrophic conflicts and respond to common existential crises. (3) Philosophically, the Personalist Social Contract recovers the logical defensibility and experiential compatibility of this shared moral foundation for our pluralistic world, upon which the UN and similar institutions facilitate a global political economic framework that manages strategic competition, reduces conflict, and builds cooperation. It does so by ethically preserving the modern social contract framework of the *UDHR* (as convergent consensus of basic political principles of justice as fairness with enhanced care for more vulnerable populations), while safeguarding its future (replacing the cracked modern nominalist metaphysical foundation with a concrete classical realist Aristotelian one, elucidating and formalizing the implicit or explicit realist foundation inherent to our diverse belief systems while making it more intelligible to modernity). This ethical system therefore can reach the conclusions which modern ethics otherwise seeks but falls short of, including articulating and proving the reality of and duty to respect intrinsic personal value and pluralist multiculturalism. It thus demonstrates for reasons inherent to our varied cultures and belief systems the basic metaphysical reality of the person as a unique member of the global human family, and therefore the need for an AI-accelerated efficient and equitable global public health ecosystem to protect, serve, and preserve it.

4. *Content*: The Personalist Social Contract provides the moral substance of the political consensus about human security–based integral sustainable development, the essence of the grand strategy of the global human ecosystem (articulated and championed by the UN and the high-level multisector and multidomain joint declarations, state constitutions, multilateral organizations, and public–private partnerships) and its derivative AI-enabled global public health ecosystem. The Chapter 3 on development analyzed how the UN's 1986 General Assembly confirmed the shared belief that "the

right to development is an inalienable human right," realized integrally (across the cultural, societal, and political economic dimensions) for "every human person and all peoples," as it is in this development process "in which all human rights and fundamental freedoms can be fully realized." Integral development (which always and everywhere occurs in community as an operation and necessity of the common good) derives from and operationalizes the dignity of the person, encompassing rights flowing from and required for the fulfillment of dignity, especially the flourishing of the human person. From dignity, the General Assembly reasoned toward development, requiring the freedoms of "self-determination" and "sovereignty" (as long as they do not harm the good of the person and peoples in the simple utilitarian pursuit of "development"). The General Assembly therefore asserted that "the human *person* [emphasis added] is the central subject of development and should be the active participant and beneficiary of the right to development." The UN's 1987 Brundtland Report provided a practical societal blueprint for realizing this moral vision, formalized as "sustainable development" conceptually as a global and local necessity for "sustainable human progress and human survival," and thus for our personal flourishing and "common future." The UN's 2015 Sustainable Development Goals as the grand strategy for the UN and the WHO (especially for AI-enabled digital health) bring this vision closer to a measurable plan and thus closer to achievable reality.

The Personalist Social Contract globally explicates and demonstrates this evolution as embedded already within and defended by our diverse cultures and belief systems (coming up from within rather than being imposed down upon our reason, experiences, cultures, and communities). In this framework, the person is the metaphysical key to understanding, being convinced by, and thus being united by this universal story making sense of what we already see and believe locally. Development is always motion toward something. The content of the Personalist Social Contract uniquely defines and defends ethically, pluralistically, and multiculturally that we are born into a global human family with unique dignity—not as nameless repeatable agents—as unique beings capable of developing *toward* our personal flourishing through love, realized *in* the common good. It gives the moral substance answering the questions of who, what, where, how, and why to the political economic consensus of the UN and the global international community, divided and united by cooperative, competitive, and conflicting world orders and stakeholders. And it notably resolves the inherent tension in equality and liberty that modern ethics otherwise struggles to address (by constraining one by the other in a zero-sum game). This framework instead seeks to maximize both in a positive sum game, by ordering them by and orientating them toward the real metaphysical interdependent relationship of personal dignity fulfilled in the common good (manifesting the reality of our human nature, purpose, meaning, and good). Rather than violating self-determination or sovereignty, the Personalist Social Contract facilitates equality in opportunity rather than in forced outcomes. Yet in contrast to the intent or at least application of most modern ethics, this framework's content does not require global allegiance to be globally relevant and useful. It shows how it is at least compatible with our diverse belief systems and provides the metaphysical structure and ethical framework (with a common language and logic) to substantively define and defend those common values from within our belief systems (as it explains the person who is central to all belief systems and cultures).

In summary, the Personalist Social Contract shows our convergent consensus on the intrinsic value of the human person as an integral and unique member of the global human family. It shows how this dignity derives from our self-evident biological and existential identity as a human being, irrespective of any arbitrary or artificial traits invoked to truncate such value in modern ethics systems or practices (such as sex, race, ethnicity, nationality, autonomy, social utility, religiously affiliated or unaffiliated belief system, etc.). Following Aristotle and refined by modern pluralistic insights, this framework focuses on the person, a dependent and vulnerable rational animal from our first to final moments. Daily life shows us our need for others to survive and flourish uniquely in community. Our personal vulnerability depends on communal virtues or habits of good ethical actions (like justice, wisdom, courage, and self-control as complementary human organs need each other), exceeding simple moral minimums and reaching rather toward love as their fulfillment. To really see another person as a person requires us to see them as a good (intrinsically) unto themselves. Doing so means we will the good (ultimately) for that person, proportional to the proximity of our relationship to that person and resources to care for her/him. As babies, we cannot raise ourselves. We depend on the good (moral) will of others. And the less good will we have for others as we age, the more we distance ourselves from the community in which otherwise we find our meaning. We experience the real difference between the above, for instance, when our physician treats us a unique person rather than just another numbered patient (i.e., the difference between holding our hand as we are dying and leaving us alone in an empty room). In this global human family, we become more uniquely and fully ourselves the more we treat others justly and thus lovingly. Concurrently, the community is fulfilled when this personal fulfillment is realized at collective scale. The personal good requires the common good and vice versa, as the person is both a unique individual and still a common member of a community. We not only have rights that must be respected for our individual good but also duties that bind us to contribute to the common good, guarding the individual good of all.

5. *Application (through moral interoperability)*: The Personalist Social Contract is applied to the AI-enabled global public health ecosystem through its unique concept of "moral interoperability" (of the real, convergent, and pluralistic conception of human dignity). It enables the institutional and data interoperability of its diverse stakeholders, and thus the overarching ecosystem interoperability that facilitates its sustainability. *How* they work together is determined by *why* they should in the first place, allowing a more durable, dynamic, and decolonized partnership. The lasting centrality and inherent embeddedness of this moral interoperability this framework clarifies and defends is echoed by the UN's 2012 General Resolution 67/18 (UN 2012a). It declares the global consensus that "human rights, the rule of law and democracy are interlinked and mutually reinforcing and that

they belong to the universal and indivisible core values and principles of the United Nations" (UN 2012a). "Democracy is a universal value" whose political legitimacy is generated from, anchored in, and exists for the "freely expressed will of people to "determine their own political, economic, social and cultural systems." The Personalist Social Contract further cites and elaborates on the UN's 2000 Millennium Declaration in which the world's nations affirmed the collective duty to "promote democracy" as the institutional means to protect human security (as freedom from fear and want), since this political regime "best assures these rights" (to the point the vast majority of nations including China and Russia officially describe themselves as democratic, even if there is a spectrum of intensity and inclusivity expressing democracy's essential features of free and open participatory governance). For this to be more than just a rhetorical shared declaration of liberal democracies (i.e., democracies) and illiberal democracies (i.e., autocracies) competing for global influence, moral interoperability is required to show and strengthen their intrinsic moral values. It is these values that animate their societal structures and cultures, while also showing how they can communicate and unify competing ideological and political economic blocs. For this global consensus to be broad enough to sustain the global human ecosystem and its derivative global public health ecosystem, it must be sufficiently deep (which the Personalist Social Contract facilitates by identifying and institutionalizing this ecosystem interoperability).

This framework shows for instance how the Confucian Chinese ambassador (Peng Chung Chang) and the Christian Lebanese ambassador (Charles Malik) drafted the core text of the *UDHR* (with the US Eleanor Roosevelt and Canadian John Humphrey) as the moral bedrock of the above seminal texts, for reasons inherent to their belief systems and cultural contexts. It recovers the common metaphysical and moral vision of the human person stretching across the world's belief systems, represented by the document's state signatories and articulated as the "Golden Rule" of doing to others what you want them to do to you. **The political economic suprastructure of the global world analyzed in the Chapter 5 is explicitly based and exists by the unifying values expressed by this *UDHR*—and the Personalist Social Contract shows how its underlying moral vision generated them then and can guard them now. This interoperability is operationalized by transparently and fairly clarifying and defending the value hierarchies of our diverse belief systems (internal to those systems and shared across them). This is concurrent with also practically, experientially, and logically refining the problematic elements of them and excluding those elements (but not entire belief systems in contrast to modern ethics) that are incompatible with our human coexistence, reality, and experience. With greater precision and justification than Rawls (but similar in how he tried to exclude "unreasonable" belief systems), this framework at the level of application must exclude such radical philosophical elements like materialism, spiritualism, individualism, and collectivism. This is because they excessively distort through extreme reduction the reality and identity of the person beyond the reach of logic and experience to correct them. The framework must similarly exclude such extreme ideological elements of continual conflict, elitism, and consumerism (like in Western Marxism and Chinese Marxist-

Leninism). While trying to maximize the rest of the elements (particularly the essentials) in our diverse belief systems, the Personalist Social Contract philosophically, anthropologically, scientifically, and so comprehensively defines and defends the reality of the human person, especially with our interdependent dignity and communality. It seeks to do so while historically explicating this moral vision in the *UDHR* and its related instruments mentioned earlier, and societally demonstrating the substantive convergence metaphysically, existentially, and ethically on the person. It is this convergence that empowers the resultant global moral interoperability for the global human and thus public health ecosystems. This vision is anchored in and echoed by our world's belief systems as expressed in their essential principles of societal application: Buddhism's *sila*, Christianity's doctrine of Jesus' incarnation and redemptive suffering and resurrection, Confucianism's *yi* and *jen*, Hinduism's *dharma*, Islam and Judaism's doctrine of the human person (also shared by Christianity understanding the person created in the image and likeness of God as Goodness and Love itself, and so made for unity with God and others through a just and so loving life), and secularism's Rawlsian-like pluralist and political "justice" as fairness.

6.7 Personalist Social Contract artificial intelligence health ethics: African "Ubuntu," global embodiment, and humanity's sustainability

This chapter explored the current progressive demographic shift from the Global North to the South, with the related AI-accelerated political economic power shift that may not be necessarily West *to* South but at least North *with* the South. The "table" of the world order is growing to make room for new stakeholders and expand the role of today's underrepresented ones. We therefore explored the decolonization of global AI ethics through the perspective of Personalist Social Contract ethics within Personalist Liberalism. Underlying these seismic trends, this global pluralistic ethics framework sought to unpack the global convergence of our diverse belief systems on the human person at the twilight of WWII—which formed the moral bedrock for our international institutions from the UN onward—and how this framework can develop this consensus for our AI transformed world orders at the twilight of the AI age. This transformation mandates "rights" and "justice" be more than superficial rhetoric and declared principles if they are to be relevant. So, we turn now to two emblematic cases of local efforts at substantive AI ethics for health which have been gaining attention and traction since the COVID-19 pandemic spotlighted the failure of relying predominantly on high-level global principles: African "Ubuntu" and classical "embodiment," developed and deployed especially for the global public health ecosystem through the AI health ethics evolution defined and defended by the Personalist Social Contract.

Ubuntu is a robustly diverse African cultural philosophy popularized by the Nobel Prize winning South African bishop, Desmond Tutu, who integrated it with his Christian theology to champion peaceful overturning of his country's apartheid political system of institutionalized racial segregation, in addition to the subsequent society-wide reconciliation by addressing apartheid's human rights abuses (Tutu 2009). Ubuntu (Zulu: *umuntu ngumuntu ngabantu*) generally refers to "humanity" or "human dignity," understood as the relational moral vision articulated with its classic formulation as "I am because we are." It expresses a dual conception metaphysically and ethically. To be a person is essentially and existentially to be a vulnerable, interdependent, unique individual in community who needs the community and who the community needs. Humanity is interdependence and thus harmony. Humanizing well-ordered societies flourish by developing toward the common good, and so caring for the good of all members of the community, who flourish individually by caring for this common good. I find myself when I care for you, who generated and empowered my "I" by caring first for me. In contrast, dehumanizing disordered societies decay by the strong dominating the weak, losing the unique "I" and common "we" by reducing the human family simply to a faceless power hierarchy of choosing agents, typically generated and preserved by coercion and violence. The Personalist Social Contract describes the convergence of Ubuntu's realist metaphysical and relational ethics with the framework's above detailed content (as an example of such an embedded vision and values in the world's belief systems without requiring them to "convert" to this framework, but rather encouraging them to "remain" in their comprehensive worldview, while seeing the substantive convergence with other belief systems).

COVID accelerated African calls especially to invoke the Ubuntu moral vision for global health to recognize our existence as a "global village" in which solidarity is not just good ethics, but also good global public health (that is undercut by failures to cooperatively sustain personal development at global scale, which in turn undermines political stability, economic prosperity, societal equality, and individual agency globally for us all; Jecker et al. 2022). Ubuntu is like a microcosm of this framework, as it is a collective vision rather than a uniform ethno-philosophical or cultural heritage the same way that i.e., European Catholicism had a more defined, consistent, and operationalized set of values that informed and framed the Scientific Revolution, Protestant Reformation, and philosophical Enlightenment (which progressively broke from it and informed and framed the Great Divergence of North and South, resulting in our current Western-dominated liberal world order). The growing post-COVID international emphasis on AI ethics (as its technical development coupled with concerns of its unethical applications) are being updated and applied in our modern moment. This is especially seen with Ubuntu's view of the Golden Rule supporting more inclusive global AI ethics for health as relational not just principal, and global not just Western, to more equitably and effectively advance toward global justice and solidarity (Gwagwa et al. 2022). The Global South faces not just digital barriers to inclusion in the global public health ecosystem, nor the ecosystem just pragmatic barriers to its sustainability if such truncated inclusivity persists. But it also must contend with ethical barriers, which the Personalist Social Contract echoing globally and anchored locally by Ubuntu (and related indigenous belief systems the world over) can serve as a bridge over. It can do so by providing concrete, coherent, compelling, and personal reasons to unite (without erasing) our "tribes" into a "global village" that is concurrently global and local existentially. This is possible because the village is constituted by persons who have concurrently communicable (common) and noncommunicable (unique) dimensions metaphysically.

The convergent vision of humanity expressed in our relational dignity that is shared by Ubuntu and the Personalist Social Contract also extends the Thomistic-Aristotelian Personalism of one of the leading public bioethics experts for global health, OC Snead. This American legal scholar served as the US chief negotiator for the UN's 2005 *Universal Declaration on Bioethics and Human Rights* as the bioethics application of the *UDHR*). His 2020 Harvard University Press book emphasizes the public health and law implications of "embodiment" (Snead 2020). Snead notes that regardless of state, culture, and belief system, the natural boundaries of our bodies mean we are most fundamentally vulnerable and thus dependent on others from our first to our last moment of existence. We are born into families and communities and learn to love as others first love us. Through this process we become most fully ourselves by giving ourselves to others in love (with the converse being true in which manipulation and abandonment increase social isolation and fragmentation, along with the increased likelihood the harmed person continues the cycle of conflict with others). Any autonomous agent (man or machine) can choose and obtain a soda from a vending machine as long as the right buttons are pushed and steps followed. But only a human person can love another in even a simple affectionate act like getting a soda for their child who asks for it (extending past the sole mechanical steps of physically obtaining it). At our core, Ubuntu and Snead argue (sharing the same metaphysical foundation and similar ethical framework of the Personalist Social Contract that shows its bridge with the world's belief systems), we are essentially loving persons. Our freedom is the means *for* love uniting us with others in the ever-expanding positive sum common good spanning material and immaterial goods—derivative from goodness itself—as our end. We are not essentially choosing agents. Our freedom is not our means *and* end, artificially and arbitrarily waging a zero-sum competition that manufactures and fights others for material "goods" that are ever shrinking. Yet modernity's dominant legal framework is a Western reduction of the person to choosing agents who have no intrinsic ties or duties to others, leaving the most vulnerable reliant on charity care or an under-resourced government. At the level of international governance including for the AI-enabled global public health ecosystem, we see how COVID exposed how richer nations simply "opted out" from any volitional duties to poorer nations by denying any deeper metaphysical and existential ties with them. In doing so they impoverished our humanity, weakened the ecosystem, and all the more highlighted why recovering our substantive moral convergence of our shared humanity (as the Personalist Social Contract defines and defends from *within* our already existent belief systems, cultures, and international institutions) may be thus key to its sustainability and our survivability (not just for that of the ecosystem dependent on it). Thus let us explore in this Chapter 7 how this ecosystem—generated following WWII from this moral foundation that is recoverable and needed for our common future—is concretely emerging, evolving, and embracing needed ethical reform and AI transformation. In doing so, we will bring together the book's chapters and concepts to assemble conceptually a real blueprint for this how this ecosystem functions and its future are already taking shape—in addition to how we can shape it to make room for all of humanity, moving us from human security to sovereignty to sustainability at the scale, speed, and scope which our global public health challenges and crises require.

References

Benchaita, S. 2023. "IBM Renews Commitment to Rome Call for AI Ethics, Applauds Muslim and Jewish Leaders Joining Call." IBM. Accessed June 20, 2023. https://newsroom.ibm.com/2023-01-09-IBM-Renews-Commitment-to-Rome-Call-for-AI-Ethics,-Applauds-Muslim-and-Jewish-Leaders-Joining-Call.

Bollyky, T.J., and A. Shendruk. 2017. "The Changing Demographics of Global Health." Council on Foreign Relations. Accessed June 23, 2023. https://www.cfr.org/article/changing-demographics-global-health.

Bremmer, I., and C. Kupchan. 2023. "Top Risks 2023." Eurasia Group. Accessed May 8, 2023. https://www.eurasiagroup.net/issues/top-risks-2023.

Cilluffo, A., and N.G. Ruiz. 2019. "World's Population is Projected to Nearly Stop Growing by the End of the Century." Pew Research Center. Accessed June 23, 2023. https://www.pewresearch.org/short-reads/2019/06/17/worlds-population-is-projected-to-nearly-stop-growing-by-the-end-of-the-century/#:~:text = By%202100%2C%20the%20world%20population,to%20more%20than%207.7%20billion.

Cowls, J., Tsamados, A., Taddeo, M., and L. Floridi. 2021. "A Definition, Benchmark and Database of AI for Social Good Initiatives." *Nature Machine Intelligence* 3 (2021): 111–115.

Cummings, M.L., H.M. Roff, K. Cukier, J. Parakilas, H. Bryce, 2018. "Artificial Intelligence and International Affairs." The Royal Institute of International Affairs: Chatham House. Accessed June 28, 2023. https://www.chathamhouse.org/sites/default/files/publications/research/2018-06-14-artificial-intelligence-international-affairs-cummings-roff-cukier-parakilas-bryce.pdf.

Duranti, M. 2020. "Anti-Colonialism and Human Rights in the French Empire." In *Decolonization, Self-Determination, and the Rise of Global Human Rights Politics*, edited by A.D. Moses, M. Duranti, R. Burke (Eds.).

Else, H. 2023. "Abstracts Written by ChatGPT Fool Scientists." *Nature*. Accessed July 4, 2023. https://www.nature.com/articles/d41586-023-00056-7.

Floridi, L., and J. Cowls. 2019. "A Unified Framework of Five Principles for AI in Society." Social Science Research Network. Accessed July 3, 2023. https://papers.ssrn.com/sol3/papers.cfm?abstract_id = 3831321.

García Saisó, S., and M. D'Agostino. 2021. *Artificial Intelligence in Public Health*. World Health OrganizationAccessed February 8, 2023. https://iris.paho.org/bitstream/handle/10665.2/53732/PAHOEIHIS21011_eng.pdf?sequence = 5.

Gwagwa, A., Kazim, E., and A. Hilliard. 2022. "The Role of the African Value of Ubuntu in Global AI Inclusion Discourse: A Normative Ethics Perspective." *Patterns* 3 (4): 100462.

Hansen, C.D. 2022. In *The Stanford Encyclopedia of Philosophy*, edited by E.N. Zalta, *The Stanford Encyclopedia of Philosophy*Redwood City, CA: Stanford University PressAccessed February 1, 2022. https://plato.stanford.edu/archives/spr2020/entries/daoism.

Hayatli, M. 2009. "Islam, International Law and the Protection of Refugees and IDPs." University of Oxford Refugees Studies Centre. Accessed February 1, 2023. https://www.refworld.org/pdfid/4c68eec82.pdf.

Jecker, N.S., C.A. Atuire, N. Kenworthy. 2022. "Realizing Ubuntu in Global Health: An African Approach to Global Health Justice." *Public Health Ethics*. phac022.

Monlezun, D.J. 2023. *The Thinking Healthcare System: Artificial Intelligence and Human Equity*. New York: Elsevier.

Monlezun, D.J. 2022. *Personalist Social Contract: Saving Multiculturalism, Artificial Intelligence, and Civilization*. Newcastle upon Tyne: Cambridge Scholars Press.

Monlezun, D.J., Sinyavskiy, O., Sotomayor, C., Peters, N., Steigner, L., Girault, M., Garcia, A., Gallagher, C., and C. Iliescu. 2022. "Artificial Intelligence-Augmented Propensity Score, Cost Effectiveness, and Computational Ethical Analysis of Cardiac Arrest and Active Cancer With Novel Mortality Predictive Score." *Medicina (CardioOncology)* 58 (8): 1039.

Myers, S.L., and D. McCabe. 2023. "Federal Judge Limits Biden Officials' Contacts With Social Media Sites." *New York Times*. Accessed July 6, 2023. https://www.nytimes.com/2023/07/04/business/federal-judge-biden-social-media.html.

Nadkarni, M.V. 2013. *Essays in Gandhian perspective*. Oxford: Oxford University Press.

Orf, D. 2023. "The Turing Test for AI is Far Beyond Obsolete." Popular Mechanics. Accessed July 7, 2023. https://www.popularmechanics.com/technology/robots/a43328241/turing-test-for-artificial-intelligence-is-obsolete/.

PASS. 2023. "The Fraternal Economy of Integral and Sustainable Development." Vatican City's Pontifical Academy of Social Sciences. Accessed April 5, 2023. https://www.pass.va/en/events/2023/fraternal_economy.html.

Paul II, J. 1995. *Evangelium Vitae*. Vatican City, Vatican: Vatican Press.

Phramaha, S. 2012. "The Buddhist Core Values and Perspectives for Protection Challenges." United Nations High Commissioner for Refugees. Accessed February 1, 2023. https://www.unhcr.org/en-us/protection/hcdialogue%20/50be10cb9/buddhist-core-values-perspectives-protection-challenges-faith-protection.html.

Rawls, J. 2005. *Political Liberalism*. New York: Columbia University Press.

Rothenberg, N. 2017. *Rabbi Akiva's Philosophy of Love*. New York: Palgrave-Macmillan.

Sachs, J.D., Karim, S.S.A., Aknin, L., Allen, J., Brosbøl, K., Colombo, F., and G.C. Barron, et al., 2022. "The Lancet Commission on Lessons for the Future From the COVID-19 Pandemic." *Lancet* 400 (10359): 1224−1280.

Shine, I. 2023. "From AI to Robot Jellyfish, Here's the Technology Protecting Biodiversity." World Economic Forum. Accessed June 27, 2023. https://www.weforum.org/agenda/2023/05/ai-technology-international-biodiversity-day/.

Silvestro, D., Goria, S., Sterner, T., and A. Antonelli. 2022. "Improving Biodiversity Protection Through Artificial Intelligence." *Nature Sustainability* 5, 415−424.

Snead, O.C. 2020. *What It Means to be Human: The Case for the Body in Public Bioethics*. Cambridge, MA: Harvard University Press.

Tsai, D.F.-C. 2005. "The Bioethical Principles and Confucius' Moral Philosophy." *BMJ Global Medical Ethics* 31, 159−163.

Tutu, D. 2009. *No Future Without Forgiveness*. New York: Doubleday.

UN. 2020. "Roadmap for Digital Cooperation: Implementation of the Recommendations of the High-Level Panel on Digital Cooperation." United Nations 74th General Assembly. Accessed June 11, 2022. https://www.un.org/en/content/digital-cooperation-roadmap/.

UN. 2015. "Transforming Our World: The 2030 Agenda for Sustainable Development." United Nations. Accessed April 5, 2023. https://sdgs.un.org/2030agenda.

UN. 2012a. "Education for Democracy: Resolution 67/18 Adopted by the General Assembly." United Nations. Accessed February 15, 2023. https://documents-dds-ny.un.org/doc/UNDOC/GEN/N12/479/68/PDF/N1247968.pdf?OpenElement.

UN. 2012b. "The Secretary-General's Address to Parliament of the Former Yugoslav Republic of Macedonia." United Nations. Accessed February 15, 2023. https://www.un.org/sg/en/content/sg/statement/2012-07-25/secretary-generals-address-parliament-former-yugoslav-republic.

UN. 1948. "Universal Declaration of Human Rights." United Nations. Accessed January 16, 2023. https://www.un.org/en/about-us/universal-declaration-of-human-rights.

UNESCO. 2020. "Dr. Dominique J. Monlezun Received the Microsoft Award for Artificial Intelligence Doctoral Dissertation." United Nations Educational, Scientific and Cultural Organization Chair in Bioethics & Human Rights. Accessed January 16, 2023. https://www.unescobiochair.org/2020/03/11/dr-dominique-j-monlezun-received-the-microsoft-award-for-artificial-intelligence-doctoral-dissertation/.

UN. "Transforming our world: The 2030 Agenda for Sustainable Development. United Nations." https://sdgs.un.org/2030agenda (accessed 05 April 2023).

UNDP. "Human development report 1994: New dimensions of human security. United Nations Development Programme." https://hdr.undp.org/content/human-development-report-1994 (accessed 15 February 2023).

Vallance C. "Artificial intelligence could lead to extinction, experts warn. BBC." https://www.bbc.com/news/uk-65746524 (accessed 30 May 2023).

van Heerden, A.C., Pozuelo, J.R., and B.A. Kohrt. 2023. "Global Mental Health Services and the Impact of artificial Intelligence–Powered Large Language Models." *JAMA Psychiatry* 80 (7): 662–664. https://doi.org/10.1001/jamapsychiatry.2023.1253.

WHO. 2023. "WHO Calls for Safe and Ethical AI for Health." World Health Organization. Accessed June 20, 2023. https://www.who.int/news/item/16-05-2023-who-calls-for-safe-and-ethical-ai-for-health.

WHO. 2021a. "Ethics and Governance of Artificial Intelligence for Health." World Health Organization. Accessed June 20, 2023. https://www.who.int/publications/i/item/9789240029200.

WHO. 2021b. "Global Strategy on Digital Health 2020–2025." World Health Organization. Accessed June 11, 2022. https://www.who.int/docs/default-source/documents/gs4dhdaa2a9f352b0445bafbc79ca799dce4d.pdf.

WHO. 2015. "Biodiversity and Health." World Health Organization. Accessed June 20, 2023. https://www.who.int/news-room/fact-sheets/detail/biodiversity-and-health.

WHO. 2002. "Health and Human Security." World Health Organization. Accessed January 16, 2023. https://apps.who.int/iris/handle/10665/122074.

7

Our common home: artificial intelligence + global public health ecosystem

7.1 Global needs, crises, and hope

In this book journey together, we explored the shared story from our first to present days focused on populations then productivity, and then purpose. In premodern times, there had to be enough people to farm, fish, hunt, and protect communities. In early modern times, we turned science into technologies into industries into global power and supply chains, bringing historic prosperity but also conflicts. In late modern times currently, purpose is taking more of center stage as being peaceful and prosperous are globally necessary—but not sufficient—goods. More states, societies, and belief systems are seeking to understand the purpose of these goods as means to a higher end, one which the United Nations (UN), World Health Organization (WHO), governments, corporations, universities, and communities increasingly describe with the convergent conception of global well-being. Sufficient security and salaries are widely described as good, not as a final end but as an instrumental means to the end of personal flourishing and the common good, equitably at scale for a healthy humanity. This modern emphasis on values not just classical political economics appears rooted both in the widespread moral claims (expressed by the world's nations in the UN's *Universal Declaration of Human Rights [UDHR]*) about our common humanity and thus dignity, rights, and duties to our common good. But they are also embodied in the pragmatic societal context that we cannot consistently achieve our individual goods without also advancing the common good (which encompasses our individual goods as well). Meanwhile, artificial intelligence (AI) appears to signal a new human epoch of unprecedented productivity for population health and renewed purpose, accelerating the emerging global public health ecosystem whose collective mission is this global well-being. Yet the path toward health through peace, prosperity, and equity appears to be going off the rails, or even running out of road. Chapter 1 opened with the somber 2022 warning of the UN Secretary-General:

> *Geopolitical tensions are reaching new highs. Competition is trumping cooperation and collaboration. Distrust has replaced dialogue and disunity has replaced disarmament...humanity is just one misunderstanding, one miscalculation away from...annihilation.*

The COVID-19 pandemic showed us our AI may not be as smart as we hoped, nor the global ecosystem as effective, or our institutions as trustworthy. Russia's 2022 full-scale invasion

Responsible Artificial Intelligence Re-engineering the Global Public Health Ecosystem. DOI: https://doi.org/10.1016/B978-0-443-21597-1.00007-X

of Ukraine and weaponization of energy and food showed us a fair and effective rules-based international order does not always stop rogue actors seizing other's land and resources by force, and that the West does not consistently care for the Global South's own conflicts while it seeks to enlist its support to stop aggression against it. And southeast Asian neighbors' alarm about China's progressive threats and use of force against Taiwan and others shows us the growing risk that world wars may not be extinct. A global UN coalition in the 1990s pushed Iraq out of Kuwait after it invaded and seized 20% of the world's oil supply (and yet China's 2020s seizure of Taiwan would give them control of 90% of the world's semiconductors and nearly 100% of the global digital economy and data on which our countries daily depend). Power is not the problem, but not using it justly for the common and individual good is. We have seen throughout this book how the AI-accelerated hope of shared survival and flourishing animates and frames the full-spectrum, multidomain, and multicultural ecosystem partners that make our common home and future still possible. And this hope suggests we can continue averting the dark days we envisioned we could permanently put behind us when we emerged from the ashes of World War II with its colonial and great power clashes. This chapter will pull together the different conceptual and concrete components of that ecosystem each chapter analyzed to do a "walk through" of this ecosystem as our common home. By considering the leading use cases, stakeholders, and their relationships in this summary chapter, we will try to simplify the size, complexity, and speed of the ecosystem into a manageable and actionable vision of that home, how it is changing, and how we can improve it.

The ecosystem and thus this chapter's structure translates the earlier chapters into the subsequent sections by showing how the latest state-of-the-art concrete health AI advances fit together according to the ecosystem's decentralized organic design (financing and integral sustainable development), framework (data architecture and political economics), inhabitants (culture and demographics), and foundation (human/national security and ethics). Notably this structure is a formula for the future frames—but does not wholly determine—the ecosystem's future. It projects its probable path by understanding its inputs or data to reasonably predict its outputs or results. We therefore assessed the trends of digitalization (connecting more sectors, people, and regions to the global digital ecosystem), deglobalization (with national security interests particularly in AI and related digital technologies prioritized over economic efficiency, narrowing supply chains more to domestic and close allies' markets), and demographics (with the growing burden of noncommunicable disease as people live longer but with less healthy behaviors, as the global population and maybe even power center shift to the Global South). As these trends frame the evolution of the global public health ecosystem, we detailed the major categories for AI use cases within them, which include population health (optimizing health at scale particularly by prioritizing lower cost and more effective prevention and early diagnosis and treatment), precision public health (providing resources proportional to need and likelihood of net benefit), and system optimization (boosting ecosystem efficiencies providing greater health benefit with lower costs and disparities).

But before we scan the full spectrum vision of the leading emblematic AI use cases in its constitutive below domains, let us first better clarify the ecosystem stakeholders advancing them now and for the foreseeable future. Hoffman and Cole generated what remains the largest and most comprehensive map of global health actors spanning 203 entities that constitute the decentralized organizational structure of the global public health ecosystem, overwhelmingly dominated by the West generally and the United States specifically (Hoffman and Cole 2018). An actor was identified as an "individual or organization that operates transnationally with a primary intent to improve health." Of these, 98.03% are from the West, including 66.50% from the United States alone. Analysis of social network strength demonstrated that the most influential actors (by degree) were the WHO (48), Global Health Council (40), Family Health International 360 (39), The Global Fund to Fight AIDS, Tuberculosis, and Malaria (38), the United States (37), and the Population Council (34). The WHO was also the top influential actor by closeness (1.87) and betweenness centrality (2987), which is nearly five times the next top ranked actor. These three network analytic metrics essentially and respectively measure each actor's connectivity (number of connections), access (distance among actors), and importance (position on the shortest path compared) to other actors. By far, the WHO is the top institutional actor, and the United States is the top government actor (and concurrently the leading AI actor). They exert the most influence on the global public health ecosystem, understood as a network that orders the flow of political influence, economic capital, data, knowledge, and AI technologies. Within this network, how is AI revolutionizing the ecosystem in its different domains?

7.2 Design: financing

Chapter 2 on finance focused on how the money that makes the ecosystem possible and shapes its design principally does so by its (1) structural and (2) strategic financing of AI advances. (1) Structurally, public–private partnerships are leveraging private innovation for public governance and its societal mandate for global public health. The higher health value generated by corporations and academics can be deployed for government provision of health goods, services, and capacity building. This value reduces the taxpayer burden of otherwise higher research and development (R&D) required to generate those innovations, while increasing the more cost-efficient provision of those goods and services (especially in population health management and virtual health assistants reducing the costly population burden of disease, medical care for failures in population health, and labor costs from a shrinking human workforce). Private players get market access, data, and recognition to improve their other profit-generating products and services, while public players get more efficient deployment of health resources and resultant global health in a mutual win. This emergent ecosystem of federated partnership networks appears to be the primary competitor to the traditional patchwork of the noninteroperable conglomerate of political or economic monopolies (costing more and delivering less population health) on one structural extreme and an interoperable centralized monopoly (with similar disadvantages but on a greater scale given the absence of financial incentives to compete, innovate, and improve; Pearl 2023). "Digital global health diplomacy" is arising from these partnerships to leverage AI digital platforms to advance cooperative global health diplomacy (Chattu 2022). But it also advances the prerequisite political economic collaboration of the involved institutions, governments, corporations, and academics to ultimately improve human security, sustainable development, and thus global well-being. The net impact of these efforts is greater interconnectedness, social network strength, system efficiencies, and ecosystem equity among populations worldwide.

(2) In strategic financing, there are a growing number of AI use cases within these partnership networks we analyzed. They build capacities at amplifying points of leverage in this structure to sufficiently fund needed boosts in the abovesaid impact areas. AI-enabled finance tracking such as with Duke University and Berlin's Open Consultants use random forest supervised AI/machine learning (ML) and natural language processing models to automatically categorize over 10,00 DAH or development assistance for health financing projects, allowing less funding redundancy and greater health impact. The "Impact Investment Matrix" with its "design hygiene" then imports standardized preinvestment screening analytics and other private R&D best practices into global public health funding, particularly by informing more equitable and decolonized program codesign (in which global funders can back local health agencies focused on local needs by maximizing impact and minimizing cost). Smarter funding can then be used to drive smarter and cheaper clinical and public health trials through AI-enabled research economies of scale, such as with the REMAP-CAP trial pairing reinforcement learning with Bayesian inference to save more critically sick COVID-19 patients through more rapid and precise identification of the proper treatment for groups sharing similar health traits. The RECOVERY trial along with simulated and real-time studies of pandemic countermeasures similarly get to better results with fewer dollars. Better finance tracking and research can then be translated to real-world use as AI is additionally projected to reduce health program and provision costs by upwards of 10% of national health expenditures through full spectrum optimization of the health cycle: value-based care (based on population need and risk stratification), continuity (guiding populations through public health and healthcare systems by need and phase of care), analytics (seamless care pathways augmented by quality clinical decision support and health worker productivity), operations (streamlining population flow served by value supply chains), safety (minimizing errors and maximizing compliance), and management (improving denials, claims, coding, allocation, profit, governance, and talent). Such provision capacities collectively shift the focus of traditional healthcare and public health from volume to value through embedded value-based funding models. A leading example of this is the NHS Wales capitation-based data infrastructure which was integrated with its financing infrastructure. Population health needs could thus determine resource allocation and provider payments to incentivize better performance (better quality health at lower costs). AI automation then enables resilient revenue cycles for healthcare systems and public health agencies separately and in concert. They do this by more accurately and reliably navigating complex intra- and interstate billing and compensation to ensure accurate charge capture, financial accounting, payments, and expanded benefits to eligible and uninsured populations. Finally, ecosystem-wide AI integration then can unite and optimize the abovementioned elements in a continuous improvement cycle across global public

health stakeholders through such advances as AI-driven Computational Ethics and policy analysis or AiCE: causal health inference, cost effectiveness, and equitable ethical and policy analyses combine with real-time health including electronic health record data (with similar applications for national health data) to guide affordable and equitable population health improvements, with related boosts in national health and productivity.

7.3 Design: integral sustainable development

AI improving the management of these dollars in turn funds better development, serving each person holistically and populations equitably. Chapter 3 on development explored how the evolution of more sophisticated technological tools and conceptual understanding of health into the 21st century (following the significant medical and public health advances of the 20th century). This crystallized in the UN General Assembly and WHO consensus of how global public health—spanning medical and health issues and measures with equitable international impact—can be achieved by integral and sustainable development. The high-profile marriage of these technological and conceptual advances culminated in the UK−US public−private−academic partnership of AI × sustainable development goals (SDGs). Oxford University's Saïd Business School with Microsoft, Google, and Facebook collaborated to operationalize the moral and pragmatic vision that AI should be used for social good globally to ultimately advance health that is ecologically responsible and equitably focused. The Oxford team chose the UN's 2015 SDGs that the world's nations universally affirmed as the optimal normative standard for this socially good and thus responsible AI as it is the broadest, oldest, and highest level empirical consensus on measuring, progressing toward, and unifying partners for equitable global well-being. All the SDGs either explicitly address health or implicitly advance broader societal determinants of and elements required for it. Leading AI use cases for the SDGs therefore address poverty and hunger (maximizing crop yields with remote sensors and robotics through "precision agriculture" minimizing labor, land, seeds, water, and pesticides), climate change (improving longer and more accurate forecasting of extreme weather, adverse climate change, and efficacy of various countermeasures especially for the most at-risk populations), energy (guiding a more precise, efficient, affordable, and accessible clean energy transition especially for lower income countries), equity (as with the public−private NHS−Google-university partnership showing how rising costs from worsening physician shortages can be improved with their artificial neural network algorithm detecting and treating breast cancer more effectively than radiologists), and partnerships (including Western government funding accelerating competitive development of private mRNA COVID-19 vaccines in record time, in addition to the UK−Africa public−private partnership on lab-on-a-chip remote testing and broader AI-augmented radiology).

Of emerging advances, generative AI and scaled learning may be the top use case expanding the efficacy and reach of such AI for SDGs. A McKinsey analysis of 63 use cases of generative AI (i.e., ChatGPT) suggest that the 2023's widespread adoption of these deep learning or DL models (using massive datasets to create high-quality images, text, video, code, and other content personalized by user prompts) is projected to annually add upwards of $4.4 trillion to the global economy in improved productivity—greater than the United Kingdom's national GDP (Chui et al. 2023). This one AI technique is projected to account for nearly half of AI's global societal impact in the near future, and nearly 80% if it is embedded in existing software outside the abovesaid use cases. Current estimates indicate generative AI by 2045—a decade faster than expected prior to ChatGPT—may automate upward of 75% of employee work, particularly for "white-collar" knowledge-based work that traditionally requires higher education and produces higher wages. This assumes there are no other major technical breakthroughs during that period, which is unlikely given the unexpected explosion of generative AI (suggesting such advances will not only occur, but will also do so at a faster and faster rate with synergistic breakout technological developments). By 2023, ChatGPT as one of the earliest publicly available generative AI models had already passed the US medical licensure exam, suggesting immediate real-world health applications of such generative AI, especially to accelerate the SDGs by extending limiting health workforce and improving their efficiency (particularly for underserved communities worst hit by such shortages and other related drags on their development; Kung et al. 2023).

Finally, such algorithm advances as generative AI for SDGs are coupled with the concurrent data architecture advances enabling more equitable, global, and thus effective AI ecosystem discoveries and deployment. Generally, the more data *from* and design *for* local communities, the more effective for human development their AI will be. A 2023 French–US *Nature* study of triple-negative breast cancer demonstrated proof-of-concept for local ML models running on local patient data (kept securely behind healthcare systems' firewalls) through a federated learning data architecture. They then accurately predicted treatment response based on histological biomarker patterns. In addition, their performance was improved through model collaboration of the federated partner sites, even achieving comparable success to the much more expensive and less available best-in-class ML models (built through time and cost intensive expert annotations; Ogier du Terrail et al. 2023). Federated learning therefore allows insight sharing through international model collaboration—but without data sharing—empowering more secure and equitable AI advances, i.e., as sophisticated AI creators in the Global North can share data expertise and resources with the Global South in local SDG efforts. Yet federated learning can struggle with digital bottlenecks especially in lower income communities with less internet connectivity that entails limited network bandwidth and utilization for both centralized and decentralized data architectures. A 2023 Chinese IEEE study demonstrated that this communication challenge may be resolved without sacrificing the convergence performance of federated learning by a novel "gossip" decentralized federated learning (Tang et al. 2023). Its superior efficient communication right-fits bandwidth based on more precise time-specific communication with relevant parties, allowing them to use only the digital resources they need at the time and for the tasks needed. This slashed communication time among partners nearly in half and traffic by nearly 40%, while notching accuracy comparable to competing state-of-the-art models.

7.4 Framework: data architecture

To operate the design driven by dollars and development, the AI-powered global public health ecosystem requires an effective global data architecture to guide cooperation through data sharing, analytics, and decision-making with speed and precision (with the WHO serving as the world leader in data, knowledge, and governance coordination of ecosystem partners). The primary AI use cases advancing this digital framework are focused on (1) interoperability, (2) integration, and (3) security. Like the abovementioned federated and gossip learning for SDGs, the United Kingdom's CO-CONNECT hybrid data architecture, India's National Digital Health Mission enterprise federated data architecture, and German swarm learning demonstrate promising solutions to leveraging the resources and data of diverse ecosystem partners through joint (1) interoperability. CO-CONNECT balanced a decentralized data architecture (keeping secure data local) with a complementary centralized data architecture (allowing queries and aggregate metaanalysis of pseudonymized data across partners). It therefore could unite an international partnership for collective real-time learning "at scale and pace" for COVID-19 best practices in population health management. To fit the needs for India, a federated architecture is progressively deployed to efficiently match nationwide resources to local needs through interoperability-by-design. This facilitates a digital and thus clinical and organizational continuum of care to optimize its population health through this "national digital health ecosystem." The German team's technical breakthrough of swarm learning architecture seeks (like gossip learning but as a narrower variation of federated learning) to right fit the unique advantages of different data architectures for partner needs (including efficiency with centralized learning and security with decentralized learning). Their approach utilizes blockchain-based edge computing to locally secure data without pseudonymization and run AI models at the point where data is first generated and stored at the partner site. This boosts knowledge sharing—collaboratively and iteratively improving the overall architecture's AI models—without data sharing. Its superior performance and lower barriers to adoption suggest it may even become the dominant data architecture for the global public health ecosystem.

Once ecosystem partners can digitally communicate with the same "language" through a unifying data architecture, they must be (2) integrated to empower collective action. Application programming interfaces (APIs), shallow learning, and precise computing (stream, batch, and quantum) mark a significant evolution in this category. The US Veterans Affair national healthcare system uses APIs to enable secure internet-based digital integration among public–private partnerships for healthcare delivery, as does the WHO Hub for Pandemic and Epidemic Intelligence to integrate, analyze, and alert partners to new global public health crises as AI "augmented public health intelligence" for local healthcare system and public health agency decisions. A 2023 Israeli academic team demonstrated that once such digital tools as APIs integrate partners' communication, shallow learning in contrast to the alternative state-of-the-art DL simplifies and boosts model efficiency, performance, and so democratization by reducing cost, hardware, software, data, energy, and time. Finally, a 2018 Moroccan academic team showed how integrating digital communication and algorithms can further be improved through precise computing using the Big Data on which the global public health ecosystem digitally runs. Batch and stream computing, respectively, bring accurate and timely insights by processing and analyzing data in chunks and flows, balancing them together to allow periodic but more complete insights, which in turn are regularly updated with lower resolution but real-time insights. Although with fewer real-world proven successes thus far but with exponentially greater promise, the emerging breakthrough of quantum health computing is widely projected to be the next major computing revolution —and even "ultimate" breakthrough—driving ecosystem integration and collective performance. An early pioneer is the US-based Cleveland Clinic and IBM as a world leading health provider and Big Tech company established in 2023 the first on-site commercialized quantum health AI computer. Their big dollar bet on heath's data future is predicated upon the reality that quantum is orders of magnitude faster and more powerful than classical computing (including batch and stream), allowing it to integrate multiomics, pharmaceutical, clinical, social media, and global health datasets to drive more rapid and effective drug, treatment, and policy advances.

Interoperability enables integration and thus efficient performance. Yet distrust from insufficient security can undermine the participation of ecosystem partners in their shared global data architecture. Thus, there are AI use cases significantly improving (3) security through zero-trust dual-defense, blockchain, data solidarity, and cloud-fog-edge computing. Zero-trust data architecture focuses on prevention (of intruders' invasion into an IT infrastructure) and containment (promptly kicking them out while halting the spread of their damage). It does so by "least-privilege access controls" along with infrastructure-wide visibility across cloud partners. Blockchain as a distributed digital ledger links data blocks with a tamper-resistant digital signature, allowing a unified security interoperability across multiple domains with no single point of security failure, unlike traditional security methods. Blockchain-based security is already being deployed in health applications like in the above-said swarm use case. It should be noted that quantum computing appears to threaten even blockchain, though there are considerable investments and development by governments and the private sector (but significantly less in health) to overhaul traditional classical computing-based security with quantum security in a new phase of quantum blockchain. Quantum entanglement and other unique properties of this computing revolution appear progressively that they may allow secure encryption and data communication among partners even in political regimes attempting to restrict the free flow of secure data or undermine its integrity on the blockhain. Aside from the technical security advances, conceptual security advances in data solidarity are accelerating the decolonization of the global data architecture to optimize collective data ownership and the balance between data risks and public value (enjoying growing global support in the Global South and the UN including the Broadband Commission). Finally, blockchain-secured cloud–fog–edge architectures using hybrid and federated architectures has been deployed for "smart cities" to optimize population health (including through integrated ecosystem partners, remote and home devices, fog nodes, and cloud data centers). Its most advanced form to date appears to be "deep reinforcement learning-aware blockchain-based task scheduling," efficiently coordinating cloud and fog communication with Internet of Things edge devices even amid diverse cost, latency, energy, and delay constraints of various partners to right-fit and time digital resources based on user needs in the health data architecture.

7.5 Framework: political economics

The primary hurdles and promises for an effective unifying data architecture for the global public health ecosystem meet in AI data governance, the intersection of technology and political economics. There are currently three competing paradigms embodied by three of the world's top power blocks in both of the abovesaid domains, as all three of whom are seeking to influence the rest of the world especially in the Global South. They manifest different institutional models to balancing national security and sovereignty with varying degrees of technical and institutional interoperability among them, which in turn determine the extent of internal and external data interoperability, integration, and security (including innovation and regulation). Europe's government-driven open model, the United States' market-driven open model, and the government-driven closed Chinese model are rapidly gaining traction in the global digital ecosystem and threatening to further balkanize or splinter the global internet into geographic, economic, and ideological fault lines (as with China's Great Firewall and Russia's related Sovereign Internet Law; Larsen, 2022). As data flows are disrupted, so too are the flows of people, ideas, and capital. Such restrictions accelerate the digital deglobalization that can be structurally fatal to an effective global public health ecosystem (and international governance addressing any shared existential threat or global crisis). It is unclear which governance model will ultimately predominate and remake the ecosystem's data architecture and larger governance system (currently fragmented) in its image. The democratic rights-based substance of the European and US models contrasts with the autocratic control-based model of the Chinese. The governance modality further differentiates them. Europe features a government-driven, top-down, by-design, regulation-focused maximization of freedom bounded by human rights guardrails. America has an individual-driven, bottom-up, organic, innovation-focused maximization of freedom bounded by those similar guardrails. China rather utilizes a government-driven, top-down, by-design, censorship-focused maximization of government control bounded by political "pressure release valves" (which blow when popular resistance is too great as with extended COVID lockdowns).

The European Union's (EU's) 2018 General Data Protection Regulation (GDPR) established the first comprehensive and stringent nationwide data protection regulation, setting the stage for the first comprehensive AI regulation with its 2023 AI Act, a risk-based governance model specifying greater restrictions on technologies posing greater public risk (Larsen, 2022). It bans excessively high-risk AI uses, including a Chinese-style social credit scoring or real-time public facial recognition. It significantly regulates high risk uses including in credit and job applications according to independent conformity assessments, while more lightly regulating limited risk uses like chatbots, which must just comply with transparency standards. Finally, it avoids regulation for low risk uses such as AI-augmented spam filters and video games. Europe additionally through its Digital Markets Act and Digital Services Act aims to respectively reduce market monopolies (by technology companies controlling significant consumer data and limiting compatibility among external digital products and services) and misinformation (requiring companies' content moderation). Concurrently, Europe seeks to expand the influence of its data governance scheme by expanding its technical and market power (through its 2022 European Chips Act to compete with the United States and China for semiconductor and AI dominance), while requiring the world's largest technology companies (based in the United States and China) to comply-by-design with its regulatory framework (in exchange for access to their large market). This balance of cooperation and competition echoes the EU's 2021 study on a shared multinational "data strategy for public health," unified with the common moral and pragmatic vision of shared well-being, operationalized by an AI-driven "health data centre," empowered to sufficiently "influence Member State[s] public-health-relevant data ecosystems," and technically equipped with an effective data architecture spanning a "central coordination and support structure with advanced digital public health functions" (Martins 2021, p. iii).

America has a different take on regulation and rights. Fearing the former will become excessive and infringe on the latter, including competitive innovation, the United States largely has avoided any national regulation on data protection, leaving California's 2020 Consumer Privacy Act based on the GDPR to become America's default national policy (Larsen, 2022). Still, various federal agencies, states, and corporations generate a patchwork of fragmented regulations, incentives, and disincentives. Proponents argue this approach maximizes as close to local as possible self-determination of digital freedom and innovation, while opponents counter it stifles both given the collective drag against them created by an excessively complex and conflicting regulatory scene. Considering the failed passage of the 2022 Algorithmic Accountability Act (as the American version of Europe's AI Act), President Biden announced the 2023 public–private partnership (the de facto American version of government regulation) on data and AI self-regulation by seven of the top AI companies including OpenAI, Microsoft, Google, Amazon, Meta, Anthropic, and Inflection (McCallum 2023). They agreed in principle on internal and external security testing, public watermark disclaimers of AI products, AI capability and limitation public reporting, and risk research in privacy, discrimination, and bias. The upside is that these world leading AI firms—which generally set the standards and norms most companies follow globally—embedded these influential self-corrective mechanisms in the global digital ecosystem through their technologies powering it. But its downside is that it relies on fragmented norms with questionable definition, defense, and enforceability. Nonetheless, consider how such organic decentralized governance may be akin to the successful modern model of nuclear deterrence. We have never had so many countries bristling with so many nuclear weapons which can destroy our common home multiple times over—with no unified enforceable law preventing their use. And yet, we have made it nearly a century without seeing our destruction (though assuming this will continue indefinitely does not in and of itself justify ambivalence and inaction toward stronger collective guardrails). This distinctive American game theory–like deterrence and decentralized governance for AI, like in nuclear weapons, trades standardized consistency for agile durability (similar to the notable domestic and foreign policy mistakes of the US governance model since its inception, which nonetheless are the implicitly accepted cost of the unprecedented technical, political, and economic growth sustained with similarly unprecedently successful self-corrective mechanisms).

Finally, China has a take on regulation that maximizes government might while minimizing individual rights. Its 2017 national AI strategy, the GDPR-informed 2021 Personal Information Protection Law and its 2022 "Internet Information Service Algorithmic Recommendation Management Provisions" progressively adopted stricter and more centralized control over digital services, products, and communication that shifted from a personal data security–focused governance into more national security–focused data governance (Larsen, 2022). The 2022 provisions specifically mandated private companies (domestic and foreign) keep and process data locally to promote content moderation through algorithmic recommender engines. Global observers describe such mechanisms as forceful government propaganda, while promoters describe rather as preservation of patriotic communist values required for national unity and security (against the supposed corrosive effects of foreign particularly American influence). Unlike the abovesaid US companies simply joining Biden for unified AI standards, the Chinese Communist Party or CCP progressively acquires ownership control of such companies (through state-run private equity funds) and management control (by placing party officials on their board of directors). And where AI is principally a European and American innovative tool for social progress, it is principally a tool for social control in China or "intelligent social construction," particularly through its "social credit system" according to its latest 5-year plan. Chinese proponents argue its version of "digital sovereignty" is superior to the American model of supposed ideological imperialism "forcing" its values on the world, with Xi Jinping concurrently asserts that "efforts should be made to build our country into a cyber power...The countries that take command of the internet will win the world" (Raymond 2023; Johnson 2023). The US, European, and wider critics of China's governance model counter that China is not seeking a positive sum multipolar world to deny the US global dominance, particularly in the global digital ecosystem (while it ironically continues its self-colonization by radical fringe Western ideologies like Marxism and fascism—repudiated by the West in the Cold War and World War II (WWII)—which featured centralization of unprecedented power into a cult of personality, as when Mao unleashed the Cultural Revolution to violently purge Chinese identity and culture to replace them with such ideologies). Rather, its end game is a zero-sum Chinese authoritarian takeover of the European−American−led democratic world order that neoimperializes the Global South and West with its expanded closed and controlling political economics and related digital governance. From withholding COVID origin, genetic, and public health data (undermining the critical initial window to successfully manage the pandemic for the world), such critics argue that China's governance model is inferior pragmatically (inefficient), politically (excessively unstable), economically (stifling innovation), and societally (denying self-determination and thus self-correction). China is already the largest trading partner with the Global South, and particularly with its Digital Silk Road within its Belt and Road Initiative. Through it, China progressively controls the majority of the South's internet by expanding its IT infrastructure (building the data centers, delivery networks, cloud services, and dependent internet platforms), service extensions (e-commerce paired with social media platforms), authoritarian venture capitalism (buying influential and controlling stakes in foreign companies to access their intellectual property and governance), global technology standard setting (reshaped according to its data governance scheme), cyberattacks (including property theft and espionage), data expansion (obtaining sovereign countries' commercial, telecommunications, government, military, health, and even genomic data to "own" other countries), and coercion (on states and companies to relinquish their data and governance through economic and military threats and force).

"Data security" for "national security" therefore is actually "party security" according to this line of critique, as the CCP seeks to maintain its controlling grip on power domestically by extending and cementing it globally—with global health as diplomatic means and AI digital technologies as technical means of furthering that ultimate aim. Failing to divide the United States and Europe especially after its partner's full-scale Ukraine invasion, China has faced growing global resistance to this governance model including global derisking from excessive Chinese reliance, Global South diversification away from Russia, India's closer ties to America, and Europe's increasingly explicit resistance to China not just for its Russian support (Ero 2023). Germany as one of the world's largest economies and most strategically conservative European democracies, noted in its 2023 China strategy that its pivot to a more muscular military defense of Ukraine against Russia will occur *with* a full-spectrum countering against a perceived excessive Chinese influence campaign on its people: "In key areas, the [European Union] must not become dependent on technologies from [non-EU] countries that do not share our fundamental values," particularly Chinese communist authoritarian ones (Ziady and Schmidt 2023). By September 2023, Germany's foreign minister joined other senior world leaders in labeling Xi as a "dictator," against the backdrop of the country's new policy labeling China as a "partner, competitor, [and] systemic rival" (Soni 2023). The United Kingdom was earlier and went further in its 2020 global data governance assessment, warning that the global zero-sum competition in global data governance systems features China pitting its imperial totalitarian model (closed and controlling) against the European and American sovereign democratic model (open and free; UK 2020).

In contrast to the abovesaid three models, a fourth was explored in the Chapter 5 on political economics—Personalist Liberalism—which may articulate the optimal (and practical) alternative by integrating the other models' less problematic and more compatible unifying elements (given the lower likelihood any unipolar power will durably dominate global data governance): European human rights—foundation, American free market orientation, Chinese sovereign—emphasis, and Indian (and larger Global South) multicultural insistence. This data governance model essentially is a human security approach bounded by national and data sovereignty, as manifested by Japan's championing of such a model at the 2023 G7 summit and its Data Free Flow with Trust framework (Habuka 2023). The 20th-century colonial empire—turned 21st-century cooperative democracy seeks reportedly to make national data governance systems interoperable (not imperial or identical) by making them globally trustworthy: maximized country's core national security necessities, minimized inter- and intrastate threats to human security, coordinated by a single international organization (such as the Organisation for Economic Cooperation and Development [OECD] or a more "neutral" institution between the West and the Rest), stewarded and accountable to global multistake-holder input, operationalized by trade (synced with the global digital economy) and regulation (syncing consensual global standards), and institutionalized into the dignity-based moral political economic framework for the global human ecosystem (Arasasingham and Goodman 2023). These structural changes ultimately are grounded and self-corrected by its moral foundation which the Japanese articulated since its 2019 "Social Principles of Human-Centric AI" as a person-centered approach, based on the metaphysical not just moral principles of human dignity (as a Japanese Buddhism development in line with the *UDHR*) and the derivative principles of inclusivity and sustainability. In the Japanese understanding, an authoritarian governance model structurally undermines these globally shared and pragmatically necessary principles more than a democratic model (while global governance historically has been more practically democratic than autocratic, as single rulers never have sustainably dominated the world's countries by consistently dictating internal and external policies). Also, an authoritarian model undermines their sustainable defense because of weaker or absent structural self-correction mechanisms for political instability, economic stagnation, and societal fragmentation from autocratic power centralization. The modern Japanese model therefore integrates the European risk-based approach (without its "holistic and hard-law elements") with the American and UK-style "sector-specific and soft-law" approach and Chinese stability-focus, along with the AI principles articulated by the G20 and OECD, to produce a fourth way of "agile governance"—preserving its moral core while adopting operations with changing technical and political economic trends and the inclusion of more sectors and stakeholders. There is thus growing multilateral interest and support in Japan's human security–based data sovereignty approach to data governance, bounding national security interests with global security interests, as excessive nationalism destabilizes the global human ecosystem and thus inadvertently undermines national security for the countries that constitute it (as the G7 argues that Russia's imperial invasion of Ukraine supposedly for its national security actually imperils it by massively reducing its allies and access to global markets for its exports and imports).

This follows the 2021 Oxford University Press analysis of how a moral foundation is required for its overarching political and economic frameworks to articulate common moral values from a shared metaphysical vision of our common humanity; accordingly, we explored the global pluralistic metaphysics uniting the world's diverse belief systems as articulated by the international consensus in the *UDHR*, defended in breadth and depth by Personalist Social Contract ethics within Personalist Liberalism political economics (Carugati and Levi 2021; Monlezun 2022). A collaborative approach to data flows follows from and requires intellectual, cultural, demographic, and population flows to reduce neocolonialism, power centralization, and destabilizing homogenization. The 2019 Pew Research Center global analysis demonstrated that democratic nations (led by Canada, Australia, the United Kingdom, Sweden, Japan, and the United States) generally are the largest migrant receiving countries and are most likely to favorably view them as a national security net benefit (through their diversity, work, and talents), instead of a net burden (by taking social benefits and jobs)—in contrast to the more autocratic Russia and China (notching negligible to no significant immigration; Gonzalez-Barrera and Connor 2019). These competing political economic and intertwined data governance models typically are centered between strong autocracies (with their often oil, commodities, and manufacturing-based economies with closed and censored politics) and advanced democracies (with their more diversified, digital, and service-based economies with open and free politics), competing for greater power over the other and influence with the Global South's emerging markets and governments navigating the Bremmer J-curve discussed earlier (Ritter 2023). The fourth model of agile governance—manifested by Japan and articulated by the Personalist Social Contract—seeks to enable managed strategic competition between both. It seeks to do so not only while preserving an existential and moral floor of human security to guard and guide the guardrails to these relationships. But it also empowers states to advance on that J-curve toward more free, open, and stable self-governing democracies should they collectively opt (without imposing this political economics scheme upon them, in contrast to how autocracies reportedly do so repeatedly and pervasively through force and coercion on their own people and spheres of influence).

This personalist approach to governance additionally safeguards against the nationalist populism in both democracies (including America's Trump and Turkey's Erdoğan) and the more forceful autocracies. The latter often have initially robust but self-limited and self-destabilizing transient support domestically and even internationally. This includes outlier advocates in democracies including the Irish Nobel Prize laureate, George Bernard Shaw, who praised Stalin as French intellectuals did for Mao, as part of a larger historical phenomenon articulated by the Irish writer, Fintan O'Toole: "There is the same impatience with the messiness and inefficiency of democracy, and it leads to the same crush on the strongman leader who can cut through the irrelevant natterings of parliaments and parties," even if it means cutting down one's people and future (Noonan 2023). Yet there is hope for a Japanese style agile cooperative governance including between democracies and autocracies, which Personalist Liberalism describes substantively and the UN Security Council's 2023 seminal meeting on AI displays concretely (Nichols 2023). The Chinese ambassador emphasized the need to balance "scientific development with security" while the US ambassador emphasized the need to ensure AI is not used to "repress or disempower people." Their convergence support how shared existential AI challenges including in health may help accelerate the shared focus on human security. Doing so may ultimately help broaden security concerns, without ignoring individual rights or states' legitimate concerns for their own security from internal instability and external coercion. Further technical advances building on this trend include the 2023 *Nature* study on DEFINED, a "rigorous and rapid," real-world, real-time, sector-specific, integrated framework to provide graduated regulatory guidance on digital health interventions, proportional to the strength of their evidence (Silberman et al. 2023). Further, the explosive growth of AI particularly with the 2023 advances in generative AI are built collaboratively in free and open data ecosystems, which resist controlled and closed data or political economic governance models. By January 2023 alone (a few weeks after its release), ChatGPT was already listed as coauthor on four scientific publications as scientists regardless of their political economic regimes used global tools for global benefit (Stokel-Walker 2023), in a process simultaneously described as democratizing and decolonizing AI depending on what political economic regime observers are in.

7.6 Families and foundation: artificial intelligence security ethics amid multicultural demographic shifts

The questions of how we use power (in technology and politics economics) and for what ends we are using them to achieve it are first answered by who is using it. And that "who" is rapidly shifting, both in terms of demographics and multicultural ethics, as the above section emphasized how the governance model is decolonizing and deimperializing to become more diverse and inclusive. In 2023, the Global South accounted for 80% of the global population and 130 of the 193 UN voting seats. By 2050, it is expected to boast six of the seven largest economies. And unlike the secular or religiously unaffiliated West which dominates the majority of international institutional governance, the global digital ecosystem, and the global public health ecosystem, the majority of the Rest is *not* secular. This portends profound implications in how those embedded cultural and religiously affiliated values and their expression in public discourse affect different governance models in the abovesaid power structures now and for our future (Raymond 2023; Monlezun 2022; Hackett et al. 2015; Taylor 2018; Künkler et al. 2018). The 16th-century European Scientific Revolution and later European–American Industrial Revolutions reshaped early modern science and political economics, setting the West up to dominate global governance for the next five centuries. They did so framed by these states' increasingly secular values in which the predominant Christianity gave way progressively to religious pluralism, the separation of church and state, and the eventual late modern resistance or restriction of religiously affiliated belief systems in public discourse and governance. As the center of gravity for global power is projected to shift away from the West, the Rest's more robust and public relationship between state and religion will profoundly reshape not just power but how it is used. In 2010, religiously affiliated belief systems accounted for 83.6% of the world population (primarily by Christianity at 31.4%, Islam at 23.2%, unaffiliated at 16.4%, Hinduism at 15.0%, and Buddhism at 7.1%). By 2050, Islam is expected to edge closer to Christianity's levels while religiously unaffiliated are expected to drop to nearly the single digits. Muslim families' fertility rate (3.1 children per woman) and that of Christians (2.7) are the only ones expected to remain well above replacement level; meanwhile, European and American unaffiliated (1.7) and Asian Buddhists (1.6) are projected to remain well under that threshold. Population decline or even collapse in the Global North (particularly in China, Russia, and East Europe) are estimated to therefore occur, while population rise or even surge accelerates in the Global South especially in Africa. The moral foundation for the global political economic structure and the families inhabiting it are only expected to continue reshaping the global public health ecosystem it manifests and serves. Justice and pragmatism thus demand a rethink of how we think and decide about managing such public goods.

The Personalist Social Contract ethics that Chapter 6 explored may uniquely be poised to not only account for our current but also our future dominant ethics. It does so by historically, culturally, and philosophically tracing how the world's dominant modern ethics (human dignity-based rights, expressed by global consent in the UN's *UDHR*) is structurally a Western secular social contract framework (agreeing to a shallow political conception of justice as fairness that is cautions of other objective truth claims) that can be made more inclusive and sustainable by recovering its classical realist metaphysical foundation (through a Thomistic-Aristotelian Personalism latent within it, bridging the world's diverse belief systems by expressing a common conception of humanity, dignity, and the common good which substantively unite us as a global human family essentially rather than artificially). It shows how for reasons inherent in our diverse culturally conditioned belief systems, we reach common conclusions about dignity, rights, and concrete ethical actions to maximize them (with greater speed, sustainability, and substance than secularism's shallower modern ethics, along with greater intelligible moral interoperability than the world's diverse belief systems separately). It uniquely therefore generates a pluralistic but substantive convergent —rather than simply superficial overlapping—consensus about the human security "floor" for global well-being, bridging the political economic divides between democracies and autocracies (whose imperial manifestations may fatally divide the global digital ecosystem and the interdependent AI-enabled global public health ecosystem), and the integral sustainable development "ceiling" without a roof. Accordingly, it has already been demonstrated to be embedded, interoperable, and efficient in substantively guiding human-in-the-loop automatic computational ethics for the global public health ecosystem, while providing a more robust breadth and depth to the international debate and dialogue on AI ethics and related research, regulation, and deployment. By recovering what it means to be human, Personalist Social Contract ethics may make AI more human. By recovering what our common good is (collectively informed by our diverse cultures and belief systems), we can revive a workable plan for preserving our common home and future.

Chapter 6 therefore explored how Personalist Liberalism political economics has an embedded Personalist Social Contract moral foundation that brings together competing political economic regimes (and laudable but insufficient attempts like shallower WHO AI ethics or related shifting global regulations). It focuses on the common overarching needs and goals of human security, sovereignty, sustainability that can serve as guard rails for the managed strategic competition between and among regimes, sectors, and stakeholders. Doing so seeks to maximize their technical and political economic cooperation required for the survivability of the AI-empowered global public health ecosystem. At scale, speed, and specificity, it uniquely may facilitate global institutionalized consensus (animating the UN and our international power structures) through philosophically sound, multiculturally plural, and pragmatically effective means to translate our common values into concrete solutions, driving our ecosystem forward to solve our existential health crises and pressing challenges. It additionally provides a "metaphysical Turing Test" (to understand what separates man/person from machine), novel global "moral interoperability,", substantive inclusivity (especially in global health AI ethics, including Africa's "Ubuntu" and existential embodiment), pragmatic effectiveness (to resolve traditionally polarizing problems like AI-fueled misinformation, which can only be broadly understood as misinformation if realist metaphysics like with the Personalist Social Contract shows how there really is an objective truth that others can misrepresent), and automatic embedded computational ethics (already interoperable with the healthcare systems and the larger global public health ecosystem as with its application in AiCE). What is more real than concepts and structures? The human person (with relational agency that is not simply a product of our societal structures and individual circumstances) and our unique experiences of our shared reality. The Personalist Social Contract attempts to show and operationalize the above for global ethical decision-making, the critical prerequisite for the durable political economic consensus underpinning the structure and operations of the AI-transformed global public health ecosystem. It plural-istically and practically shows how the common good (securing our individual flourishing) is our common end or objective to which integral sustainable development is orientated (oper-ationalizing our human dignity and multicultural diversity). In parallel, it demonstrates how justice (as metaphysical not simply political or rhetoric) and its derivative equity (as we are relational members of the global human family bounded by justice and bound for unity) serve as guardrails and self-corrective mechanisms to our science-driven political economics, in which intermediary goods like health, prosperity, and stability facilitate humanity's devel-opment toward the ultimate or common good.

There are key concrete AI ecosystem trends that integrate and advance the related use cases and concepts under the Personalist Social Contract umbrella of human security in (1) global localizing, (2) personalizing, (3) embedding, and (4) rehumanizing AI health ethics.

7.6.1 Globalizing and localizing artificial intelligence health ethics

The Personalist Social Contract shows how the *UDHR* translated classical Thomistic-Aristotelian Personalism into modern global institutionalized capitalist liberal democracy, transitioning from the historical international relations paradigm of nationalist imperialism to the emergent model of local globalism (balancing subsidiarity and solidarity, networks and hierarchies, vertical and horizontal governance, and the individual and community to leverage global resources for local needs, driven by local agency and voices)—and how the world's 2015 SDGs echoed this global moral political economy. Recently, the SDGs operatio-nalized as a WoW or whole-of-world approach (integrating whole-of-government and whole-of-society approaches) has been applied to population health and equity at the local com-munity level (Ortenzi et al. 2022). The most robust local demonstration of this approach may be seen in Ukraine: structurally with communities and sectors nationally mobilizing (to sur-vive what they describe as an existential threat of a foreign power seeking to eliminate them, with the invaders unleashing internationally harmful effects particularly on the Global South) and technically using AI to operationalize that societal mobilization (maximizing their health sector's resilience and resource management, while increasing the efficient lethality of its defense forces by shortening the "kill chain" from invader target acquisition to elimination through more rapid, precise, and complex Big Data battlefield intelligence, spanning a massive range of sensors, drones, videos, and personal reports; Maçães 2023). The private US AI company, Palantir, is providing a potent demonstration of the future of defense through this AI-accelerated algorithmic warfare with important implications for health. This paradigm shows the ecosystem power of self-optimizing processes embedded in a global interoperable data architecture (with real-time complex orchestration of the abovementioned diverse data streams through a central intelligent platform). Accordingly, the US Chairman of the Joint Chiefs of Staff, Mark Milley, as the country's top ranking military leader points to this technological revolution as the most transformative milestone in the complex and ancient human phenomenon of conflict. War is increasingly about digitalization and deterrence rather than physical domination and destruction. But in the other complex and ancient human phenomenon of health fighting disease and disparities rather than ourselves and each other, an AI-enabled approach—that is about WoW marshalling of interdependent and integral sustainable development for human security—seeks to maximize cooperation and minimize conflict, while shortening the "life chain" between (prediction and early) identification of global health threats to generation of rapid, precise, and equitable countermeasures eliminating (or at least mitigating) them.

7.6.2 Personalizing artificial intelligence health ethics

The Personalist Social Contract seeks to demonstrate that human security is applied AI health ethics, both substantively (as to secure the basic goods necessary for relational human flourishing is to satisfy the demands of justice in human relations) and practically (as the growing global consensus and emphasis especially through the UN and WHO on it requires collective ethics-informed agile regulation and cooperation in ecosystem governance on global public health goods). In our politically divided but digitalized interdependent world, this may mean AI is not so much democratized as it is decolonized or personalized. This may help transcend traditional rigid conceptions of democracies versus autocracies (though the latter does historically underperform with optimizing liberty, equality, stability, and prosperity) to maximize the personal protection of individuals and communities, which is required for safeguarding human security and thus sustainable development at global scale. Toward personalizing AI health ethics globally, a significant emblematic MIT breakthrough in 2023 generated an end-to-end AI platform, BioAutoMATED, that automatically processed multiomics data, selected the appropriate analytic model, and designed biological sequences for it (Valeri et al. 2023). It used an open-source ML platform to personalize AI for biologists globally with limited AI experience, while accurately predicting synthetic biology components, gene regulation, and peptide–drug interactions that can accelerate drug and vaccine design. Accordingly, it lowers the cost and expands the health AI benefit especially for lower income communities and diverse sectors lacking advanced AI capacities. Similarly, Google's DeepMind in 2023 deployed "circuit neural networks," a DL approach to better decolonize and personalize the AI supply chain, particularly using powerful AI to make the historically specialized process of AI-based chip design more automated, affordable, and accessible to the world (Lin 2023). Its approach is also significantly more efficient—up to 30% more than the related competition's winner the prior year. This is particularly notable as current processes are vastly dependent on a small number of geographically concentrated power players controlling the manufacturing of this bedrock modern technology (particularly China and the United States along with its allies). In addition, DeepMind reached a landmark 2022 discovery in synthetic biology in which its AlphaFold algorithm accurately predicted nearly all known protein structures, translating biology's basic building blocks into explosive data-driven insights into how to use them for drug discovery, food insecurity, sustainability, and so on. The US digital and semiconductor company, Qualcomm, points to such "opening up" of AI to the larger world within the larger strategic tend in which the "future of AI is hybrid": strong edge computing (not just cloud) pushes more and more computing and AI analytic power to the point of users of the ecosystem, enabling a personalization of AI for the local user through a global digital ecosystem (Qualcomm 2023). The more open a society is, the more personalized, pervasive, and powerful the AI can advance its local needs.

7.6.3 Embedding artificial intelligence health ethics

Effective ethics can only be so if they are embedded in global power structures, influential institutions, and agile operation as laws, regulations, and declarations will always be late with limited enforceability. The Lancet Commission's strategic postmortem report on the highest level failure of modern global public health—the COVID-19 pandemic—concluded its 2022 technical assessment with an ethical admonition, invoking the *UDHR* on its 75th anniversary as the world's "moral charter" already embedded in and unifying our global human family and public health ecosystem, the safeguards for the hope of a better collective response and future (Sachs et al. 2022). In the report's run-up, the WHO published the "Health Systems for Health Security" framework to operationalize the already latent common values about our duties to the common good and thus the practical need to "minimize vulnerability to acute public health events that endanger the collective health of populations," including our own, and so to integrally link human security and sustainable development for health and fairness (Brown et al. 2022). Yet from 2000 to 2020, there were only 204 publications on health systems and health security worldwide, generally focused on security over systems and security mostly for acute health emergencies, while conflating "state" with human security. As healthcare and public health become more expensive amid rising debt crises and aging populations, the top performing healthcare systems and public health agencies (especially in West Europe) increasingly are struggling to sustain that high level of population health. Up to this point, it has been achieved through its hallmark WHO-endorsed UHC or universal health coverage financed, prevention-focused, and healthy lifestyles—enabled approach to public—private partnerships for population health (empowering lower income countries to adopt and personalize this blueprint for their communities). Although embedded, the values still require better ethical elucidation and technical and governance operationalization. Even in the world's richest country, America's human security health programs that are expanding essential healthcare access and social safety net services are rapidly approaching insolvency, while there is widespread empirical documentation of non-profit health providers exploiting taxpayer-provided charity funds without commensurate public benefit (Economist 2023; Glassman 2023). Wanting to help people is not enough—it requires effective, efficient, and continuous actualization of common moral values through continuous technical and governance optimization.

Thus there are notable recent hybrid advances that bring together the science and ethics. Google's DeepMind in 2023 published the technical translation of modern Kantian-informed Rawlsian social contract ethics into AI algorithms in the *Proceedings of the National Academy of Sciences*, one of the world's top-cited comprehensive multidisciplinary scientific journals (Weidinger et al. 2023). It used this ethical system to derive fair AI ethical principles in a pluralistic world from commonly held embedded values informing our overlapping consensus of fairness, regardless of whether such principles would definitely benefit any one individual. Their responsible AI assistant was then bound by algorithmic rules that balance a "maximizing principle" (optimizing total performance achieving an objective, typically by focusing on more productive stakeholders) with a "prioritizing principle" (supporting disadvantaged stakeholders for more equitable performance). Diverse human subjects chose the latter if they were behind the "veil of ignorance" and would not know in advance of a game if they would be an advantaged or disadvantaged individual in the game. The study therefore showed how this modern social contract framework may be an effective mechanism to guide distributive justice ethical principles in responsible AI, while the Personalist Social Contract shows how such contract-based ethics can be elevated to and deepened within the personal dimension with global not just Western application. Although early, the controversial yet still globally influential American—South African technology titan, Elon Musk, argued in 2023 in a similar line of reasoning but on the ultimate end of the AI evolution spectrum that superintelligent AI would be the safest approach to AI development (Shin 2023). He argues that it would technically maximize curiosity and truth-seeking, as the AI would feature embedded ethical values infused into the AI from its human creators' own embedded (even if latent) moral world vision. Because "humanity is much more interesting than not humanity," the superintelligent AI according to this understanding would minimize the existential threat of it harming us, even when it becomes more powerful than us. Yet there at least appears to be widespread multisector and multicultural global consensus that such existential and current human security threats should not be left to chance—more work is required to collectively go from embedded to effective health AI values given such high stakes.

7.6.4 Rehumanizing artificial intelligence health ethics

This requires ensuring AI fairly reflects the global population it is meant to serve according to our global values, expressed by and informing human security and sustainable development, particularly with influential trends in culturally sensitive demographic support and resocialization of social media. The COVID-19 pandemic and India's population eclipsing China by 2023 accelerated global concerns about our global aging population and the related health and health financing challenges it entails, for which AI may accelerate countermeasures. Based on data from the former UN Population Division (articulating consensus demographic findings), there are growing efforts in the Global North (where demographic decline is particularly severe) to reverse racial and gender inequalities in marriage and the related economic and birth inequalities which disproportionately and negatively impact lower income communities (Chamie 2021; Yamaguchi 2023). Certain nations are taking it many steps further for enhanced funding and focus on full-spectrum demographic challenges and even crises, including in Japan as a global AI leader and the third largest economy. Its government asserted they are facing their "last chance" to reverse their collapsing already record-low birth rate "by supporting individuals' pursuit of happiness" for those wanting more children, while also encouraging immigration. Yet it reports having daunting headwinds for doing so, including difficulties reported by their own people finding self-identified compatible mates/spouses and supportive education, jobs, maternal care, work leave, and cultural acceptance of their family choices. Concurrent with the OECD and the Global North's cultural rise of the religiously unaffiliated into the 21st century, there have been historic declines in births and long-term child rearing and marriage (with African Americans and Hispanics experiencing nearly double the decline of marriage rates compared to Caucasians). Significant political economic inequalities for singles versus married—including the former versus latter being poorer, sicker, and sadder—are cited to support the increasing Northern policies designed to financially and culturally support couples opting for shared lives including with children (Grover and Helliwell 2017; Greenstone and Looney 2012). Rehumanizing may be advanced not just with repopulation but also by retooling. AI automation appears to hold global rehumanizing benefit, particularly for racial minorities and lower income community, by boosting their efficiency and thus livable wages amid worsening labor shortages (Bove 2023). A 2021 MIT analysis even demonstrated that up to 35% of robotic and automation adoption is driven by population aging (with Japan, South Korea, and Germany already leading this technical trend with their worsening demographic trends).

Significantly greater efforts are underway rehumanizing AI health ethics through the resocialization of social networks. Following the global COVID lockdowns, the US Surgeon General went so far as to warn of the emergent "epidemic of loneliness" as a growing global public health crisis (HHS 2023; Bollyky et al. 2023). As families shrink, along with the prospect of finding meaningful friendships, liveable wages, and compatible partners, the abovesaid trends are worsening societal fragmentation and isolation. According to the Surgeon General's report, people using media users for over 2 hours daily double their self-reported isolation. Mortality doubles with this loss of social connection, which has since been demonstrated as an independent mortality predictor (controlling for age, health, socioeconomic, and health behavior status). Loneliness worsens heart disease by 29% and dementia by 50%, while driving up COVID-19 mortality and remaining the top predictor of suicide. Conversely, survival surges by 50% with enhanced social connections according to 148 studies with a mean follow-up of 7.5 years. The Surgeon-General's report additionally highlights how social media is a potent driver of social isolation, polarization, fragmentation, and weaponization, as it is itself primarily driven by AI-accelerated economic incentives for profit and control, generating the net result of near-term worsening of inequality and authoritarian and elitist power centralization, according to 305 global experts through the Pew Research Center (Anderson and Rainie 2023). AI can worsen social connections, job displacement, human rights, human knowledge, governance, institutions, and thus health and well-being. Therefore, person-centered revamping of AI digital technologies is meant to respond to these challenges. The main means are fostering an ethically grounded critical mass of global social pressure to optimize human security, while generating sufficient political economic disincentives to governments and companies misusing the technical power of AI. Concrete advances in this area include the shift from authoritarian abuses like in China (including making corporations explicit arms of the communist party including owning their data) and overreliance on individual rights (like with US-driven corporations dominating social media, especially through their AI algorithms predominantly maximizing individual engagement through anger and other tribal instincts at the expense of surging societal fragmentation; Lewis and Moorkens 2020). Instead, this Irish analysis generating the abovementioned results supported the pivot to collective rights (following the UN, WHO, and Japan's agile data governance) by balancing industry self-regulation with industry–state coregulation, informed by continuous public discourse actualizing our common embedded values to make the AI algorithms (technically creating and determining our digital social networks) more trustworthy and transparent. This is meant to make them more human and social, rather than artificial and divisive.

7.7 The future of the artificial intelligence + global public health ecosystem: just power, serving a humanity worth saving

7.7.1 Personal(ist) ecosystem and responsible artificial intelligence reengineering

The abovesaid structural elements together allow us to understand the emergent future of AI-powered global public health as a personal(ist) ecosystem, re-engineered by responsible AI explored progressively through this book. The formula for this integral vision—structurally, principally, and strategically—will be formalized in the next section. It is this blueprint that is enabled by the moral interoperability, data interoperability, and thus ecosystem interoperability empowering the effective cooperation of the diverse culturally conditioned belief systems, sectors, and partners constituting the ecosystem. This capacity to operate together is facilitated by the essential integrating factor of human security at scale, scope, and specificity—through the three-level global context of the political economics which drives the societal frame and function of the ecosystem, along with the technical dimension of its data architecture enabling the data flow and augmented intelligence shared among these partners. We therefore explored (1) Personalist Liberalism as the interoperable political economic framework and language to understand these three levels—of the suprastructure of international institutions, structure of state relationships, and substructure of common values. In addition, we sought to use (2) Personalist Social Contract ethics as the moral inter-operable framework and language to understand and facilitate the decolonization of these structures by recovering our common humanity, values, and vision of a fair future we can pragmatically achieve amid competing powers. Accordingly, (1) and (2) may further enhance the success of the abovesaid formula for how to realize the WHO digital strategy for health's future (as an ecosystem of public–private and democratic–autocratic partnerships), the landmark Declaration of Alma Ata (as health for all through equitable efficiency, technologi-cally enabled, pragmatically driven, and morally grounded), the Great COVID Reset (as a sustainable global social contract, made so by being metaphysically grounded in human dig-nity), and thus the *UDHR* (as the moral charter for a decolonized modern world order that moves from premodern imperialism of unchecked power to modern international law and justice that bounds power competition with moral and pragmatic guardrails).

Responsible AI is the essential enabler of human security integrating the partners and their values, resources, objectives, and data to generate (and reengineer) the global public health ecosystem. It is itself an integrated product of science and ethics, in which the former is bounded by the latter to orientate it toward the common good. Responsible AI thus fosters the transparent trust and agile cooperation needed to accelerate the ecosystem toward that ultimate strategic end. Collectively, this integral ecosystem vision of (or systems approach to integral ecology at the global level for) health and AI moves the current organizational evolu-tion—from limited or project focused AI to enterprise-wide or mature AI—ultimately to eco-system AI. Chapter 3 on development analyzed how the Sustainable Development Goals or SDGs are our modern world's UN-driven, consensus-based political economic grand strate-gic plan for equitable prosperity. We also considered how the WHO applied them as its comprehensive ecosystem strategy for AI-enabled health, in which equitable public health + human security = responsible political economics + national security. Personalist Liberalism articulates how responsible AI in this historic context is thus meant to catalyze the transition from *democratic* to *human* globalization, in which human security is structur-ally scaled globally and equitably through just political economic structures and effective data architectures, while limiting the traditional cooperation hurdles of competing value blocks such as democracies versus autocracies or the West versus the East versus the South. Dignity-grounded development driving the global public health ecosystem generates this responsible health AI, operationalized as accountable and effective governance (institution-ally and technically through the WHO and other key suprastructure coordinators, maximiz-ing global resources for local-defined, driven, and led programs and operations).

We considered how development is the roofless ceiling of this ecosystem with human secu-rity as the floor, defined by the 2000 UN Commission as freedom from fear and want through protection and empowerment. These essential rights were articulated first by the 1948 *UDHR*, flowing from the other two essential rights of freedom of speech and belief. As the ash and dust settled following the carnage and chaos unleashed by the WWII clashes of imperial powers, the UN's moral charter asserted through collective democratic consensus that rules not rulers should ultimately predominate rather than dominate, that we can be more than ani-mals as predators and prey in shifting power dynamics. We can recover the reality that we are persons and communities that can be in sustainable justice relationships. This global pluralistic political consensus, realized economically through globalized capitalism rather than imperialism, is morally grounded in our common values uniting our diverse belief systems and unique experiences—human dignity, rights, and duties to the common good, safeguarding our individual good and in which our individual good is realized. This unifying vision of just power protecting the human family animates the current empowerment of our global public health ecosystem with a responsible AI that can help move us from a simple logic of utility to dignity, social contracts to social communion, transaction to transformation, and exchange to love. Markets and alliances are meant to secure justice: you give me something that I want for something that you want just as much. Communities and cooperation are meant to surpass even justice to approximate mercy. Game theory gets us only so far to construct pragmatic pressure toward global cooperation such as in pandemics, poverty, climate change, and conflict reduction. But to make human development sustainable, we may need to move from the logic of exchange to the logic of the gift in which debt forgiveness, collective defense, and decolonized solidarity supercharge how the AI-enabled global public health ecosystem facilitates how we move from mutual survival through shifting social contracts to common flourishing through substantive social communion—for reasons inherent to our belief systems, by means that respect our communal cultures and individual identity. When just power gives way to enduring love, when united nations give way to a global civilization of love, then fragmented networks of agencies and healthcare systems may give way to a responsible AI-revolutionized global public health ecosystem that is personalized to protect and empower every person. To save humanity, it may mean that we must first recover who we are and why we are worth saving in the first place. Admittedly, this vision is ambitiously aspirational. But so was the *UDHR*. So is every time a patient walks or is wheeled into any hospital. For both, survival is so essential and urgent that it defines the aspirational simply as practical, and then gets down to the details of making the probability a reality.

7.8 Conclusion

These pages were written in between seeing my patients, the existential concrete center of gravity this book revolves around. It requires theory grounded in practice and strategic structures grounded in the reality of the human person—entailing the common good and the responsible health AI meant to accelerate it. The empirical research and patients' experiences globally suggest this is practically and strategically key: to explore a firsthand account of these AI health trends, while also recognizing the strategic context in which the local hospital nearest us may be the most sensitive and specific marker if population and public health is failing. The healthy and healthy rarely need a hospital, while the sick and poor often do (and frequently without much sustainable health being achieved at those hospitals). Historically, this is where health was defined narrowly as medical care for acute diseases. But increasingly, we see how health is more than just organs and medications, and how it is more than just what happens in institutional walls. It is about global, public, digitalized, and comprehensive well-being that requires full-spectrum, multisector, multicultural, decolonized, and comprehensive approaches that bring together scientific, ethical, and governance best practices. It requires AI technically, a global public health ecosystem institutionally, and human security–based integral sustainable development ethically—because it requires all of us as a WoW approach. The structure and content of this book therefore focused on building not just a better hospital, but a better common home by recovering our common humanity and common good, and the effective ways that power can be justly redirected to serve it through efficient and equitable health at scale, speed, and specificity. This is because the AI-empowered global public health ecosystem increasingly taking shape (and being reengineered according to this security and development) is essentially just power, embodied as freedom at scale seeking the common good (by maximizing individual health which can only be realized communally and equitably as global public health at scale). Now and for the foreseeable future, AI can augment much and automate some. But as a tool, we need to have a shared moral and strategic vision of how to use it based on what is the "why" we are using it. Personalist Liberalism political economics and its embedded Personalist Social Contract ethics attempted to define, defend, and deploy this ecosystem vision of the emergent future for global public health.

This then brings us to formalizing the projections of that mutually desired future, and the path to accelerating its realization through responsible AI. The 2023 *Thinking healthcare system* outlined the novel "AI Health" model for the future's integrated healthcare (Monlezun 2023):

$$AIHealth_{\text{Mathematical}} = \left(\text{HealthBD} \times \left[\overline{Delivery} \right. \right.$$

$$\left. \left. + \sum_{n=1}^{\infty} \left\{ \text{PrMed}\langle \cos Delivery \rangle + \text{PubHealth}\langle \sin Delivery \rangle \right\} \right] \right)^{AI-VBHC}$$

AI Health thus is the product of health Big Data (HealthBD) and the dynamic relationship balancing precision medicine (PrMed) and public health (PubHealth), all raised to the exponential power of AI-enabled Value-Based Healthcare (AI-VBHC). This in turn was simplified to the essence of the future's thinking healthcare system embodying AI Health: health (H) generated as the product of AI (A) and equity (E) squared, similar to Einstein's $E = MC^2$ as the AI-augmented human energy powering the future. This book attempted to broaden this model for the overarching global public health ecosystem spanning healthcare, public health, and global public health by showing how *individual resilience* at global scale (realized through the minimum of human security paired with the maximum of integral sustainable development) can be achieved through local *community reliance* (in relational ethics anchored in our common humanity, embodied interdependencies, and orientated to our common good in which we find our unique flourishing). Therefore, we return to the formula formalizing these relationships introduced in Chapter 1, expressed in its three dimensions structurally, principally, and strategically:

$$\text{Globalpublichealthecosystem}_{\text{structurally}} = \left(\frac{\text{Globalhealth} + \text{Healthcare}}{\text{Digitalecosystem}} \right)^{\text{Humansecurity} \times \text{AI}}$$

$$\text{Globalpublichealthecosystem}_{\text{principally}} = \text{PersonalistLiberalism}^{\text{HealthAI}}$$

$$\text{Globalpublichealthecosystem}_{\text{strategically}} = \left(\frac{\text{AI} \times \text{Equity}^2}{\text{Globalpublichealth}} \right)$$

The book thus explored the structural formula for the AI-empowered global public health system in which the design of financing and development was actualized through the framework of data architecture (technically) and political economics (societally), anchored in the ethical foundation (of the global, pluralistic, multicultural Personalist Social Contract approach to human security) and inhabited by the families of our world's changing cultures and demographics. The sum of global health and local healthcare integrated within the global digital ecosystem therefore is raised to the power of AI-enabled human security to reengineer and generate this global public health ecosystem. We explored how principally this ecosystem may be understood through the ethically grounded political economics of Personalist Liberalism, raised to the power of health AI, since strategically the ecosystem is the AI Health of the future's thinking healthcare system above, operating at the scale of global public health. Rather than a rigid roadmap, this agile formula projects the future by understanding how changing inputs through a known network of relationships can be reliably predicted, understood, and so optimize emergent outputs of concrete trend-setting AI health advances. Ultimately, we can only achieve global well-being together practically, AI technically, and a common vision ethically. Global public health requires power to actualize it, justice to do it sustainably, and ethics to do it together. Our journey into this common ecosystem home opened with a storm slamming into a pandemic, sandwiching our hospital in between. And like in that health and security crisis, we explored how this ecosystem is rapidly transforming and being reengineered (both organically and strategically) in the rehumanizing recovery of our common humanity that eclipses even these crises: we made it out together, and we can make it into a common future worthy of our dignity and responsive to our needs, together. In 2023, this book's first edition was published as a blueprint for the future of health as the AI-transformed global public health ecosystem, the same year we mark the 75th anniversary of the WHO, founded by the world's nations to give global health the chance of a future so humanity would have one. And in August of 2023, Prime Minister Modi invoked this vision when India became the first country to land on the moon's south pole where water is hypothesized to dwell, critical for space survival (Williams 2023). He declared that "India's successful Moon mission is not India's alone," but rather it is for all of humanity, achieved by a "human-centric approach" in which its moral vision of "one Earth, one family, one future is resonating around the world." Could it be that such milestones as humanity's voyage to a lifeless moon may help boldly resurrect our hope of bringing life back to our shared planetary home, solving not just climate and pandemic challenges but also advancing toward a health and peace that seems always distant? But not as far off as we once feared. Until then, whether we be patients or providers, shifting back and forth from needing more help to being able to give more of it in our shared journey, I look forward to seeing you at the bedside. Because all of us are worth saving. And it will take all of us to do it.

References

Anderson, J., and L. Rainie. 2023. "The Most Harmful or Menacing Changes in Digital Life That are Likely by 2035." Pew Research Center. Accessed July 31, 2023. https://www.pewresearch.org/internet/2023/06/21/themes-the-most-harmful-or-menacing-changes-in-digital-life-that-are-likely-by-2035/.

Arasasingham, A., and M.P. Goodman. 2023. "Operationalizing Data Free Flow with Trust. Center for Strategic and International Studies." Accessed July 29, 2023. https://www.csis.org/analysis/operationalizing-data-free-flow-trust-dfft.

Bollyky, T.J., Castro, E., Aravkin, A.Y., Bhangdia, K., Dalos, J., Hulland, E.N., and S. Kiernan, et al., 2023. "Assessing COVID-19 Pandemic Policies and Behaviours and Their Economic and Educational Trade-Offs Across US States From Jan 1, 2020, to July 31, 2022." *Lancet* 401 (10385): 1341−1360.

Bove, T. 2023. "A.I. Could Help With Demographic Aging Crisis." Fortune. Accessed July 31, 2023. https://fortune.com/2023/05/24/artificial-intelligence-ai-eric-schmidt-demographic-crisis-babies-labor-shortage/.

Brown, G.W., Bridge, G., Martini, J., Um, J., Williams, O.D., and L.B.T. Choupe. 2022. "The Role of Health Systems for Health Security: A Scoping Review Revealing the Need for Improved Conceptual and Practical Linkages." *Globalization and Health* 18 (1)51.

Carugati, F., and M. Levi. 2021. *A Moral Political Economy: Present, Past, and Future*. Cambridge, UK: Cambridge University Press.

Chamie, J. 2021. "The End of Marriage in America? The Hill. Accessed June 19, 2023. https://thehill.com/opinion/finance/567107-the-end-of-marriage-in-america/.

Chattu, V.K. 2022. "Digital Global Health Diplomacy' for Climate Change and Human Security in the Anthropocene." *Health Promotion Perspectives* 12 (3): 277−281.

Chui, M., E. Hazan, R. Roberts, A. Singla, K. Smaje, A. Sukharevsky, L. Yee, and R. Zemmel. 2023. "The Economic Potential of Generative AI." McKinsey & Company. Accessed June 21, 2023. https://www.mckinsey.com/capabilities/mckinsey-digital/our-insights/the-economic-potential-of-generative-ai-the-next-productivity-frontier#introduction.

Economist. 2023. "America's Entitlement Programmes are Rapidly Approaching Insolvency. *The Economist.* Accessed May 8, 2023. https://www.economist.com/united-states/2023/04/09/americas-entitlement-programmes-are-rapidly-approaching-insolvency.

Ero, C. 2023. "The World Isn't Slipping Away From the West. Foreign Policy. Accessed July 29, 2023. https://foreignpolicy.com/2023/03/08/russia-ukraine-war-west-global-south-diplomacy-un-putin-g20/.

Glassman, J.K. 2023. "Health Care Providers are Raking in Profits by Exploiting Programs Meant for the Poor." The Hill. Accessed July 23, 2023. https://thehill.com/opinion/healthcare/4101826-health-care-providers-are-raking-in-profits-by-exploiting-programs-meant-for-the-poor/.

Gonzalez-Barrera, A., and P. Connor. 2019. "Around the World, More Say Immigrants are a Strength Than a Burden." Pew Research Center. Accessed July 12, 2023. https://www.pewresearch.org/global/2019/03/14/around-the-world-more-say-immigrants-are-a-strength-than-a-burden/.

Greenstone, M., and A. Looney. 2012. "The Impact of Economic and Technological Change on Marriage Rates." The Brookings Institute. Accessed May 11, 2023. https://www.brookings.edu/blog/jobs/2012/02/03/the-marriage-gap-the-impact-of-economic-and-technological-change-on-marriage-rates/.

Grover, S., and J.F. Helliwell. 2017. "New Evidence on Marriage and the Set Point for Happiness." *Journal of Happiness Studies* 20 (2019): 373−390.

Habuka, H. 2023. "Japan's Approach to AI Regulation and Its Impact on the 2023 G7 Presidency." Center for Strategic and International Studies. Accessed July 29, 2023. https://www.csis.org/analysis/japans-approach-ai-regulation-and-its-impact-2023-g7-presidency.

Hackett, C., P. Connor, M. Stonawski, and V. Skirbekk, 2015. "The Future of World Religions: Population Growth Projections, 2010−2050." Pew Research Center. Accessed July 30, 2023. https://www.pewresearch.org/religion/2015/04/02/religious-projections-2010-2050/.

HHS. 2023. "Our Epidemic of Loneliness and Isolation." United States Department of Health and Human Services. Accessed May 12, 2023. https://www.hhs.gov/sites/default/files/surgeon-general-social-connection-advisory.pdf.

Hoffman, S.J., and C.B. Cole. 2018. "Defining the Global Health System and Systematically Mapping its Network of Actors." *Globalization and Health* 14 (1)38.

Johnson, M., 2023. "China's Grand Strategy for Global Data Dominance." Stanford University Hoover Institution Press. Accessed July 2023. https://www.hoover.org/research/chinas-grand-strategy-global-data-dominance.

Kung, T.H., Cheatham, M., Medenilla, A., Sillos, C., De Leon, L., and C. Elepaño. 2023. "Performance of ChatGPT on USMLE: Potential for AI-Assisted Medical Education Using Large Language Models." *PLOS Digital Health* 2 (2): e0000198.

Künkler, M., Madeley, J., and S. Shankar. 2018. *A Secular Age Beyond the West: Religion, Law and the State in Asia, the Middle East and North Africa.* Cambridge: Cambridge University Press.

Lewis, D., and J. Moorkens. 2020. "A Rights-Based Approach to Trustworthy AI in Social Media." *Social Media + Society* 6 (3). https://doi.org/10.1177/2056305120954672.

Larsen, B.C., 2022. The Geopolitics of AI and the Rise of Digital Sovereignty. Brookings Institute. Accessed July 27, 2023. https://www.brookings.edu/articles/the-geopolitics-of-ai-and-the-rise-of-digital-sovereignty/.

Lin, B. 2023. "In Race for AI Chips, Google DeepMind Uses AI to Design Specialized Semiconductors. *Wall Street Journal.* Accessed July 30, 2023. https://www.wsj.com/articles/in-race-for-ai-chips-google-deepmind-uses-ai-to-design-specialized-semiconductors-dcd78967?mod = hp_minor_pos6.

Maçães, B. 2023. "How Palantir is Shaping the Future of Warfare." Time. Accessed July 11, 2023. https://time.com/6293398/palantir-future-of-warfare-ukraine/.

Martins, H. 2021. "EU Health Data Centre and a Common Data Strategy for Public Health." European Union Parliament. Accessed April 22, 2023. https://www.europarl.europa.eu/RegData/etudes/STUD/2021/690009/EPRS_STU(2021)690009_EN.pdf.

McCallum, S., 2023. "Seven AI Companies Agree to Safeguards in the US." BBC. Accessed July 23, 2023. https://www.bbc.com/news/technology-66271429.

Monlezun, D.J. 2022. *Personalist Social Contract: Saving Multiculturalism, Artificial Intelligence, and Civilization.* Newcastle upon Tyne: Cambridge Scholars Press.

Monlezun, D.J. 2023. *The Thinking Healthcare System: Artificial Intelligence and Human Equity.* New York: Elsevier.

Nichols, M. 2023. "UN Security Council Meets for First Time on AI Risks." Reuters. Accessed July 23, 2023. https://www.reuters.com/technology/un-security-council-meets-first-time-ai-risks-2023-07-18/.

Noonan, P. 2023. "May Trump Soon Reach His Waterloo." *The Wall Street Journal.* Accessed July 12, 2023. https://www.wsj.com/articles/may-trump-soon-reach-his-waterloo-race-election-president-2024-candidate-campaign-97310a7f?st = mn6tslqbpph6gnk&reflink = desktopwebshare_permalink.

Ogier du Terrail, J., Leopold, A., Joly, C., Béguier, C., Andreux, M., Maussion, C., et al., and B. Schmauch, et al., 2023. "Federated Learning for Predicting Histological Response to Neoadjuvant Chemotherapy in Triple-Negative Breast Cancer." *Nature Medicine* 29 (1): 135–146.

Ortenzi, F., Marten, R., Valentine, N.B., Kwamie, A., and K. Rasanathan. 2022. "Whole of Government and Whole of Society Approaches: Call for Further Research to Improve Population Health and Health Equity." *BMJ Global Health* 7 (7): e009972.

Pearl, R. 2023. "U.S. Healthcare: A Conglomerate of Monopolies." Forbes. Accessed July 23, 2023. https://www.forbes.com/sites/robertpearl/2023/01/16/us-healthcare-a-conglomerate-of-monopolies/?sh = 4f30165a2e4d.

Qualcomm. 2023. "The Future of AI is Hybrid." Qualcomm. Accessed July 11, 2023. https://www.qualcomm.com/content/dam/qcomm-martech/dm-assets/documents/Whitepaper-The-future-of-AI-is-hybrid-Part-1-Unlocking-the-generative-AI-future-with-on-device-and-hybrid-AI.pdf.

Raymond, P. 2023. "Re-Platformed Planet? Implications of the Rise and Spread of Chinese Platform Technologies." Center for Strategic and International Studies. Accessed July 15, 2023. https://www.csis.org/analysis/re-platformed-planet-implications-rise-and-spread-chinese-platform-technologies.

Ritter, D. 2023. "Fueling Failure: A Global Power Shift From the West to China." National Interest. Accessed July 23, 2023. https://nationalinterest.org/feature/fueling-failure-global-power-shift-west-china-206642.

Sachs, J.D., Karim, S.S.A., Aknin, L., Allen, J., Brosbøl, K., Colombo, F., and G.C. Barron, et al., 2022. "The Lancet Commission on Lessons for the Future From the COVID-19 Pandemic." *Lancet* 400 (10359): 1224–1280.

Shin, R. 2023. "Elon Musk Wants to Create a Superintelligent A.I. Because He Thinks a Smarter A.I. is Less Likely to Wipe out Humanity." Fortune. Accessed July 23, 2023. https://fortune.com/2023/07/17/elon-musk-superintelligent-a-i-less-likely-to-wipe-out-humanity-chatgpt-openai/amp/.

Silberman, J., Wicks, P., Patel, S., Sarlati, S., Park, S., and I.O. Korolev. 2023. "Rigorous and Rapid Evidence Assessment in Digital Health with the Evidence DEFINED Framework." *Nature Digital Medicine* 6 (1)101.

Soni, M. 2023. "German Minister Calls Xi Jinping 'dictator'. 'Dissatisfied' Beijing Complains." *Hindustan Times*. Accessed September 20, 2023. https://www.hindustantimes.com/world-news/annalena-baerbock-german-minister-calls-xi-jinping-dictator-dissatisfied-beijing-complains-101695027540754.html.

Stokel-Walker, C., 2023. ChatGPT Listed as Author on Research Papers: Many Scientists Disapprove. Nature. Accessed June 24, 2023. https://www.nature.com/articles/d41586-023-00107-z.

Tang, Z., Shi, S., Li, B., and X. Chu. 2023. "GossipFL: A Decentralized Federated Learning Framework With Sparsified and Adaptive Communication." *IEEE Transactions on Parallel and Distributed Systems* 34, 909–922.

Taylor, C. 2018. *A Secular Age*. Cambridge, MA: Harvard University Press.

UK. 2020. "Evidence and Scenarios for Global Data Systems: The Future of Citizen Data Systems." United Kingdom Government Office for Science. Accessed May 8, 2023. https://assets.publishing.service.gov.uk/government/uploads/system/uploads/attachment_data/file/927547/GOS_The_Future_of_Citizen_Data_Systems_Report__2_.pdf.

Valeri, J.A., Soenksen, L.R., Collins, K.M., Ramesh, P., Cai, G., and R. Powers. 2023. "BioAutoMATED: An End-To-End Automated Machine Learning Tool for Explanation and Design of Biological Sequences." *Cell Systems* 14 (6): 525–542.

Weidinger, L., McKee, K.R., Everett, R., Huang, S., Zhu, T.O., Chadwick, M.J., et al., Summerfield, C., et al., and I. Gabriel 2023. "Using the Veil of Ignorance to Align AI systems With Principles of Justice." *Proceedings of the National Academy of Sciences of the United States of America* 120 (18)e2213709120.

Williams, N. 2023. "India Makes History as Chandrayaan-3 Lands Near Moon's South Pole." BBC. Accessed August 26, 2023. https://www.bbc.com/news/live/world-asia-india-66576580/page/2.

Yamaguchi, M. 2023. "Japan Unveils Proposal to Promote Marriage, Raise Birthrate." Associated Press. Accessed May 11, 2023. https://apnews.com/article/japan-declining-birthrate-reverse-plan-fd5c77386b0f85e9f4d993265070781b.

Ziady, H., and N. Schmidt. 2023. "'China Has Changed.' Germany Unveils Strategy to Cut Reliance on World's No. 2 Economy." CNN. Accessed July 13, 2023. https://www.cnn.com/2023/07/13/economy/germany-china-strategy/index.html.

Further reading

Singhal, K., Azizi, S., Tu, T., Mahdavi, S.S., Wei, J., Chung, H.W., and N. Scales, et al., 2023. "Large Language Models Encode Clinical Knowledge." *Nature* 620, 172–180. https://doi.org/10.1038/s41586-023-06291-2.

Abbreviations

AAMC	Association of American Medical Colleges
ACO	accountable care organization
A.D.	Anno Domini
ADHD	Attention-deficit/hyperactivity disorder
ADR	adverse drug reactions
AFL-CIO	American Federation of Labor/Congress of Industrial Organizations
AGI	artificial general intelligence
AI	artificial intelligence
AI4PH	artificial intelligence for public health
AI4SG	AI for social good
AiCE	AI-driven Computational Ethics and policy analysis
AIDS	acquired immunodeficiency syndrome
AI-EII	AI-driven Efficiency-Inequity Index
AI-HealthBD	AI-accelerated healthcare Big Data
AI-VHBC	AI-enabled Value-Based Healthcare
AJPH	American Journal of Public Health
AMA	American Medical Association
ANI	artificial narrow intelligence
ANN	artificial neural network
ANSI	American National Standards Institute
API	application programming interface
ASI	artificial super intelligence
ATE	average treatment effect
AUKUS	Australia, United Kingdom, and the United States
B.C.	Before Christ
bk	book
bk.	book
BRI	Belt and Road Initiative
BRICS	Brazil, Russia, India, China, and South Africa
BSI	British Standards Institution
CCP	Chinese Community Party
CD	communicable disease
CDC	Centers for Disease Control and Prevention
CfC	closed-form continuous-time
CGM	continuous glucose monitors
ch.	chapter
CHAID	Chi-square automatic interaction detection
CMS	Centers for Medicare and Medicaid Services
CNS	central nervous system
CPG	clinical practice guideline
CPT	Current Procedural Terminology
CSIS	Center for Strategic and International Studies
CTAD	Conference on Trade and Development

CUGH	Consortium of Universities for Global Health
CV	cardiovascular
CVD	cardiovascular disease
DAH	development assistance for health
DALY	disability adjusted life year
D-CCC	digital health–enabled community-centered care
DL	deep learning
DNGC	Danish National Genome Center
DoD	Department of Defense
DRLBTS	deep reinforcement learning-aware blockchain-based task scheduling
EBM	evidence-based medicine
ECG	electrocardiograms
ECOWAS	Economic Community of West African States
eCQM	electronic clinical quality measure
ED	Emergency Department
EHR	electronic health record
EIT	European Institute of Innovation and Technology
EMS	emergency medical service
Endo	endocrine
EOIS	Epidemic Intelligence from Open Sources
EU	European Union
FAO	Food and Agriculture Organization
FDA	Food and Drug Administration
FHIR	Fast Healthcare Interoperability Resources
FSMB	Federation of State Medical Boards
FTC	Federal Trade Commission
G7	Group of 7
G20	Group of Twenty
GAI	generative artificial intelligence
GBD	Global Burden of Disease
GCC	Gulf Cooperation Council
GDP	gross domestic product
GDPR	General Data Protection Regulation
gen	generation
GeoAI	geospatial AI
GeoARK	Geospatial Analytical Research Knowledgebase
GI	gastrointestinal
GIH	Global Health Initiative
GIS	geographic information systems
GIZ	Gesellschaft für Internationale Zusammenarbeit
GSMA	Global System for Mobile Communications Association
HAC	hospital-acquired condition
HAI	healthcare-associated infection
HealthBD	healthcare Big Data
HFrEF	heart failure with reduced ejection fraction
HGP	Human Genome Project
HHS	Department of Health and Human Services
HICs	high-income countries
HIMSS	Healthcare Information and Management Systems Society

HIPAA	Health Insurance Portability and Accountability Act
HIT	health information technology
HIV	human immunodeficiency virus
HRO	high reliability organization
ibid.	*ibidem* (in the same place)
ICC	International Criminal Court
ICD	International Classification of Diseases
ICL	Imperial College London
ICT	information and communication technology
ICU	intensive care unit
IEEE	Institute of Electrical and Electronics Engineers
i.e.,	*id est* (in other words)
IHR	International Health Regulations
IMF	International Monetary Fund
IPEF	Indo-Pacific Economic Framework for Prosperity
IoT	Internet of Things
IoM	Institute of Medicine
IP	internet protocol
IPO	initial public offering
IT	information technology
KPI	key performance indicator
LAN	local area network
LICs	low-income countries
LMICs	low- and middle-income countries
LNG	liquified natural gas
MCO	managed care organization
MDG	Millennium Development Goals
MEC	multi-access edge computing
MICs	middle-income countries
ML	machine learning
MRI	magnetic resonance images
N	number
NAS	National Academies of Sciences
NATO	North Atlantic Treaty Organization
NCD	noncommunicable disease
NCI-MATCH	National Cancer Institute Molecular Analysis for Therapy Choice
NEJM	*New England Journal of Medicine*
NHS	National Health Service
NICE	National Institute for Health and Clinical Excellence
NIH	National Institutes of Health
NLP	natural language processing
NTN	nonterrestrial networks
OECD	Organisation for Economic Cooperation and Development
OIP	Office of the Inspector General
OWS	Operation Warp Speed
p.	page
para	paragraph
PCP	primary care provider
PHI	public health intelligence

PHEIC	Public Health Emergency of International Concern
PopHealth	population health
pp	page
PPIE	Patient and public involvement and engagement
PPR	pandemic preparedness and response
PSC	Personalist Social Contact
QALY	quality adjusted live years
Quad	Quadrilateral Security Dialogue
R&D	research and development
REACH	Realizing Equity, Access, and Community Health
RF	random forest
RNN	recurrent neural networks
ROCAUC	receiver operating curve area under the curve
ROI	return on investment
SaMD	Software as a Medical Device
SCD	sudden cardiac death
SCO	Shanghai Cooperation Organization
SDG	sustainable development goals
sect	section
SOA	service orientated architecture
SPAC	special purpose acquisition company
STEMI	ST segment myocardial infarction
SVM	secure virtual machine
SWIFT	Society for Worldwide Interbank Financial Telecommunications
TAC	Trustworthy deep learning AI Co-Design
telemed	telemedicine
TFR	total fertility rate
TMLE	targeted maximum likelihood estimation
tPA	tissue plasminogen activator
UAE	United Arab Emirates
UAV	unmanned aerial vehicle
UCL	University College London
UDBHR	Universal Declaration on Bioethics and Human Rights
UDHR	*Universal Declaration of Human Rights*
UHC	universal health
UHRI	Universal Human Rights Index
UI	uncertainty interval
UK	United Kingdom
U/L	units per liter
UN	United Nations
UNDP	United Nations Development Programme
UNICEF	United Nations International Children's Emergency Fund
URI	Uniform Resource Identifier
US	United States
US	The United Nations (of America)
USAID	United States Agency for International Development
USCDI	United States Core Data for Interoperability
VA	Veterans Affair
VHS	value-based healthcare system

VieWS	VitalPac Early Warning Score
vol.	volume
VR	virtual reality
VRT	variable-rate technology
WAN	wide area network
WDO	World Data Organization
WEC	World Economic Forum
WHO	World Health Organization
WoG	whole-of-government
WoS	whole-of-society response
WTO	World Trade Organization
WWI	World War I
WWII	World War II

Index